I0882515

Vision Language Models for Next-Generation Healthcare

Pethuru Raj
https://orcid.org/0000-0001-5220-0408
Reliance Jio Platforms Ltd., Bangalore, India

B. Sundaravadivazhagan
University of Technology and Applied Sciences-Al Mussana, Oman

Venkatesh Kavitha
https://orcid.org/0000-0003-0566-8619
Sri Ramakrishna College of Arts and Science, India

M. Baby Nirmala
https://orcid.org/0000-0003-2849-9133
Holy Cross College, India

IGI Global
Scientific Publishing
Publishing Tomorrow's Research Today

Vice President of Editorial Melissa Wagner
Director of Acquisitions Mikaela Felty
Director of Book Development Jocelynn Hessler
Production Manager Mike Brehm
Cover Design Jose Rosado

Published in the United States of America by
IGI Global Scientific Publishing
701 East Chocolate Avenue
Hershey, PA, 17033, USA
Tel: 717-533-8845 | Fax: 717-533-7115
Website: https://www.igi-global.com E-mail: cust@igi-global.com

Copyright © 2026 by IGI Global Scientific Publishing. All rights reserved. No part of this publication may be reproduced, stored or distributed in any form or by any means, electronic or mechanical, including photocopying, without written permission from the publisher. Use of this publication to train generative artificial intelligence (AI) technologies is expressly prohibited. The publisher reserves all rights to license its use for generative AI training and machine learning model development.

Product or company names used in this set are for identification purposes only. Inclusion of the names of the products or companies does not indicate a claim of ownership by IGI Global Scientific Publishing of the trademark or registered trademark.

Library of Congress Cataloging-in-Publication Data

Names: Raj, Pethuru editor | Sundaravadivazhagan, B. editor | Kavitha, V. editor | Baby Nirmala, M., 1973- editor
Title: Vision language models for next-generation healthcare / edited by: Pethuru Raj, B. Sundaravadivazhagan, Venkatesh Kavitha, M Baby Nirmala.
Description: Hershey PA : IGI Global Scientific Publishing, [2026] | Includes bibliographical references. | Summary: "This book explores the transformative potential of Vision Language Models (VLMs) in healthcare, detailing their role in multimodal diagnostics, medical report generation, and clinical decision-making. It consolidates research, showcases practical applications, and outlines challenges and future directions for integrating VLMs into next-generation healthcare systems"-- Provided by publisher.
Identifiers: LCCN 2026003228 (print) | LCCN 2026003229 (ebook) | ISBN 9798337373157 hardcover | ISBN 9798337373164 paperback | ISBN 9798337373171 ebook
Subjects: LCSH: Artificial intelligence--Medical applications | Generative artificial intelligence | Machine learning
Classification: LCC R859.7.A78 V57 2026 (print) | LCC R859.7.A78 (ebook)
LC record available at https://lccn.loc.gov/2026003228
LC ebook record available at https://lccn.loc.gov/2026003229

British Cataloguing in Publication Data
A Cataloguing in Publication record for this book is available from the British Library.

All work contributed to this book is new, previously-unpublished material.
The views expressed in this book are those of the authors, but not necessarily of the publisher.
This book contains information sourced from authentic and highly regarded references, with reasonable efforts made to ensure the reliability of the data and information presented. The authors, editors, and publisher believe the information in this book to be accurate and true as of the date of publication. Every effort has been made to trace and credit the copyright holders of all materials included. However, the authors, editors, and publisher cannot assume responsibility for the validity of all materials or the consequences of their use. Should any copyright material be found unacknowledged, please inform the publisher so that corrections may be made in future reprints.

Table of Contents

Detailed Table of Contents

Healthcare systems in low-resource settings face persistent challenges, including limited clinical expertise, inadequate diagnostic infrastructure, and unreliable connectivity. While artificial intelligence offers promise in addressing these gaps, cloud-based solutions often fail to meet the privacy, latency, and infrastructure constraints of underserved environments. This chapter examines agentic, on-device vision-language models (VLMs) as a viable framework for real-time, privacy-preserving clinical decision support. The chapter reviews key technical foundations, including reasoning-capable large language models, multi-agent architectures, memory-augmented systems, and multimodal perception. Emphasis is placed on adapting medical VLMs for edge deployment through model optimization techniques and hardware-aware design. Integrated architectures comprising imaging, language, and planning agents coordinated via shared memory and orchestration layers are discussed as enablers of robust clinical reasoning and contextual awareness.

The leading cause of mortality in children, it is crucial that clinicians immediately arrive at an accurate diagnosis. The suggested deep learning algorithm can automatically detect pneumonia using chest X-rays with a 97.7% accuracy rate. EfficientNetB4 provides an optimal trade-off between fast processing and diagnostic precision. The model's sensitivity to identify small lung abnormalities is enhanced by using Architectural Convolutional Layers (TCLs). These layers extract morphological and connecting data that is not captured by ordinary convolutional

multimodal big language models in radiology. It assesses cutting-edge radiology-specific models like CXR-LLaVA, MAIRA, and MRG-LLM and examines the technological underpinnings of multimodal architectures, such as visual encoders, language models, and fusion processes. The chapter delves deeper into developments that go beyond simple report creation, such as segmentation-aware modelling and longitudinal image interpretation.

This article proposes persistent homology as a model-agnostic audit lens for vision–language medical systems whose fluent reports can mask structural inconsistencies. An end-to-end pipeline computes cubical persistence on reference images and model-mediated outputs, derives Betti-curve signatures on a shared filtration grid, and measures drift via bottleneck and Wasserstein distances in H0 and H1. Conventional baselines (reconstruction, segmentation, and semantic agreement) establish nominal adequacy, while topology reveals silent failures such as spurious holes, merged components, or fragmented regions. Topological signals are aggregated into a diagnostic index for ranking cases, setting alarms, and tracking stability. Outputs include figures, tables, and evaluation scripts.

Vision–Language Models (VLMs) are transforming healthcare by integrating visual and textual understanding for medical image analysis and clinical decision-making. Incorporating computer vision and natural language processing, vision-language models (VLMs) can manage multimodal inputs ranging from radiographic images to pathological slides and medical reports. The essence of VLMs lies in multimodal fusion, vision grounding, and medical know-how alignment, which enable reliable medical report creation, disease prediction, and anomaly discovery. The application of pre-trained models, such as CLIP, BLIP, and MedCLIP, has provided strong support for zero-shot learning and cross-modal retrieval, whereas domain-aware fine-tuning has further improved their medical adaptability and functionality. However, there are challenges related to data privacy, interpretability, and bias that need to be addressed. This paper reviews VLM architectures, training methods, and tasks, as well as challenges and directions for developing secure and clear AI for medical applications.

Vision Language Models (VLMs) can be viewed as one of the most important developments in artificial intelligence where visual and linguistic modalities are combined to improve the analysis of medical imaging and the clinical decision-making process. This chapter is an in-depth discussion of the importance of VLMs in future healthcare, and the fact that such systems are capable of handling complex multimodal information like medical images and related clinical texts. The discussion outlines the disruptive value of VLMs in enhancing the accuracy of diagnoses, automatic generation of reports, and individualising treatment planning. Nevertheless, the application of VLMs to healthcare is followed by significant challenges. Limitations to technical issues are low and nonhomogeneous medical data, large computational costs, and interpretable domain-specific model adaptation.

Vision language models (VLMs) represent a transformative paradigm in medical artificial intelligence, enabling joint reasoning over clinical images and textual information. Their ability to integrate radiology scans, pathology slides, ultrasound frames and structured/unstructured medical text positions them at the center of the next generation of intelligent diagnostic systems. This chapter provides a comprehensive and unified exploration of VLMs for medical imaging, beginning with foundational principles, covering architectural advances, discussing clinical applications, identifying challenges such as hallucination risks and mapping future research directions. The chapter integrates conceptual explanations, empirical trends and clinically informed insights with detailed figures, diagram sketches and tables. The aim is to equip researchers, clinicians and developers with a complete understanding of how vision language models can responsibly and effectively support next-generation medical imaging pipelines.

This chapter explores the emerging role of Vision Language Models (VLMs) in healthcare, focusing on their ability to integrate visual and textual data to improve medical imaging analysis and clinical decision-making. It examines the key components of VLMs, including vision and language models, their fusion techniques, and their applications in tasks like disease detection, report generation, and visual question answering. The chapter also addresses challenges such as data scarcity, privacy concerns, and model interpretability. Additionally, it highlights future directions for enhancing model generalization, improving explainability, and ensuring seamless integration into clinical workflows, while emphasizing the importance of ethical considerations and real-world validation for safe deployment in healthcare environments.

Vision–Language Models (VLMs) have emerged as a powerful paradigm for medical imaging by jointly learning from visual data and clinical language. Unlike traditional vision-only approaches, VLMs integrate medical images with radiology reports, clinical notes, and textual prompts, enabling richer semantic understanding, improved generalization, and enhanced interpretability. This chapter presents a comprehensive overview of VLMs for medical imaging, covering their motivation, fundamental architectures, training data requirements, optimization strategies, and evaluation methodologies. A detailed taxonomy of medical VLMs is discussed, including contrastive, generative, and foundation-based models. The chapter further explores

Preface

INTRODUCTION

The landscape of artificial intelligence is evolving at an extraordinary pace. What began as a focus on predictive systems has rapidly expanded into the era of generative intelligence, where models are no longer limited to forecasting outcomes but are capable of creating, interpreting, and reasoning across diverse forms of data. Among these advances, language models have emerged as a central pillar, powering a wide spectrum of applications across domains. Today, the proliferation of large, small, vision-enabled, and multimodal language models—along with specialized domain-specific variants—signals a transformative moment in the way knowledge is processed and utilized.

Within this dynamic progression, Vision Language Models (VLMs) represent a particularly compelling innovation. By enabling the simultaneous understanding of textual and visual information, VLMs establish a crucial bridge between two traditionally distinct data modalities. Their ability to learn deep associations between images and language has opened up new frontiers for intelligent systems, fostering capabilities such as visual question answering, advanced image captioning, and context-aware interpretation. As a result, VLMs are increasingly being recognized as both pervasive and persuasive technologies, gaining traction across industries seeking to deliver more intelligent and responsive solutions.

The healthcare sector, in particular, stands to benefit profoundly from these developments. The integration of visual and textual intelligence aligns naturally with the data-rich environment of modern medicine, where clinical notes, diagnostic images, and patient records coexist. VLMs offer promising avenues for enhancing medical imaging interpretation, supporting diagnostic accuracy, and enabling more comprehensive clinical decision-making. From analyzing X-rays and MRI scans to generating detailed medical reports and uncovering insights through multimodal data analytics, these models hold the potential to redefine how healthcare services are delivered and accessed. Importantly, they also address critical demands for precision, timeliness, affordability, and broader accessibility in healthcare systems worldwide.

This edited volume, *Vision Language Models for Next-Generation Healthcare*, is conceived as a timely and comprehensive resource that brings together diverse perspectives on this rapidly advancing field. The book seeks to consolidate fragmented research efforts, bridge theoretical foundations with practical applications, and provide a structured exploration of how VLMs can be effectively leveraged in healthcare contexts. It highlights both the opportunities and the challenges inherent in adopting such transformative technologies.

Contributions in this volume span multiple disciplines, reflecting the inherently interdisciplinary nature of the subject. By integrating insights from computer science, biomedical engineering, and clinical practice, the book offers a unified reference tailored to healthcare applications. It presents real-world use cases, including radiology reporting, multimodal diagnostics, and emerging areas such as drug discovery, while also addressing critical concerns related to interpretability, ethics, and policy. In doing so, it not only documents the current state of the art but also outlines future research directions and innovation pathways.

This book is intended for a broad audience. Researchers, academicians, and graduate students in fields such as computer science, biomedical engineering, and healthcare informatics will find it a valuable guide to understanding and advancing multimodal AI. At the same time, healthcare professionals, clinicians, and medical researchers can gain insights into how VLMs can augment diagnostics, treatment planning, and patient engagement. Industry practitioners, developers, and policymakers will also benefit from the practical perspectives and forward-looking discussions presented throughout the volume.

As editors, we hope this book serves as both a foundational reference and a catalyst for interdisciplinary collaboration. By bringing together technical rigor and applied relevance, we aim to support the development of next-generation healthcare systems that are more intelligent, inclusive, and impactful.

ORGANIZATION OF THE BOOK

In this volume, the chapters collectively present a rich and multidimensional exploration of Vision Language Models (VLMs), reflecting both their transformative potential and the complexities involved in their adoption within healthcare systems.

The opening chapter introduces a compelling paradigm centered on agentic, on-device VLMs designed for real-time clinical decision support in low-resource settings. It highlights how decentralized, privacy-preserving AI systems—powered by edge deployment, multi-agent coordination, and memory-augmented reasoning—can overcome persistent barriers such as limited infrastructure and unreliable connectivity. By emphasizing adaptive architectures that integrate imaging, language, and planning capabilities, the chapter sets the tone for inclusive and context-aware healthcare innovation.

Building on the clinical applicability of AI, the second chapter presents a highly specialized deep learning framework for pediatric pneumonia detection using chest X-rays. By leveraging EfficientNet-based architectures enhanced with topological convolutional layers, the work demonstrates how advanced feature extraction techniques can significantly improve diagnostic sensitivity, particularly in detecting subtle abnormalities. The inclusion of interpretability tools and robustness analysis underscores the readiness of such systems for real-world clinical deployment.

A comprehensive examination of multimodal fusion strategies is presented in the third chapter, where various integration architectures for clinical VLMs are systematically analyzed. Through empirical evaluation across multiple medical domains and benchmark datasets, the chapter highlights the performance advantages of cross-modal attention and adaptive gating techniques. It also identifies key research gaps, offering practical guidance for designing clinically viable multimodal systems.

The fourth chapter delves into one of the most impactful applications of VLMs in healthcare: radiology report generation. It explores how multimodal large language models can move beyond traditional computer-aided systems to produce structured, context-aware narratives that closely resemble expert interpretations. By examining state-of-the-art models and emerging capabilities such as longitudinal analysis and segmentation-aware reasoning, the chapter underscores the potential for both automation and augmentation in radiological workflows.

In the fifth chapter, the discussion takes a novel methodological turn by introducing persistent homology as a diagnostic audit tool for vision–language systems. This topological approach provides a unique lens for identifying structural inconsistencies that may be overlooked by conventional evaluation metrics. By quantifying differences in spatial and structural representations, the chapter contributes an important perspective on model validation and reliability.

A broader architectural and conceptual overview of VLMs in healthcare is provided in the sixth chapter, which synthesizes their foundational components, capabilities, and associated challenges. It discusses key concepts such as multimodal fusion, vision grounding, and domain adaptation, while also addressing critical concerns related to privacy, bias, and interpretability—issues that are central to the responsible deployment of AI in medicine.

The seventh chapter offers a critical lens on the challenges surrounding VLM adoption. It examines technical, ethical, and operational constraints, including data scarcity, annotation complexity, computational demands, and regulatory considerations. By systematically outlining these limitations, the chapter emphasizes the need for robust, fair, and interpretable systems, while also pointing toward future research directions that can enable sustainable integration into healthcare ecosystems.

In the eight chapter, the focus returns to medical imaging, presenting VLMs as foundational models for diagnostic reasoning and clinical workflow intelligence. The chapter provides a unified and comprehensive treatment of architectural advances, clinical applications, and emerging risks such as hallucinations. It effectively bridges conceptual understanding with practical insights, offering a roadmap for integrating VLMs into end-to-end medical imaging pipelines.

The ninth chapter further explores the multimodal nature of VLMs, emphasizing their role in enhancing disease detection, report generation, and clinical decision-making. It balances technical discussion with practical considerations, including ethical concerns, real-world validation, and workflow integration, thereby reinforcing the importance of deploying VLMs in a safe and clinically meaningful manner.

Finally, the tenth chapter presents a structured and comprehensive overview of VLMs for medical imaging, including their architectures, training strategies, and evaluation methodologies. By introducing a taxonomy of models and detailing a wide range of applications—from diagnosis to visual question answering—the chapter consolidates the field's current state while outlining pathways toward more robust, human-centered, and clinically validated systems.

Taken together, these chapters provide a cohesive and forward-looking narrative that captures the breadth and depth of Vision Language Models in healthcare. They not only illustrate the remarkable progress achieved thus far but also illuminate the path ahead for researchers, practitioners, and policymakers committed to advancing next-generation healthcare through multimodal artificial intelligence.

CONCLUSION

As we bring this volume to a close, it becomes evident that Vision Language Models (VLMs) are not merely an incremental advancement in artificial intelligence, but a foundational shift in how complex, multimodal information can be understood, synthesized, and applied within healthcare. The convergence of visual and linguistic intelligence marks a decisive step toward more holistic, context-aware, and human-aligned computational systems.

Throughout this book, we have sought to illuminate both the promise and the responsibility that accompany such transformative technologies. The contributions collectively demonstrate how VLMs can enhance diagnostic accuracy, streamline clinical workflows, expand access to care, and enable more personalized and data-driven medical decision-making. At the same time, they underscore the importance of addressing critical challenges, including data limitations, interpretability, ethical considerations, and regulatory constraints. These are not peripheral concerns but central determinants of whether these technologies can be trusted and widely adopted in real-world clinical environments.

A recurring theme across the chapters is the necessity of interdisciplinary collaboration. The successful development and deployment of VLMs in healthcare demand the combined expertise of computer scientists, clinicians, biomedical engineers, policymakers, and industry practitioners. Only through such collaboration can we ensure that these systems are not only technically robust but also clinically meaningful, ethically sound, and socially responsible.

Looking ahead, the evolution of VLMs will likely be shaped by advances in model efficiency, explainability, and domain adaptation, as well as by the growing emphasis on privacy-preserving and edge-based intelligence. Equally important will be the development of standardized evaluation frameworks and regulatory guidelines that can support safe and equitable implementation across diverse healthcare settings, including those that are resource-constrained.

As editors, we hope this volume serves as both a reference point and a catalyst—encouraging deeper inquiry, fostering innovation, and inspiring new lines of research at the intersection of multimodal AI and healthcare. The journey toward next-generation healthcare systems is well underway, and Vision Language Models are poised to play a central role in shaping that future. It is our sincere expectation that the insights presented here will contribute meaningfully to this ongoing transformation and support the creation of more intelligent, accessible, and patient-centered healthcare solutions worldwide.

Chapter 1

Agentic, On-Device Vision-Language Models for Real-Time Clinical Decision Support in Low-Resource Settings

Aanal Sanjivbhai Raval
http://orcid.org/0000-0003-3848-0882
Gujarat Technological University, India

Vaishnavi Narendrasinh Solanki
http://orcid.org/0009-0003-8087-0347
Gujarat Technological University, India

Himani Prajapati
Gujarat Technological University, India

ABSTRACT

Healthcare systems in low-resource settings face persistent challenges, including limited clinical expertise, inadequate diagnostic infrastructure, and unreliable connectivity. While artificial intelligence offers promise in addressing these gaps, cloud-based solutions often fail to meet the privacy, latency, and infrastructure constraints of underserved environments. This chapter examines agentic, on-device vision-language models (VLMs) as a viable framework for real-time, privacy-preserving clinical decision support. The chapter reviews key technical foundations, including reasoning-capable large language models, multi-agent architectures, memory-augmented systems, and multimodal perception. Emphasis is placed on

DOI: 10.4018/979-8-3373-7315-7.ch001

nt © 2026, IGI Global Scientific Publishing. Copying or distributing in print or electronic forms without written permission of IGI Global Scientific Publishing is prohibited. Use of this chapter to generative artificial intelligence (AI) technologies is expressly prohibited. The publisher reserves all rights to license its use for generative AI training and machine learning model development.

adapting medical VLMs for edge deployment through model optimization techniques and hardware-aware design. Integrated architectures comprising imaging, language, and planning agents coordinated via shared memory and orchestration layers are discussed as enablers of robust clinical reasoning and contextual awareness.

1. INTRODUCTION AND BACKGROUND

1.1 Context and Motivation

Although digital health technologies have advanced rapidly, a pronounced global healthcare disparity persists, most notably between high-income regions and low- and middle-income countries. Healthcare systems operating under resource constraints continue to experience shortages of trained clinicians, diagnostic infrastructure, specialist availability, and timely clinical decision support, particularly within primary care and emergency medicine. The COVID-19 pandemic and similar global health crises have further intensified these challenges, as limited infrastructure and delayed diagnostic capacity measurably influenced patient outcomes (Raval & Maheriya, 2023).

Artificial intelligence has demonstrated measurable potential to mitigate documented disparities through the provision of scalable, data-driven clinical decision support. Contemporary literature reports progressive expansion of AI applications in domains such as disease surveillance, diagnostic imaging, predictive analytics, and unified decision-support architectures (Kumar et al., 2025; Bae et al., 2023). Notwithstanding these advances, prevailing implementations presuppose sustained access to cloud-based computational resources and high-throughput infrastructure; consequently, they remain ill-suited for settings marked by intermittent network availability, constrained processing capacity, and stringent data-privacy constraints (Nissen et al., 2025). This discrepancy motivates the development of on-device, real-time, and autonomous artificial intelligence systems that are capable of operating directly at the point of care within resource-constrained environments.

1.2 Agentic Artificial Intelligence in Healthcare

Emerging developments in agentic artificial intelligence have established a framework for systems capable of autonomous reasoning and decision-making. Agentic AI denotes a class of models that manifest goal-oriented behavior, structured reasoning, and adaptive action by coordinating multiple reasoning agents rather than relying on a single monolithic architecture (Dernbach et al., 2024; Plaat et al., 2025). These systems demonstrate particular applicability in complex and uncertain environments, including clinical decision-making scenarios characterized by incomplete information (Raval & Borisagar, 2022).

Empirical studies have identified several representational mechanisms that constitute the prevailing basis for autonomous, agent-based reasoning. These include the explicit articulation of intermediate inference steps achieved through chain-of-thought prompting (Zhang et al., 2022), the tight coupling of reasoning and acting exemplified by the ReAct framework (Yao et al., 2022), the delegation of sub-tasks among multiple agents to sustain coherence in extended contexts (Zhang et al., 2024), and deliberative exploration of solution spaces by means of tree-structured search (Yao et al., 2023). Building upon these mechanisms, recent contributions incorporate diffusion-based generative processes that admit stochastic sampling during inference, thereby facilitating probabilistic revision and self-correction of previously generated reasoning traces (Ye et al., 2024; Hersche et al., 2025).

Within the theoretical literature, agentic reasoning has been examined through neuroscience-informed frameworks, which emphasize correspondences between multi-agent artificial systems and human cognitive operations including abstraction, concurrent hypothesis assessment, and adaptive control (Liu et al., 2025; Yamada et al., 2025; Huang et al., 2025). Accordingly, agentic AI has moved rapidly beyond language-centric applications into domains such as scientific discovery, laboratory automation, and integrated biomedical research workflows (Gridach et al., 2025; Patel et al., 2025; Hartung, 2025).

1.3 Vision–Language Models in the Service of Clinical Decision Support

Vision-language models constitute a significant advance in multimodal artificial intelligence because they jointly process visual and textual information. Within medicine, these models permit the simultaneous interpretation of radiologic images, structured electronic health records, and free-text clinical notes, thereby supplying the representational substrate for prospective clinical decision support frameworks (Ardic & Dinc, 2025; Kamrul et al., 2025).

Recent multimodal corpora, exemplified by EHRXQA and MIMIC-CXR-VQA, have advanced clinical visual question answering and image-centric inference by establishing correspondences between chest radiographs and structured electronic health record entries alongside diagnostic enquiries (Bae et al., 2024; Dombrowski et al., 2024). Such compilations have subsequently promoted empirical investigation into interpretable, interactive diagnostic systems whose capacities extend beyond conventional static classification frameworks.

A substantial body of narrative and systematic reviews indicates that multimodal clinical artificial intelligence systems generally achieve superior performance relative to their unimodal counterparts, especially when diagnostic tasks demand contextual interpretation and reasoning across heterogeneous data sources (see citations (Ardic & Dinc, 2025; Das & Akter, 2025; Ahmed & Naji, 2025; Maheriya, 2025; Saini & Sunil, 2025)). These reviews concurrently identify persistent challenges concerning interpretability, potential algorithmic bias, data heterogeneity, and the requirement for rigorous clinical validation.

1.4 On-Device, Real-Time AI in Low-Resource Environments

On-device artificial intelligence constitutes a technically viable strategy for introducing clinical decision-support capabilities in settings characterised by restricted computational and network infrastructure. Executing model inference locally on consumer-grade smartphones or resource-constrained embedded devices permits immediate diagnostic recommendations and obviates the requirement for sustained Internet access. Furthermore, localised data processing limits the transmission of identifiable patient information beyond the device, thereby strengthening privacy protections, and concurrently reduces dependence on external services, contributing to overall system resilience in operational clinical environments (Kumar et al., 2025).

Recent empirical investigations have established that optimized deep-learning architectures for diagnostic objectives—including the identification of brain neoplasms and the interpretation of chest radiographs—can be executed locally on resource-limited mobile hardware (Abdelrahman, 2025; Bareja et al., 2025). Parallel assessments of compressed large-language-model variants further indicate that clinically pertinent inferential capacities remain attainable under the memory, energy, and computational ceilings imposed by handheld platforms, provided that meticulous algorithmic pruning, quantization, and task-specialized architectural adjustments are implemented (Tran et al., 2025).

When on-device vision–language models are augmented with agentic reasoning and multimodal perception capabilities, they can function as clinical assistants that provide triage, explanatory feedback, and adaptive decision support at the point of care. Empirical evaluations indicate that the greatest utility of these systems occurs among community health workers, primary-care facilities, and emergency-response units operating within underserved regions (Dangi et al., 2025; Reddy et al., 2019).

1.5 Chapter Objectives and Scope

This chapter aims to:

- Conceptual Integration of Agentic AI and Clinical Decision Support: The chapter undertakes a systematic synthesis of recent advances in large language models that exhibit explicit reasoning capabilities, multi-agent coordination protocols, and memory-augmented architectures, situating these developments within the specific requirements of clinical reasoning tasks such as triage, differential diagnosis generation, and adaptive workflow planning.

- Technical Foundations for On-Device Multimodal Intelligence: It offers a detailed exposition of vision-language model topologies pretrained on paired medical imagery and textual corpora, and it delineates the optimization trajectories—quantization, structured pruning, and knowledge distillation—that are necessary to achieve executable latency and memory footprints on resource-constrained edge devices including smartphones and embedded neural processing units.
- Architectural Design Patterns for Healthcare Applications: The contribution introduces modular system backbones in which task-specialized agents (imaging, natural-language, and hierarchical planning modules) interact through a unified working memory store and an orchestration layer; the resultant architecture is shown to enhance fault tolerance, maintain conversational and episodic context, and support continuous human-in-the-loop governance.
- Application Scenarios in Low-Resource Clinical Settings: Via illustrative deployments in point-of-care ultrasound interpretation, dermatological screening, infectious-disease triage, and smartphone-based diagnostic workflows, the chapter empirically illustrates that agentic vision-language models can raise clinical decision quality while remaining compatible with intermittent connectivity and minimal institutional infrastructure.
- Deployment, Ethical, and Sustainability Considerations: The discussion critically reviews operational impediments encountered in field deployment, among them training-data scarcity, post-deployment model drift, algorithmic bias, patient privacy constraints, and jurisdiction-specific regulatory mandates, and it proposes mitigation protocols consistent with principles of equitable and trustworthy healthcare AI.
- Future Research Directions and Impact: The chapter concludes by mapping prospective research avenues toward compact foundation models, heterogeneous edge accelerators, and environmentally sustainable deployment pipelines, thereby positioning on-device, agentic vision-language systems as a potentially scalable mechanism for building resilient and globally inclusive healthcare delivery networks.

2. AGENTIC VISION LANGUAGE MODELS

Figure 1. Agentic reasoning layers for clinical vision language models

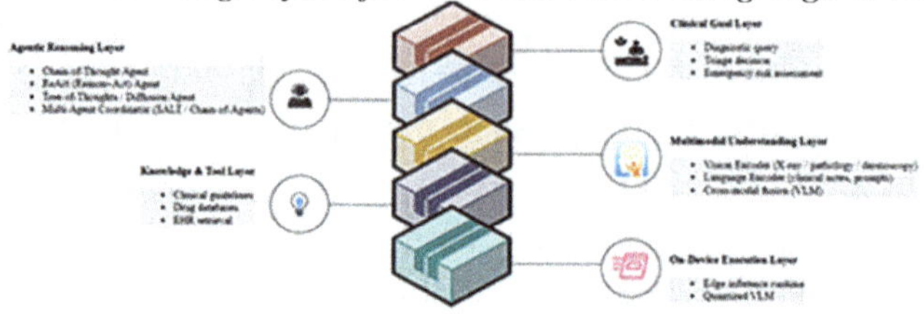

The modules in this section are represented as layers in Figure 1. The figure illustrates how multiple reasoning agents such as chain-of-thought, ReAct, Tree-of-Thoughts, diffusion-based operate above a shared vision language perception layer, enabling planning, self-correction, and knowledge grounded clinical decision support on device.

2.1 Reasoning Mechanism for Agentic AI

Agentic AI represents a change from static, fixed-parameter models to systems capable of independent judgment, planning and adaptive decision making. At its core, agentic AI breaks complex tasks into sequences of reasoning steps, often distributed across multiple interacting agents each having a specialized roles or competencies (Dernbach et al., 2024; Plaat et al., 2025).

Early foundations of agentic reasoning in large language models (LLMs) were established through chain-of-thought (CoT) prompting, which enables models to explicitly generate intermediate reasoning steps before producing final outputs (Zhang et al., 2022). Self-operating models further reduce human intervention by allowing models to self-generate reasoning, improving concepts across complex tasks (Zhang et al., 2022). In reference to healthcare, CoT-style reasoning enhances transparency and enables models to formulate diagnostic logic, thereby supporting clinician trust and interpretability.

Building on the concept of Chain-of-Thought (CoT), the ReAct framework merges critical thinking with practical application. It helps AI models connect their internal logic to real-world tasks like using external tools, finding information, or interacting with a system (Yao et al., 2022). This method is especially useful in medical fields, specifically for clinical decision support. In these situations, healthcare professionals need to access a variety of data sources such as searching medical databases, analysing patient scans, and reviewing health records to make informed choices.

Several sophisticated methods are being developed to make artificial intelligence mimic the way humans think and solve problems.

The technique Tree-of-Thoughts (ToT), works by the creation of a branching, search-like process which builds on traditional linear thinking (Yao et al., 2023). "This method lets the AI try out a bunch of different ways to think through a problem in such a way that it can toss aside the ones that don't work as well. Being able to fix its own mistakes and still make good calls, even when it doesn't have all the facts, is super important for critical situations like those you'd find in a hospital. "Diffusion" is the name of another set of newer methods. These methods approach the reasoning process as if it were an exploration of a concealed realm of potential answers. This allows the AI to manage ambiguity and refine its answers progressively (Ye et al., 2024; Hersche et al., 2025).

Researchers are also creating systems where multiple AIs work together much like a team of people. Frameworks like Chain-of-Agents show how a group of language models can collaborate on complex tasks by sharing their intermediate thinking processes (Zhang et al., 2024). One alternative strategy is known as SALT (Thinking Fast and Laterally), which draws on a variety of parallel reasoning methods inspired by the diverse ways human minds operate; this approach enables rapid and creative exploration when tackling new problems. Research rooted in neuroscience indicates that these types of multi-agent systems are actually more effective at mirroring human thought processes, including elements such as the use of abstract ideas, feedback loops, and adaptable control mechanisms.

Ultimately, these various AI "thinking" strategies are providing the necessary groundwork for future clinical AI systems that can plan ahead, fix their own mistakes, and effectively integrate new knowledge to assist in medical decision-making.

Figure 2. Reasoning paradigms in clinical decision support

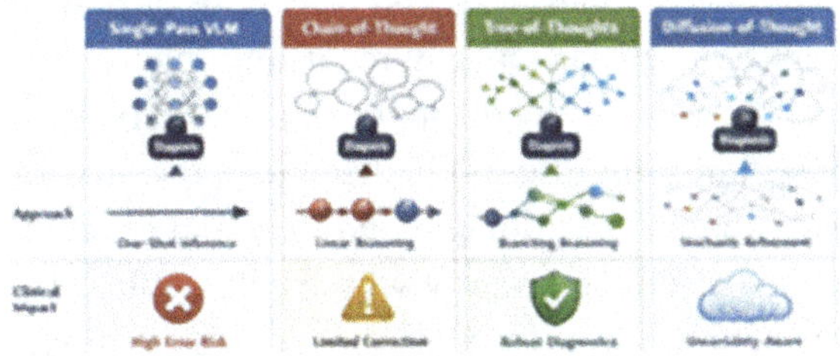

The above Figure 2 shows a side-by-side comparison of different thinking styles used in AI systems. It shows how we've moved from simple, one-shot processing to more complex, organized ways of thinking methods that can actually handle uncertainty. These advanced, multi-step systems are the kind we use now to help make crucial decisions in healthcare settings.

2.2 Vision Language Models in Healthcare

Vision Language Models (VLMs) merge sight and sound information by processing how images and words connect which helps line up the meaning between what we see and what we read (Das & Akter, 2025; Ahmed & Naji, 2025). In the medical field, this ability is key for activities like writing descriptions for medical images, creating reports, answering questions based on pictures and thinking through patient information using different sources. (Kamrul et al., 2025; Maheriya, 2025).

Clinical Vision Language Models (VLMs) often require paired datasets, which match a medical image like a chest X-ray or pathology slide with its corresponding report or electronic health record (EHR) text. Large and multimodal datasets like EHRXQA and MIMIC-CXR-VQA provide realistic scenarios for testing how well these VLMs can reason using both image and text information in the medical field (Bae et al., 2023; Bae et al., 2024).

Recent progress in artificial intelligence shows that medical imaging models known as foundation models benefit greatly from being initially trained on diverse types of data at a large scale (Raval et al., 2024). Extensive pretraining reduces the necessity for manual annotation as the models can more effectively adapt to new tasks.

Further studies and reviews confirm the increasing importance of AI systems that can interpret multiple types of information at once, in helping doctors make clinical decisions. They point out that diagnostic accuracy improves when imaging data is combined with relevant patient notes and structured clinical information (Kamrul et al., 2025; Das & Akter, 2025; Maheriya, 2025; Saini & Sunil, 2025; Kurz et al., 2025).

Clinical Vision Language Models (VLMs) have a lot of potential but they need to overcome significant hurdles particularly regarding inherent data bias, shifts in medical domains, and the crucial need for transparent explanations of their reasoning. Research consistently highlights the necessity for ongoing validation and monitoring once these models are implemented in actual clinical environments to detect issues like data drift. This is exactly why Explainable AI (XAI) techniques are being rapidly integrated into multimodal systems, it's essential for building trust and encouraging their broader adoption among medical professionals.

2.3 Model Optimization and On-Device AI Hardware

Running powerful Vision Language Models (VLMs) as agents in healthcare settings often requires processing these models locally on the device itself, rather than depending on cloud services especially where internet connectivity is limited. This on-device inference is essential for ensuring swift performance, patient privacy and reliable operation in environments with fewer resources. The technology that enables this typically involves common edge computing platforms such as Modern Smartphones equipped with specialized components like Neural Processing Units (NPUs), built-in Graphics Processing Units (GPUs), and energy-efficient micro-controllers (Sharshar et al., 2025).

Today's mobile devices boast remarkable power but they still have limitations such as including restricted memory, battery life and thermal management (heat). Consequently, the large and complex artificial intelligence models we rely on for tasks like interpreting images, text and voice or functioning as smart agents, cannot simply be deployed in their original form, they require substantial optimization and fine-tuning to run efficiently within this constraint. Here are the key ways by which the developers optimize these models:

- Quantization: This strategy is like using a simpler scale for numbers. By reducing the numerical precision needed for calculations the models use less memory and computational power.
- Pruning: Developers remove redundant parts or connections within the model that don't significantly affect performance.
- Knowledge Distillation: This involves training a smaller and more efficient "student" model to mimic the performance of a much larger "teacher" model. The goal is to transfer the essential smarts to a package better suited for running directly on your phone.

These techniques help ensure that powerful AI features work seamlessly on the device in your pocket (Sharshar et al., 2025).

Recent research indicates that advanced AI specifically optimized deep learning models can be successfully run directly on smartphones for medical diagnoses like identifying brain tumours and analysing chest X-rays (Nissen et al., 2025; Huang et al., 2025). These models perform well enough for clinical use and operate in real-time right on the device. Furthermore, evaluations of on-device large language Models (LLMs) suggest that lighter weight AI reasoning models can effectively aid clinical decision making, provided they are carefully adjusted to work within the limitations of smartphone hardware (Tran et al., 2025).

Due to several software frameworks, it is now possible to run powerful AI applications directly on user devices. This feature that enables for rapid analysis without constant internet connectivity, is essential for effective healthcare AI particularly in places with limited resources. TensorFlow Lite, Apple's Core ML and more recent additions like Apple's powerful MLX are important frameworks supporting this effort. These tools are specifically engineered to execute compressed AI models effectively on edge devices like smartphones and tablets offering several critical features such as:

- Hardware Acceleration: They utilize devices with specialized internal components such as Graphics Processing Units (GPUs) and Neural Processing Units (NPUs) to significantly speed up complex mathematical calculations necessary for AI.
- Memory Optimization: The frameworks incorporate smart memory management to allow sophisticated models to run smoothly even on devices with constrained memory preventing system crashes.
- Privacy Preserving Inference: A crucial feature for sensitive healthcare applications as all data processing occurs locally on the device. This ensures private patient information remains under the user's control and never leaves the device thus maintaining confidentiality and complying with privacy regulations.

These combined features create the scalable and efficient infrastructure needed to make advanced healthcare AI widely accessible and practical.

Figure 3. On-device deployment pipeline for agentic vision language model

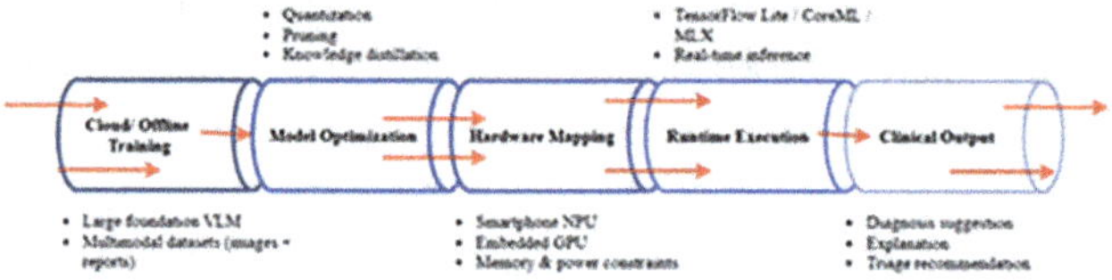

Large AI models that can understand different kinds of data (like images, text and sound) are being made smaller and tailored to work directly on devices with limited power such as a smartphone or a small computer in a hospital room. This allows them to analyse medical information instantly and keep it private because the data never has to leave the device (Figure 3). In plain terms, powerful diagnostic AI is being built to run quickly and securely *on* the device itself providing instant insights while protecting patient privacy.

3. DESIGNING AGENTIC ARCHITECTURES FOR HEALTHCARE

Agentic architectures augment traditional vision–language or language-only foundation models through the incorporation of goal-directed reasoning, tool invocation, persistent memory, and sequential decision-making capabilities that are requisite for complex clinical workflows. Within healthcare deployments, and notably in settings characterized by limited computational and data resources, these architectures are required to maintain a trade-off among reasoning accuracy, robustness, and computational efficiency while simultaneously satisfying stringent privacy and latency requirements. The present section examines three principal design axes: (i) models that support reliable reasoning, (ii) memory and grounding mechanisms, and (iii) frameworks for multi-agent collaboration.

3.1 Reasoning-Capable Models for Clinical Decision Support

Conventional end-to-end neural networks typically conduct inference in a single pass and do not retain an explicit reasoning trace; this characteristic limits their utility in safety-critical medical contexts. Agentic large language models mitigate the limitation by embedding structured reasoning techniques such as chain-of-thought prompting, ReAct-style cycles of reasoning and action, and tree-based search procedures (Dernbach et al., 2024; Liu et al., 2025; Zhang et al., 2024). Within clinical settings, these models can be operationalized through several configurations: (1) chained architectures that sequence multiple language-model invocations to decompose complex objectives—patient triage, for instance, may be segmented into symptom summarization, risk stratification, and recommendation synthesis; (2) tool-augmented agents that call external resources, for example pharmaceutical interaction databases, diagnostic criteria repositories, or scoring calculators, while reasoning (Liu et al., 2025); and (3) self-correcting loops that assess intermediate conclusions against clinical guidelines or predefined uncertainty thresholds, allowing iterative refinement prior to final output generation (Zhang et al., 2024). In emergency triage, an illustrative pipeline might first process patient-reported symptoms, subsequently query a knowledge base to identify high-risk indicators, and finally output a prioritized list of recommended actions accompanied by justifications. Empirical evaluations indicate that such multi-step reasoning yields markedly higher reliability relative to single-pass inference (Yao et al., 2022).

3.2 Memory and Grounding for Clinical Context Awareness

A critical limitation of standalone LLMs is their lack of persistent memory and grounding in patient-specific data. In healthcare, effective decision support requires reasoning that is contextualized to patient history, institutional protocols, and validated medical knowledge.

3.2.1 Retrieval-Augmented Generation (RAG)

Retrieval-augmented generation incorporates an external retrieval component that locates pertinent documents—clinical guidelines, research articles, or patient records—and appends them to the language model's context window (Zhang et al., 2022). This procedure decreases hallucination, increases factual accuracy, and permits prompt knowledge updates without retraining the base parameters. In settings with limited computational resources, lightweight vector databases or compressed knowledge stores can be instantiated on-device or on proximal edge servers to provide the grounding substrate required for RAG (Raval & Maheriya, 2023).

Retrieval-Augmented Generation conjoins parametric language models with external corpora to enhance factual precision, personalisation, and contextual continuity. We systematically examine RAG's deployment for two complementary objectives: memory, which supports durable retention and re-use of user-specific information, and grounding, which restricts generated content to externally verifiable evidence. Architectural configurations, data pipelines, and retrieval protocols for both objectives are delineated, together with error-mitigation techniques. Figure 4 Memory and grounding mechanisms for agentic clinical decision support. Retrieval-augmented generation, when anchored in electronic health records, facilitates patient-specific reasoning that remains consistent with established knowledge and diminishes hallucination probability.

Figure 4. Memory and grounding mechanisms for agentic clinical decision support

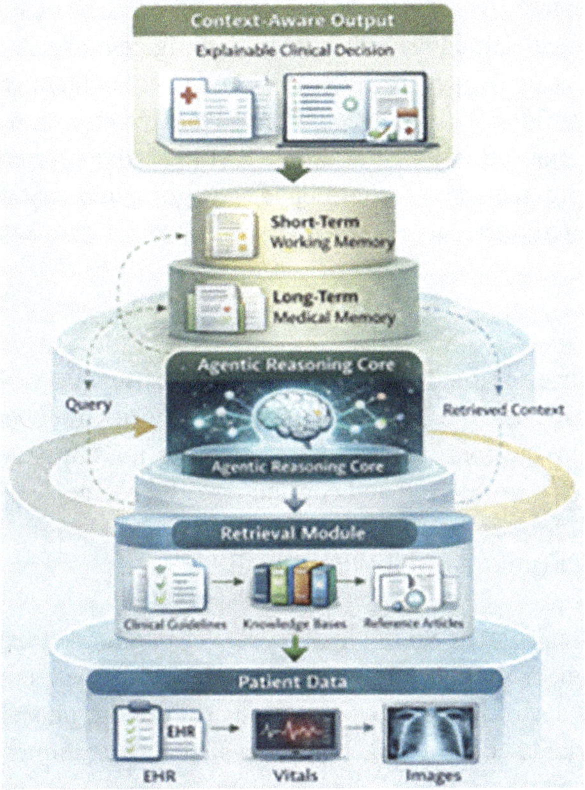

3.2.1.1 Retrieval-Augmented Memory

The scope of retrieval-augmented memory encompasses user preferences, historical interaction traces, and distilled factual knowledge accumulated across successive sessions. In contrast to short-term conversational context, these representations remain persistent and undergo incremental modification over time.

> <u>RAG-Based System Architecture:</u> A retrieval-augmented memory subsystem extends the language model with an external, vector-indexed store. The architecture comprises (i) a memory extraction component, (ii) an embedding model, (iii) a vector database, and (iv) a retrieval mechanism invoked during inference. Formally, for an interaction instance x_t, the extractor f_m generates a set of memory items $M_t=\{m_1,\ldots,m_k\}$. Each item is transformed by encoder $E(\cdot)$ into an embedding and subsequently stored in the vector database.

Memory Storage (Write Path): Following each interaction, durable information is isolated via constrained prompting or classification. Transient or low-confidence elements are discarded to mitigate noise. A memory entry is expressed as c_i, τ_i, γ_i, where c_i denotes the textual content, τi the timestamp, and γi the confidence score in equation 1. Dense vector representations of the content are indexed in a vector store (FAISS, Milvus, or equivalent), while accompanying metadata—confidence, category, recency—are retained to support filtered retrieval.

$$m_i=(c_i,\tau_i,\gamma_i) \qquad (1)$$

Memory Retrieval (Read Path): At inference, the user query q is embedded and employed to retrieve the top-K most similar memories by cosine similarity. The retrieved items are concatenated into the prompt, thereby providing contextual grounding for personalized and continuous response generation (equation 2).

$$sim(q,m_i) = E(q)*E(mi) / [||E(q)|| \cdot ||E(mi)||] \quad (2)$$

Memory Management Strategies: To curtail unbounded expansion and the accumulation of outdated information, relevance is attenuated through an exponential decay function by equation 3. Periodic clustering of episodic memories yields compressed, higher-level semantic summaries, decreasing redundancy while retaining salient content.

$$w_i=\gamma_i \cdot e^{-\lambda \Delta t} \qquad (3)$$

3.2.1.2 RAG for Grounding

Grounding denotes the practice of restricting generated outputs to information retrieved from authoritative external sources. In contrast to memory mechanisms, grounding data are not user-specific; rather, they function as a reference standard for factual accuracy. Source documents are divided into partially overlapping chunks so as to preserve semantic coherence while simultaneously maximising retrieval recall. Every chunk is annotated with structured metadata that typically includes document identifiers and temporal markers. Hybrid retrieval strategies that integrate dense vector similarity with sparse lexical matching—most frequently BM25, as indicated in equation 4—are routinely adopted. Grounding is implemented by means of explicit prompt constraints that proscribe the incorporation of information lying beyond the retrieved context. When the available evidence is judged insufficient, the model is directed to withhold a response.

$$score=\alpha \cdot dense(q,d)+\beta \cdot BM25(q,d) \qquad (4)$$

Advanced grounding techniques encompass multi-hop retrieval and reranking procedures. Multi-hop retrieval is characterized by queries of elevated complexity; such queries, which necessitate reasoning across more than one document, are resolved through successive retrieval iterations in which intermediate entities direct subsequent retrieval cycles. Cross-encoder reranking models are subsequently applied to refine the relevance of the retrieved evidence prior to generation. Table 1 presents a comparative overview of memory and grounding within retrieval-augmented generation. Figure 5 shows the failure modes with their analysed solutions

Figure 5. Failure modes

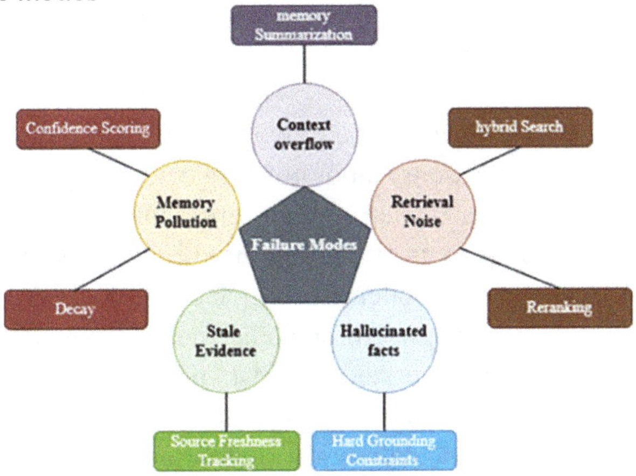

Table 1. Comparative overview of memory and grounding within retrieval-augmented generation

Dimension	Memory-Oriented RAG	Grounding-Oriented RAG
Objective	Personalization and continuity	Factual correctness
Data scope	User-specific	Global / authoritative
Persistence	Long-term	Query-time
Error impact	Low to moderate	High
Update cycle	Incremental	Periodic or real-time

3.2.2 EHR-Grounded Agentic Reasoning

Conventional clinical decision support (CDS) architectures are generally classified into three groups. Although these implementations can attain strong task-specific performance, they offer limited visibility into intermediate reasoning and are not readily transferable to multi-condition clinical settings.

- The first group comprises rule-based systems that encode guideline-derived alerts through if then logic.
- The second encompasses statistical risk models such as logistic regression or Cox proportional-hazard models for outcome forecasting.
- The third consists of machine-learning predictors—for example, gradient-boosted tree ensembles or neural networks—trained on structured electronic health record (EHR) features.

Agentic models may be anchored directly in EHRs by temporally ordering patient data summaries (medications, laboratory trajectories, prior diagnoses). The agent performs inference over this structured representation while satisfying privacy constraints, because raw data are not required to leave the local environment (Yao et al., 2023). Memory components can include short-term working memory for episode-level reasoning, long-term episodic memory for patient history, and semantic memory derived from curated medical knowledge bases. This anchoring supports personalized recommendations and preserves traceability and explanatory capacity (Ye et al., 2024). EHR data contain structured components (laboratory results, medication records, ICD- or SNOMED-coded diagnoses) and unstructured textual elements (progress notes, discharge summaries). An EHR-anchored agent usually integrates:

- FHIR-based extraction pipelines that provide standardized access to structured data;
- Clinical natural-language-processing modules for entity recognition, negation identification, and temporal alignment within narrative text;
- Patient-state representations, frequently expressed as time-indexed feature graphs or serialized clinical summaries.

These representations constitute the substrate upon which downstream reasoning operates. The system's central component is a reasoning agent, typically instantiated as a large language model supplemented with external tools. The agent follows an iterative loop that enables sequential clinical reasoning rather than a single inference pass:

1. State assessment: interpreting the present patient context from EHR-derived representations;
2. Hypothesis generation: formulating diagnostic, prognostic, or management hypotheses;
3. Evidence evaluation: querying EHR data, clinical guidelines, or computational calculators to test hypotheses;
4. Planning and action selection: determining subsequent reasoning steps or therapeutic suggestions;
5. Reflection and revision: updating internal beliefs when contradictions or new evidence arise.

3.3 Multi-Agent Collaboration in Healthcare Systems

Complex clinical decision-making often involves multiple specialized competencies, such as image interpretation, language understanding, and treatment planning. Multi-agent systems address this by decomposing tasks across cooperating agents, each optimized for a specific role (Hersche et al., 2025; Plaat et al., 2025). Figure 6 shows Multi-agent collaboration framework for healthcare decision support. Specialized agents communicate through structured protocols to jointly perform perception, reasoning, and planning tasks.

Figure 6. Multi-agent collaboration framework for healthcare decision support

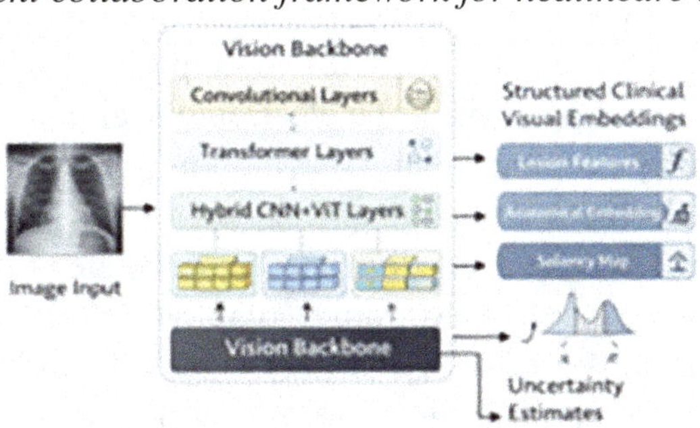

3.3.1 Specialized Clinical Agents

A prototypical EHR-grounded, agent-centric healthcare architecture decomposes clinical reasoning into a collection of functionally specialized agents whose respective optimisation targets are aligned with particular data modalities and inferential objectives. Such a modular configuration permits scalable reasoning over heterogeneous clinical inputs while simultaneously facilitating interpretability and enforcing safety constraints.

Imaging Analysis Agent: The imaging-analysis agent assumes responsibility for the processing of radiological, pathological, or point-of-care imaging data. It is typically implemented through deep convolutional neural networks or transformer-based visual encoders that have been pretrained on large-scale medical imaging corpora. Contemporary implementations increasingly favour vision–language models in which a visual encoder such as Vision Transformer or Swin Transformer undergoes joint training with a language decoder so as to generate structured findings together with textual interpretations. Formally, given an imaging input x_{img}, the agent derives a latent representation according to equation 5, where f_{θ} denotes the pretrained visual encoder. The resulting representation is subsequently mapped to clinically meaningful outputs, including probabilistic labels, region-level annotations, or free-text reports, each of which is explicitly grounded in imaging-derived evidence and forwarded to downstream agents.

$$z_{img}=f,(x_{img}) \qquad (5)$$

Language Reasoning Agent: The language-reasoning component ingests heterogeneous clinical text such as progress notes, discharge summaries, and patient-authored reports. Ordinarily it is implemented as a large language model fine-tuned on domain-specific corpora and supplemented by retrieval routines that query structured portions of the electronic health record. The supported operations encompass named-entity recognition, temporal relation extraction, differential diagnosis formulation, and explanatory text synthesis. To ensure factual anchoring, the agent conditions every generated token on a structured patient state vector s_t computed from available EHR features; it additionally applies constrained decoding or citation layers to attribute individual claims to concrete data points. Formally, the agent's output is produced according to Equation 6, where K represents external medical knowledge bases such as clinical guidelines or biomedical ontologies.

$$y_{text}=g_{\phi}(x_{text},s_t,K) \qquad (6)$$

Planning and Orchestration Agent.: The planning or orchestrative agent aggregates multimodal evidence generated by domain-specific agents and concurrently manages uncertainty, temporal dependencies, and clinically relevant objectives. Implementation may rely on a deliberative planning framework, policy models derived from reinforcement learning, or symbolic planners whose search is guided by neural scoring functions. The agent retains an explicit belief state over alternative clinical hypotheses and chooses actions—such as soliciting supplementary information, querying external instruments, or issuing recommendations—by optimizing an expected-utility function while satisfying predefined safety and scope constraints. This capacity supports adaptive reasoning along dynamically changing patient trajectories rather than restricting inference to a single, static decision step.

3.3.2 Communication and Coordination

Coordinated interaction among functionally specialized agents constitutes a prerequisite for coherent and clinically defensible decision support. Communication is conventionally realized through structured message-passing protocols, shared vectorised memory regions, or planner-mediated schemes that retain full provenance and uncertainty metadata.

Centralized Orchestration: Under centralized control, a single controller agent orchestrates every specialist, maintains a global state vector, and adjudicates conflicts. While this arrangement simplifies governance and facilitates audit, the controller can become a throughput bottleneck as the population of agents increases.

Decentralized Negotiation: Decentralised coordination enables agents to operate with partial autonomy, exchanging messages that encode beliefs, confidence values, or partial plans. When conflicts emerge, consensus or voting mechanisms reconcile divergent outputs, thereby enhancing robustness in clinical contexts characterised by noisy or incomplete data.

Hierarchical Planning: Hierarchical planning structures stratify agents into abstraction tiers. Higher-level agents formulate high-level clinical goals—diagnostic clarification, for example—whereas lower-level agents implement modality-specific sub-tasks. Such hierarchies map readily onto established clinical workflows and enable temporally extended, decomposable reasoning (Plaat et al., 2025). Independently of the chosen coordination paradigm, strict interface specifications and validation layers ensure that inter-agent discourse remains anchored to verifiable electronic health-record data and that the final recommendations are interpretable and clinician-facing.

4. ARCHITECTURAL BACKBONES AND SYSTEM DESIGN FOR AGENTIC CLINICAL AI

Each agent in the framework is instantiated using a domain-optimized backbone, selected based on modality characteristics, computational constraints, and clinical interpretability requirements.

4.1 Backbone Models for Specialized Clinical Agents

Imaging Agent: Vision Backbone: The imaging agent employs deep visual backbones tailored to medical imaging modalities such as X-ray, ultrasound, fundus photography, or histopathology. Common architectural choices include Convolutional Neural Networks (CNNs) for spatially localized feature extraction in low-resolution or noisy images. Vision Transformers (ViTs) for global context modeling and improved representation of anatomical structures. Hybrid CNN, Transformer architectures, balancing inductive bias and long-range dependency modeling. These backbones are typically pretrained on large-scale medical datasets or initialized from vision foundation models before task-specific fine-tuning. Intermediate outputs such as abnormality embeddings, saliency maps, or uncertainty estimates are exposed to downstream agents rather than raw logits, enhancing interpretability and robustness. Figure 7 shows basic structure of vision backbone multiagent clinical AI.

Figure 7. Structure of vision backbone multiagent clinical AI

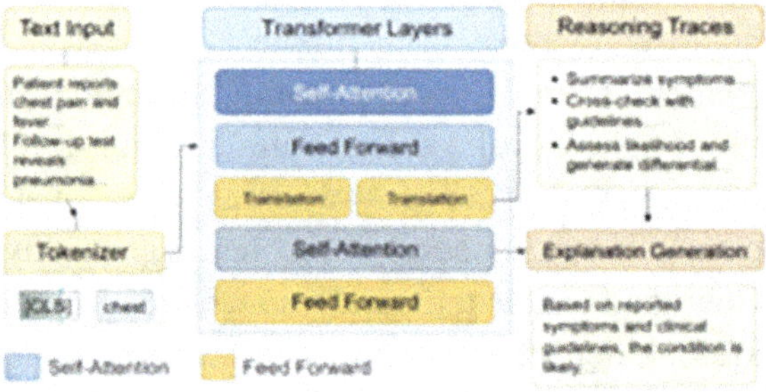

Language Agent: Clinical NLP Backbone: The language agent is built upon transformer-based large language models adapted for healthcare text. Its responsibilities include Parsing unstructured clinical notes and radiology reports,

Mapping free-text descriptions to standardized medical concepts, Generating clinician-facing explanations and summaries. Domain adaptation is achieved via continued pretraining on biomedical corpora and instruction tuning using clinical question–answer pairs. Chain-of-thought and tool-augmented prompting strategies enable the language agent to perform multi-step reasoning and integrate external medical knowledge. Figure 8 shows language backbone for clinical AI agent

Figure 8. Language backbone for clinical AI agent

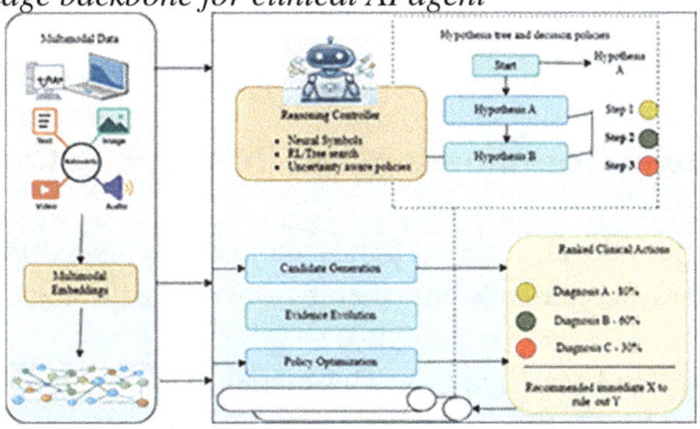

<u>Planning and Reasoning Agent: Decision Backbone:</u> The planning agent orchestrates decision synthesis across modalities. Unlike purely neural predictors, this agent integrates Neural-symbolic reasoning, combining learned policies with rule-based constraints, Reinforcement learning or tree-search mechanisms for exploring diagnostic hypotheses, Uncertainty-aware decision policies to trigger deferral or human review. This agent operates on structured evidence produced by other agents and generates ranked diagnostic or triage recommendations with confidence scores. Figure- 9 shows architecture for planning and reasoning agent for clinical decision support system.

Figure 9. Architecture for planning and reasoning agent for clinical decision support system

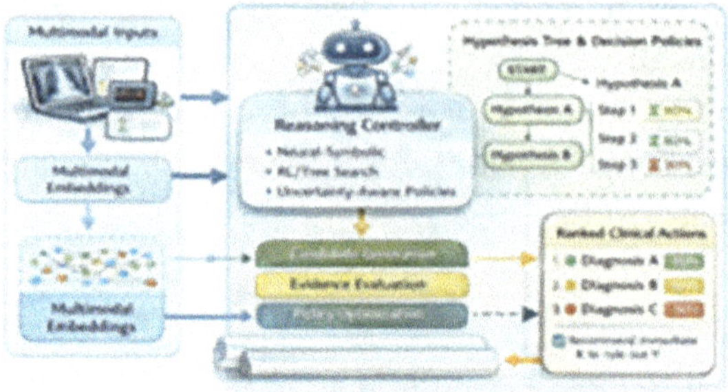

4.2 System-Level Coordination and Communication Backbone

At the architectural level, coordination is realised by a shared-memory substrate coupled with a message-passing bus, thereby obviating the requirement for end-to-end fusion.

Shared Memory and Message Bus: The shared-memory component retains intermediate agent outputs, temporal patient-context information, and metadata that encode confidence scores and provenance. This arrangement facilitates asynchronous agent execution, isolates faults, and supports longitudinal reasoning that extends across successive patient encounters.

Orchestration and Control Logic: A lightweight orchestration layer supervises the invocation order of agents, adjudicates conflicts among their outputs, and enforces safety checks together with fallback mechanisms. The explicit control scheme is indispensable for ensuring clinical reliability and for satisfying applicable regulatory obligations.

4.3 End-to-End Backbone Architecture: Integrated View

To consolidate the above components, an end-to-end backbone diagram is strongly recommended. Figure 10 shows the base architectural diagram of Agentic Clinical AI backbone which unifies agentic reasoning, multimodal perception, and clinical workflow integration. This includes different input modalities like images, vitals and text. The figure shows a specialized agent backbone which has shared memory and communication pathways. This forms the core idea for planning and arbitration logic.

Figure 10. Backbone of agentic clinical AI backbone

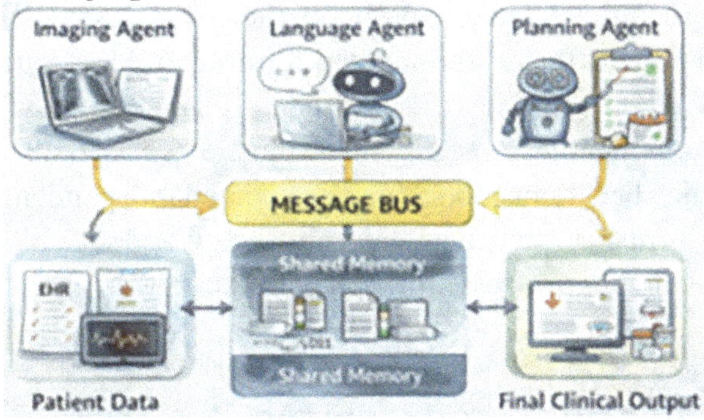

Input layer: The Imaging Agent ingests visual data through a vision encoder whose backbone can be instantiated as convolutional neural networks, vision transformers, or hybrid convolutional-transformer variants. It derives high-level diagnostic embeddings enumerating anatomical deviations, lesion attributes, or uncertainty measures and translates these embeddings into structured diagnostic tokens rather than retaining raw pixel intensities.

Language Agent: The Language Agent rests on a transformer-based large language model that has been further fine-tuned on medical corpora. It parses clinical narratives, compresses patient histories, and emits reasoning chains and natural-language explanations that comply with standard clinical lexicons. Additionally, the agent operates as the primary locus for clinician interaction and system interpretability.

Planning agent: The Planning Agent embeds decision-oriented learning modules, exemplified by reinforcement-learning policies or symbolic-neural controllers. It assimilates evidence furnished by upstream agents, maintains an intermediate reasoning buffer, and performs task decomposition, risk stratification, and recommendation ranking while satisfying applicable clinical constraints.

Shared memory: Agent communication is mediated by a Shared Memory / Message Bus that persistently stores patient histories, external knowledge bases, and intermediate reasoning states. This common substrate permits asynchronous message passing, longitudinal context retention, and auditable information flow—attributes necessary for sustained patient monitoring and post-hoc explanation.

Orchestration and Arbitration Layer: Subjacent to the memory layer, the Orchestration and Arbitration Layer enforces system-wide coordination. Its control logic resolves priority contentions, enforces safety assertions, and adjudicates conflicts among agent outputs, thereby ensuring that final recommendations conform to predetermined clinical protocols and ethical guidelines and that errors remain localized rather than propagating.

Clinical output: The system culminates in a Final Clinical Output that packages context-sensitive recommendations, probabilistic risk assessments, and annotated decision traces. These artifacts are intended for human-AI co-operation, allowing clinicians to inspect, corroborate, or supersede AI suggestions within established clinical workflows. Collectively, the schematic illustrates a decoupled yet harmonized architecture in which backbone models can be updated independently and the agent-based framework furnishes robustness, interpretability, and scalability—capabilities regarded as prerequisites for real-time decision support in resource-constrained environments.

4.4 Design Rationale and Advantages

The proposed backbone-centric architecture consists of a number of advantages relative to monolithic models. Modularity permits individual backbones to be updated or replaced without necessitating system-wide alterations. Interpretability is enhanced because agent-specific outputs generate structured, traceable explanations. Scalability is preserved through the straightforward incorporation of additional agents (for instance, genomics or wearable-derived modules) without wholesale redesign. Deployment feasibility is maintained under resource constraints by accommodating both edge and hybrid deployment schemes. Collectively, these characteristics render the architecture well-suited to low-resource and safety-critical healthcare settings.

5. MULTIMODAL CLINICAL DECISION SUPPORT USE CASES

5.1. Point-of-Care Imaging and Triage

A principal application domain for autonomous vision–language models is point-of-care medical imaging, encompassing chest radiography, ultrasonography, and retinal photography. Within this framework, vision encoders derive structured visual representations from the acquired images, and language models subsequently situate these representations within the context of associated clinical text—for example, symptom descriptions, triage documentation, and historical diagnoses (Ahmed & Naji, 2025; Raval & Borisagar, n.d.). In emergency and primary-care environments, multimodal systems are capable of the following functions:

(i) automated triage of chest radiographs for pathological indicators such as pneumonia or tuberculosis,
(ii) generation of structured radiological reports or visual question-answering outputs, and

(iii) ranking of cases according to estimated clinical urgency (Sharshar et al., 2025; Abdelrahman, 2025).

Empirical benchmarking indicates that multimodal foundation models achieve higher diagnostic accuracy and enhanced robustness compared with unimodal convolutional pipelines, an advantage that is especially pronounced when imaging data are degraded by noise or incomplete acquisition (Kurz et al., 2025; Edirisinghe et al., 2025).

5.2 Dermatology and Ophthalmology

Dermatologic evaluation of skin lesions and retinal assessment for diabetic retinopathy represent clinical tasks that are particularly compatible with mobile or edge-based artificial intelligence implementations, primarily because both tasks rely on static images as the principal data modality. Architectures that couple deep convolutional feature extractors examples include MobileNetV2 and EfficientNet with parsimonious language-oriented reasoning components that can execute interpretative and explanatory functions directly on the device (Reddy et al., 2019). Empirical evaluations of smartphone-driven fundus photography and dermoscopic inspection indicate that, in low-resource environments, such systems can attain sensitivity and specificity values that compare favourably with conventional specialist-dependent pathways, thereby mitigating constraints imposed by limited specialist availability (Dangi et al., 2025; Bareja et al., 2025). When supplementary inputs such as concise symptom narratives and concise historical details are incorporated, vision–language models that exhibit agentic properties can issue screening recommendations conditioned on estimated risk, yielding measurable gains in the proportion of cases identified at earlier stages.

5.3 Infectious Disease Diagnosis and Symptom Reasoning

Multimodal symptom checkers integrate Patient-reported symptoms (text or speech), Vital signs and Contextual epidemiological information. Agentic reasoning models can sequentially infer disease likelihoods, query relevant medical knowledge bases, and refine hypotheses through self-correction loops (Raval & Maheriya, 2023; Yao et al., 2023). During infectious disease outbreaks, such systems support rapid decision-making in resource-constrained environments, as demonstrated in COVID-19–related multimodal AI systems (Raval & Maheriya, 2023; Raval et al., 2024).

5.4 Integration of Agentic VLMs into Clinical Workflows

For measurable clinical utility, agentic vision–language models must interface with pre-existing clinical workflows while preserving human supervisory control. Rather than functioning as autonomous diagnostic engines, these systems are intentionally positioned as decision-support instruments that output ranked recommendations, calibrated confidence intervals, and explicit lines of reasoning in lieu of conclusive diagnoses (Kamrul et al., 2025; Das & Akter, 2025).

5.4.1 Mobile and Telemedicine Deployment

In settings characterised by limited infrastructure, agentic VLMs can be instantiated as smartphone applications utilised by community health workers; the architecture tolerates intermittent or fully offline connectivity. Corresponding embedded components integrated into telemedicine platforms supply remote clinicians with multimodal case synopses and differential suggestions (Raval et al., 2024). Real-time inference is attainable through device-level optimisation strategies such as quantisation-aware training, knowledge distillation, and hardware acceleration on mobile neural processing units or embedded graphics processors (Tran et al., 2025; Raval & Oza, 2025).

5.4.2 Human–AI Collaboration and Explainability

Human & AI interaction continues to constitute a prerequisite for dependable deployment. The models emit intermediate reasoning traces (for example, chain-of-thought textual summaries), visually demarcated regions of interest, and natural-language justifications mapped to prevailing clinical guidelines (Bae et al., 2023; Merkow et al., 2023). Explainable artificial intelligence methodologies enhance clinician trustworthiness and streamline post-hoc auditing, particularly within medical imaging contexts where algorithmic bias and dataset drift represent extensively documented liabilities (Bae et al., 2024; Dombrowski et al., 2024).

5.5 Designing for Low-Resource Clinical Contexts

5.5.1 Edge and Offline Functionality

Low-resource settings typically exhibit limited network reliability and computational infrastructure. Consequently, agentic vision-language models intended for deployment in such contexts emphasize on-device inference, offline reasoning and retrieval, and minimal demands on memory and power consumption (Tran et al., 2025; Reddy et al., 2019). Edge-compatible vision-language models and compressed multimodal architectures support sustained operation without recourse to cloud services, thereby safeguarding patient privacy and reducing latency (Nissen et al., 2025).

5.5.2 Minimalist Interfaces and Multilingual Support

User interfaces must remain intelligible and accessible to individuals who lack specialist training. Effective interface designs therefore favor visual cues over dense textual information, support multilingual natural-language interaction, and present simple confidence indicators rather than detailed probability distributions (Huang et al., 2025; Raval et al., 2024). These principles are essential for adoption by community health workers and primary-care providers in low- and middle-income countries.

5.5.3 Evidence from Low-Resource Deployments

Empirical investigations have established the feasibility of artificial-intelligence-supported screening and diagnostic procedures in constrained environments. Representative examples include smartphone-based brain-tumor detection via optimized convolutional neural networks (Reddy et al., 2019), large-scale primary-care chest radiography interpretation (Bareja et al., 2025), and community-based diabetic-retinopathy screening programs assisted by artificial intelligence (Miró Catalina et al., 2024). Collectively, these implementations underscore the capacity of agentic multimodal systems to address clinical requirements when operational constraints are explicitly incorporated into model design (Raval & Oza, 2025; Raval et al., 2024).

6. DEPLOYMENT CHALLENGES AND SOLUTIONS

Deploying autonomous, on-device vision–language models to provide clinical decision support in settings with limited infrastructure introduces a distinct constellation of infrastructural, data-related, and operational difficulties. Progress in this domain necessitates coordinated improvements in system architecture, model resilience, and end-to-end lifecycle governance.

6.1 Connectivity and Power Constraints

Regions characterised by intermittent internet access and unreliable electricity render cloud-dependent artificial intelligence solutions impractical. Sustained transmission of data to distant servers increases latency, raises operational expenditure, and amplifies privacy exposure, whereas power-intensive inference stages conflict with the energy constraints inherent to mobile clinical routines (Raval & Oza, 2025; Raval et al., 2024).

Offline-First and Edge-Centric Architectures:

To accommodate these constraints, offline-first deployment patterns are gaining traction. Such architectures emphasise local inference executed with compressed representations, asynchronous synchronisation scheduled whenever intermittent connectivity permits, and graceful degradation that sustains partial functionality when resources are restricted. Advances in mobile artificial intelligence accelerators including smartphone neural processing units, embedded graphics processing units, and specialised machine-learning chips facilitate efficient execution of quantised and distilled vision–language models within stringent power envelopes (Tran et al., 2025; Raval & Oza, 2025). Empirical comparisons of on-device large language models indicate that meticulously optimised edge deployments can deliver reasoning accuracy acceptable for clinical purposes while markedly lowering energy expenditure (Bareja et al., 2025).

6.2 Data Scarcity, Domain Shift, and Model Robustness

Limited and Heterogeneous Medical Data: A continuing obstacle for artificial intelligence in low-resource healthcare is the limited availability of labelled local data alongside pronounced heterogeneity in imaging conditions, acquisition hardware, and patient demographics. Models trained on corpora collected in high-income settings frequently incur performance penalties attributable to domain shift (SHarshar et al., 2025; Kurz et al., 2025).

Robust Pretraining and Adaptation Strategies: Recent developments in foundation-scale models and large-scale multimodal pretraining alleviate data scarcity by enabling transfer learning across divergent domains (Edirisingh et al., 2025; Raval & Oza, 2025). Principal methodological components include domain adaptation via fine-tuning on modest local datasets, self-supervised and weakly supervised learning to exploit unlabelled instances, and synthetic data generation or augmentation to emulate varied acquisition circumstances. Diffusion-based reasoning frameworks and agentic architectures further bolster robustness by supporting stochastic exploration and uncertainty-aware inference, thereby diminishing brittle behaviour under distributional shift (Ye et al., 2024; Hersche et al., 2025).

6.3 Monitoring, Maintenance, and Continuous Learning

In contrast to static clinical software, artificial-intelligence-driven clinical decision support systems necessitate ongoing monitoring to preserve safety and performance characteristics as conditions evolve. Data drift, demographic shifts, and revisions to clinical protocols can insidiously erode model reliability (Dombrowski et al., 2024).

Model Drift Detection and Evaluation: Procedures for bias evaluation, data-drift identification, and performance auditing constitute prerequisites for sustained deployment. Implementations such as CheXStray exemplify real-time monitoring pipelines tailored for multimodal medical imaging, permitting early identification of performance anomalies (Merkow et al., 2023).

Safe Model Updating: Within resource-constrained environments, retraining pipelines must remain computationally economical, interpretable, and consonant with regulatory stipulations. Federated and incremental learning strategies permit model enhancement through decentralised data while safeguarding privacy and limiting communication overhead (Raval et al., 2024). Nonetheless, stringent safeguards are required to forestall catastrophic forgetting and inadvertent behavioural divergence. The deployment of agentic AI in healthcare raises critical ethical, legal, and societal questions, particularly when systems are introduced in vulnerable or underserved communities.

7. ETHICAL, LEGAL, AND SOCIAL CONSIDERATIONS

The deployment of agentic AI in healthcare raises critical ethical, legal, and societal questions, particularly when systems are introduced in vulnerable or underserved communities.

7.1 Privacy and Security

On-device inference confers a measurable privacy benefit by obviating the transmission of sensitive patient data to external cloud infrastructures, thereby diminishing the probability of data breaches and instances of regulatory non-compliance (Bareja et al., 2025; Raval & Oza, 2025). Nonetheless, the retention of data and models on the local device introduces distinct security challenges, including secure model execution, encrypted storage of patient information, and fine-grained device-level access control. Consequently, edge deployment must be accompanied by security mechanisms of demonstrated robustness in order to satisfy prevailing healthcare data-governance standards.

7.2 Bias, Fairness, and Equity

Models trained on datasets that do not capture the full demographic spectrum may exhibit systematically inferior performance for specific subgroups, thereby amplifying extant healthcare disparities (Dombrowski et al., 2024; Miró Catalina et al., 2024). Sources of bias encompass class imbalance within training data, heterogeneity in imaging protocols, and socio-demographic covariates. Mitigation approaches include the deliberate curation of diverse and inclusive datasets, calibration procedures applied across subpopulations, and the institution of continuous bias audits throughout the deployment lifecycle (Kurz et al., 2025; Edirisinghe et al., 2025). Agentic reasoning frameworks additionally facilitate explicit uncertainty quantification, permitting systems to withhold automated decisions or to solicit human review when confidence metrics fall below predefined thresholds.

7.3 Trust, Transparency, and Regulation

Trust constitutes a necessary precondition for the clinical uptake of decision-support technologies. Explainability methods—including visual attention maps, structured reasoning traces, and natural-language rationales—provide clinicians with the evidentiary basis required to interpret and critically appraise AI-generated recommendations (Bae et al., 2023; Bae et al., 2024). From a regulatory standpoint, agentic clinical decision-support systems may be classified as medical devices under existing frameworks such as FDA or CE marking regimes, thereby necessitating clearly delineated accountability structures, fully traceable decision logic, and rigorous validation coupled with systematic post-market surveillance (Das & Akter, 2025; Maheriya, 2025).

7.4 Human–AI Collaboration and Cultural Acceptance

Empirical observations indicate that agentic systems achieve optimal utility when conceptualised as assistive instruments rather than as autonomous agents exercising independent clinical authority. Continued clinician oversight remains indispensable, particularly within high-acuity contexts. Educational programmes and participatory design initiatives contribute to the formation of accurate mental models regarding system capabilities and limitations, an outcome that supports cultural acceptance, including in settings historically underserved by technological interventions (Huang et al., 2025; Raval et al., 2024)

8. CASE STUDIES AND IMPLEMENTATION INSIGHTS

8.1 Field Deployments in Low-Resource Settings

Empirical field evaluations indicate that AI-assisted diagnostic tools remain operationally viable within resource-constrained settings. Representative implementations include smartphone-adapted retinal screening modules for diabetic retinopathy, compressed convolutional-network pipelines for intra-cranial tumour identification on handheld devices, and primary-care chest-radiograph interpretation systems operating distal to tertiary referral centres (Reddy et al., 2019; Miró Catalina et al., 2024). Outcomes from these feasibility studies document increased screening coverage and reduced diagnostic turnaround intervals, while concurrently identifying usability constraints centred on interface minimisation and alignment with established clinical workflows.

8.2 Agentic and Multi-Agent Systems in Practice

Although comprehensive clinical roll-out of fully autonomous multi-agent architectures is still comparatively restricted, experimental prototypes illustrate the analytical utility of collaborative agent assemblies. Configurations that integrate imaging specialists, language-reasoning agents, and hierarchical planning modules demonstrate measurable gains in diagnostic consistency and error-rate reduction within multi-step clinical processes (Dernbach et al., 2024; Zhang et al., 2024; Plaat et al., 2025).

8.3 Deployment Infrastructure Models

Contemporary healthcare AI deployments generally adopt one of three architectural paradigms: (i) edge-only execution, emphasising data privacy and minimal latency; (ii) edge–cloud hybridisation, facilitating intermittent parameter synchronisation; or (iii) federated learning, enabling joint model refinement without raw-data exchange (Raval et al., 2024). Each paradigm entails distinct trade-offs among scalability, governance overhead, and operational expenditure.

9. FUTURE DIRECTIONS

Although the proposed framework furnishes a foundational structure, multiple research trajectories remain open to systematic extension.

- Clinical validation and real-world deployment- Prospective studies conducted across heterogeneous clinical sites, ranging from tertiary referral centres to resource-limited facilities, are required to quantify clinician trust, decision concordance with standard care, and measurable patient outcomes prior to translational adoption.
- Federated and privacy-preserving extensions -Embedding federated learning protocols and secure multi-party computation within the multi-agent architecture would permit inter-institutional collaboration without transferring identifiable patient data, thereby satisfying prevailing regulatory and ethical constraints.
- Adaptive agent learning and role evolution- Agents presently operate under fixed role definitions; subsequent iterations may incorporate reinforcement or continual learning mechanisms that allow behavioural adaptation, iterative refinement of collaboration policies, and dynamic redistribution of responsibilities informed by evolving clinical contexts.
- Explainability and accountability mechanisms- Augmenting explainability at both the component and system levels remains an objective of high priority. Future investigations should delineate structured rationale generation, quantified confidence estimation, and fully traceable decision paths to support clinical accountability and auditability.
- Integration with clinical knowledge graphs and guidelines- Linking agents to curated medical knowledge graphs, standard ontologies, and evidence-based guidelines can anchor recommendations within established biomedical knowledge and facilitate guideline-aware reasoning.
- Scalability to multi-disease and longitudinal care scenarios- Extending the framework to encompass chronic disease management, longitudinal patient trajectories, and the interaction of multiple comorbidities constitutes a potentially fruitful avenue for broadening clinical relevance.

10. CONCLUSION

This study introduced a Multi-Agent Collaboration Framework for Clinical Decision Support that integrates heterogeneous information sources through functionally specialised agents dedicated to imaging interpretation, language understanding, and decision planning. Coordination is effected via a shared memory layer and message-passing protocol, enabling structured reasoning over multimodal clinical data while preserving modularity and interpretability. In contrast to monolithic clinical AI architectures, the proposed design decomposes complex diagnostic and therapeutic tasks into discrete agent-level competencies; each agent operates strictly within its domain of expertise while contributing to a unified clinical output. Such collaboration enhances transparency, supports incremental system evolution, and aligns with existing clinical workflows. The framework is explicitly intended for contexts that demand synthesis of multimodal evidence, retention of longitudinal patient context, and adaptive decision support.

Collectively, the results indicate that agent-based collaboration can augment the robustness, scalability, and explainability of clinical AI systems, thereby constituting a viable direction for the development of next-generation decision support tools.

REFERENCES

Abdelrahman, A. Y. M. (2025). Deep Learning-Based Brain Tumor Diagnosis on Smartphones Using Optimized MobileNetV2 Models. *Journal of Information Technology*, *5*(13), 1–13. DOI: 10.70619/vol5iss13pp1-13-698

Ahmed, Y. K., & Naji, A. N. (2025). Smart feature extraction using deep learning for early diagnosis of chronic diseases in next-generation medical decision support systems. *Network Modeling and Analysis in Health Informatics and Bioinformatics*, *14*(1), 140. DOI: 10.1007/s13721-025-00641-y

Ardic, N., & Dinc, R. (2025). Emerging trends in multi-modal artificial intelligence for clinical decision support: A narrative review. *Health Informatics Journal*, *31*(3), 14604582251366141. DOI: 10.1177/14604582251366141 PMID: 40808352

Bae, S., Kyung, D., Ryu, J., Cho, E., Lee, G., Kweon, S., & Choi, E. (2023). Ehrxqa: A multi-modal question answering dataset for electronic health records with chest x-ray images. *Advances in Neural Information Processing Systems*, *36*, 3867–3880. DOI: 10.52202/075280-0170

. Bae, S., Kyung, D., Ryu, J., Cho, E., Lee, G., Kweon, S., ... & Choi, E. (2024). Mimic-ext-mimic-cxr-vqa: A complex, diverse, and large-scale visual question answering dataset for chest x-ray images.

Bareja, R., Carrillo-Perez, F., Zheng, Y., Pizurica, M., Nandi, T. N., Shen, J., . . . Gevaert, O. (2025). Evaluating Vision and Pathology Foundation Models for Computational Pathology: A Comprehensive Benchmark Study. medRxiv, 2025-05. DOI: 10.1101/2025.05.08.25327250

Dangi, R. R., Sharma, A., & Vageriya, V. (2025). Transforming healthcare in low-resource settings with artificial intelligence: Recent developments and outcomes. *Public Health Nursing*, *42*(2), 1017–1030. DOI: 10.1111/phn.13500 PMID: 39629887

Das, D. C., & Akter, M. S.Debashis Chandra DasMst Shahana Akter. (2025). AI-Powered Multimodal Diagnostics in Modern Healthcare: A Shift Toward Integrative Intelligence. *Asia Pacific Journal of Medical Innovations*, *2*(3), 47–57. DOI: 10.70818/apjmi.v02i03.027

Dernbach, S., Michel, A., Agarwal, K., Brissette, C., Gupta, G., & Choudhury, S. (2024). Thinking Fast and Laterally: Multi-Agentic Approach for Reasoning about Uncertain Emerging Events. arXiv preprint arXiv:2412.07977.

Dombrowski, M., Prenner, A., & Kainz, B. (2024). Bias assessment and data drift detection in medical image analysis: A survey. arXiv preprint arXiv:2409.17800.

Edirisinghe, D., Nimalsiri, W., Hennayake, M., Meedeniya, D., & Lim, G. (2025). [-Ray Report Generation Using Abnormality Guided Vision Language Model. IEEE Access.]. *Chest*, •••, X.

Gridach, M., Nanavati, J., Abidine, K. Z. E., Mendes, L., & Mack, C. (2025). Agentic ai for scientific discovery: A survey of progress, challenges, and future directions. arXiv preprint arXiv:2503.08979.

Hartung, T. (2025). AI, agentic models and lab automation for scientific discovery–the beginning of scAInce. *Frontiers in Artificial Intelligence*, *8*, 1649155. DOI: 10.3389/frai.2025.1649155 PMID: 40951330

Hersche, M., Moor-Smith, S., Hofmann, T., & Rahimi, A. (2025). Soft-Masked Diffusion Language Models. arXiv preprint arXiv:2510.17206.

Huang, L., Koutra, D., Kulkarni, A., Prioleau, T., Wu, Q., Yan, Y., . . . Zhou, D. (2025, May). Towards Agentic AI for Science: Hypothesis Generation, Comprehension, Quantification, and Validation. In Companion Proceedings of the ACM on Web Conference 2025 (pp. 1639-1642).

Huang, S. C., Jensen, M., Yeung-Levy, S., Lungren, M. P., Poon, H., & Chaudhari, A. S. (2025). A systematic review and implementation guidelines of multimodal foundation models in medical imaging. *Research Square*, rs-3. DOI: 10.21203/rs.3.rs-5537908/v1

Kamrul, S. M., Jobair, H. F. M., Bofan, H., Cheng, J. Q., & Huanying, G. (2025). Multimodal Models in Healthcare: Methods, Challenges, and Future Directions for Enhanced Clinical Decision Support. *Information (Basel)*, *16*(11), 971. DOI: 10.3390/info16110971

Kumar, R., Sporn, K., Gowda, C., Paladugu, P., Alnemri, A., Khanna, A., & Zaman, N. (2025). *Integrating Multi-Modal Predictive Modeling*. Imaging Biomarkers, and EHR-Linked Decision Support Systems in Spine-Focused Biomedical Informatics.

Kurz, C. F., Merzhevich, T., Eskofier, B. M., Kather, J. N., & Gmeiner, B. (2025). Benchmarking vision-language models for diagnostics in emergency and critical care settings. npj. *Digital Medicine*, *8*(1), 423. PMID: 40640347

Liu, Z., Li, H., Lu, J., Ma, G., Hong, X., Iacca, G., . . . Wang, L. (2025). Nature's Insight: A Novel Framework and Comprehensive Analysis of Agentic Reasoning Through the Lens of Neuroscience. arXiv preprint arXiv:2505.05515.

. MAHERIYA, A. (2025). BRIDGING THE GAP: XAI FOR TRUSTWORTHY AI-POWERED MEDICAL IMAGING ARPITA MAHERIYA, SHAILESH PANCHAL, AANAL RAVAL AND KOMAL BORISAGAR. Clinical Imaging Diagnosis: Data-Driven Techniques, Analytical Frameworks and Practical Applications, 242.

Merkow, J., Soin, A., Long, J., Cohen, J. P., Saligrama, S., Bridge, C., . . . Lungren, M. P. (2023, October). CheXstray: a real-time multi-modal monitoring workflow for medical imaging AI. In International Conference on Medical Image Computing and Computer-Assisted Intervention (pp. 326-336). Cham: Springer Nature Switzerland. DOI: 10.1007/978-3-031-43898-1_32

Miró Catalina, Q., Vidal-Alaball, J., Fuster-Casanovas, A., Escalé-Besa, A., Ruiz Comellas, A., & Solé-Casals, J. (2024). Real-world testing of an artificial intelligence algorithm for the analysis of chest X-rays in primary care settings. *Scientific Reports*, *14*(1), 5199. DOI: 10.1038/s41598-024-55792-1 PMID: 38431731

Nissen, L., Zagar, P., Ravi, V., Zahedivash, A., Reimer, L. M., Jonas, S., . . . Schmiedmayer, P. (2025). Medicine on the edge: Comparative performance analysis of on-device LLMs for clinical reasoning. arXiv preprint arXiv:2502.08954.

Patel, J., Patel, D., & Raval, A. (2025). Artificial Intelligence for Predictive Modeling in CRISPR/Cas9 Gene Editing: A Survey of Methods and Design Strategies. *The Journal of Gene Medicine*, *27*(12), e70061. DOI: 10.1002/jgm.70061 PMID: 41367203

Plaat, A., van Duijn, M., van Stein, N., Preuss, M., van der Putten, P., & Batenburg, K. J. (2025). Agentic large language models, a survey. arXiv preprint arXiv:2503.23037.

Raval, A., & Borisagar, K. (2022, March). A Survey on Techniques and Methods of Recommender System. In *International Conference on Computational Intelligence in Data Science* (pp. 97-114). Cham: Springer International Publishing. DOI: 10.1007/978-3-031-16364-7_8

Raval, A., & Maheriya, A. (2023). A Survey on Deep Learning Methods for Addressing COVID-19 Issues. In *Information and Communication Technology for Competitive Strategies (ICTCS 2022) Intelligent Strategies for ICT* (pp. 61–73). Springer Nature Singapore. DOI: 10.1007/978-981-19-9304-6_7

Raval, A., Maheriya, A., Panchal, S., & Borisagar, K. (2024, August). Disentangled Attention Based Multi-Task Learning with Structural Estimations for Audio Feature Processing and Identification. In 2024 4th Asian Conference on Innovation in Technology (ASIANCON) (pp. 1-7). IEEE. DOI: 10.1109/ASIANCON62057.2024.10837983

Raval, A., & Oza, R. (2025). Advancing AI with Quantum Computing: Synergies Between Quantum Neural Networks and Quantum Reinforcement Learning. In *Quantum Machine Learning in Industrial Automation* (pp. 305–332). Springer Nature Switzerland. DOI: 10.1007/978-3-031-99786-0_14

. Raval, A. S., & Borisagar, K. R. (n.d.). Document Recommendation: An anatomization of neoteric advancements, problems and potential scope.

Reddy, C. L., Mitra, S., Meara, J. G., Atun, R., & Afshar, S. (2019). Artificial Intelligence and its role in surgical care in low-income and middle-income countries. *The Lancet. Digital Health*, *1*(8), e384–e386. DOI: 10.1016/S2589-7500(19)30200-6 PMID: 33323217

Saini, S. K., & Sunil, D. (2025). A Comprehensive Review Of Methodologies In Clinical Data-Driven Decision Support Systems For Healthcare. *International Journal of Environmental Sciences*, *11*(24s), 4204–4218. DOI: 10.64252/0e30q322

Sharshar, A., Khan, L. U., Ullah, W., & Guizani, M. (2025). Vision-language models for edge networks: A comprehensive survey. *IEEE Internet of Things Journal*, *12*(16), 32701–32724. DOI: 10.1109/JIOT.2025.3579032

Tran, J., Estevez, J. J., Howard, N. J., & Kumar, S. (2025). Barriers and Enablers Influencing the Implementation of Artificial Intelligence for Diabetic Retinopathy Screening in Clinical Practice: A Scoping Review. *Clinical & Experimental Ophthalmology*, *53*(7), 791–802. DOI: 10.1111/ceo.14567 PMID: 40515637

Yamada, Y., Lange, R. T., Lu, C., Hu, S., Lu, C., Foerster, J., . . . Ha, D. (2025). The ai scientist-v2: Workshop-level automated scientific discovery via agentic tree search. arXiv preprint arXiv:2504.08066.

Yao, S., Yu, D., Zhao, J., Shafran, I., Griffiths, T., Cao, Y., & Narasimhan, K. (2023). Tree of thoughts: Deliberate problem solving with large language models. *Advances in Neural Information Processing Systems*, *36*, 11809–11822.

Yao, S., Zhao, J., Yu, D., Du, N., Shafran, I., Narasimhan, K. R., & Cao, Y. (2022, October). React: Synergizing reasoning and acting in language models. In The eleventh international conference on learning representations.

Ye, J., Gong, S., Chen, L., Zheng, L., Gao, J., Shi, H., & Kong, L. (2024). Diffusion of thought: Chain-of-thought reasoning in diffusion language models. *Advances in Neural Information Processing Systems*, *37*, 105345–105374.

Zhang, Y., Sun, R., Chen, Y., Pfister, T., Zhang, R., & Arik, S. (2024). Chain of agents: Large language models collaborating on long-context tasks. *Advances in Neural Information Processing Systems*, *37*, 132208–132237.

Zhang, Z., Zhang, A., Li, M., & Smola, A. (2022). Automatic chain of thought prompting in large language models. arXiv preprint arXiv:2210.03493.

Chapter 2

Deep Learning–Based Pediatric Pneumonia Detection Using EfficientNetB4 With Topological Convolutional Layers

N. Raghu
http://orcid.org/0000-0002-2091-8922
Jain (Deemed to be) University, India

M. Inbalatha
Jain (Deemed to be) University, India

R. N. Ojashwini
Global Academy of Technology, India

ABSTRACT

The leading cause of mortality in children, it is crucial that clinicians immediately arrive at an accurate diagnosis. The suggested deep learning algorithm can automatically detect pneumonia using chest X-rays with a 97.7% accuracy rate. EfficientNetB4 provides an optimal trade-off between fast processing and diagnostic precision. The model's sensitivity to identify small lung abnormalities is enhanced by using Architectural Convolutional Layers (TCLs). These layers extract morphological and connecting data that is not captured by ordinary convolutional layers. The approach improves model accuracy using MixUp, CutMix, and adaptive distortion

DOI: 10.4018/979-8-3373-7315-7.ch002

t © 2026, IGI Global Scientific Publishing. Copying or distributing in print or electronic forms without written permission of IGI Global Scientific Publishing is prohibited. Use of this chapter to enerative artificial intelligence (AI) technologies is expressly prohibited. The publisher reserves all rights to license its use for generative AI training and machine learning model development.

approaches to handle tiny imbalanced pediatric datasets. To verify results, radiologists employ Grad-CAM graphics to examine model predictions, which highlight clinically significant areas. Sensitivity study shows that the model remains stable when presented with noisy or imbalanced data, indicating that it is ready for use in real-world clinical settings.

1. INTRODUCTION

The majority of individuals think of pneumonia as a terrible illness that kills a lot of kids. The illness manifests abruptly in sporadic bouts that, if left untreated, may be lethal. Thousands of children under the age of five die each year from pneumonia, making it the top cause of mortality in this age group. The prevalence of pediatric pneumonia is still too high, even though medical technology has come a long way. This is especially true in underdeveloped nations where people lack access to adequate healthcare and diagnostic resources (O'Grady, 2022). When it comes to diagnosing pneumonia, chest radiography (also known as a chest X-ray) is still among the most dependable methods. Radiologists with the necessary training must be able to differentiate between minor changes in lung patterns in order to interpret these pictures, which is no easy task even for seasoned experts. Misinterpretation of X-rays may lead to diagnostic delays or incorrect diagnoses, which can have catastrophic consequences for young children, yet radiologists are in limited supply in many underprivileged regions (Sodero et al., 2025).

In the last ten years, medical imaging has been revolutionized by Deep Learning (DL) and other types of AI. Because of their superior pattern recognition skills, deep learning algorithms can match or surpass human performance in some image classification tasks. Problems abound when trying to use these algorithms to detect pediatric pneumonia. The development of AI systems confronts different problems due to small pediatric datasets, varying image quality requirements, and mild pneumonia symptoms in children. The study aims to address these difficulties (Mehra et al., 2024). To succeed, you need to design a deep learning system that works well, produces comprehensible results, and has a high-performance rating. To construct a diagnostic system that will aid clinicians, reduce diagnostic mistakes, and make sophisticated medical treatment accessible to underprivileged groups, the study integrates EfficientNetB4 with Topological Convolutional Layers (TCLs) and improved augmentation approaches (Jalnnavar et al., 2023).

The unequal allocation of diagnostic knowledge and the global epidemic of pediatric pneumonia highlight the necessity of our effort. AI-powered solutions could overcome this issue by giving quick and precise second readings of CXRs and thereby cutting down the use of overworked specialists (Kermany et al., 2018).

Current options are neither affordable nor suitable for low-quality images, nor are they transparent in their decision-making. This project focuses directly on these obstacles with a model architecture especially made for children's anatomy, a preprocessing pipeline adjusted to the differences in real-life imaging, and interpretability features that are in sync with clinical workflows (Raghu et al., 2025). Figure 1 presents a selection of images taken from the original dataset for this research.

Figure 1. Sample images of pneumonia and normal

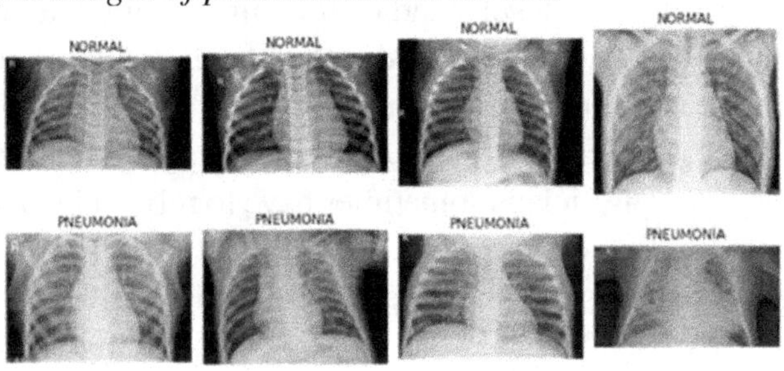

1.1 Global Burden of Pediatric Pneumonia

According to the World Health Organization (WHO), pneumonia is responsible for approximately 14% of all deaths among children under five, killing an estimated 700,000 children every year. The disease does not discriminate, but its impact is felt most profoundly in low- and middle-income countries, particularly across South Asia and Sub-Saharan Africa, where children are often malnourished, healthcare systems are under strain, and access to early diagnostic tools is limited. The effects of pneumonia on communities and families extend well beyond the short-term danger to lives (Xu et al., 2023). Recurrence of respiratory problems and impaired immunity are potential consequences for children who do manage their recovery from severe diseases. The ripple effect of parents missing work due to sick children may be devastating: less income, which exacerbates family health problems. It is critical to quickly create reliable automated diagnostic methods that do not need extensive clinical infrastructure, since the COVID-19 pandemic exposed significant deficiencies in pediatric respiratory treatment (George et al., 2022). Developing a diagnostics system powered by artificial intelligence that can reliably identify infections from lung X-rays is both a technical and ethical need in this worldwide setting (Swarup et al., 2024). Especially in places with little medical care or in remote regions, this technology makes faster evidence-based choices possible, which directly impacts increasing child survival rates (Alabdulqader et al., 2024).

1.2 Challenges in Early and Accurate Diagnosis

Radiographic imaging has the potential to diagnose pneumonia; nevertheless, clinicians face a number of interrelated challenges that hinder them from making an accurate early diagnosis.

- Even highly experienced radiologists have trouble identifying small chest X-ray abnormalities since their findings are frequently contradictory. Image contrast settings, lighting levels, and overlapping bodily features all contribute to making infection patterns harder to discern, which in turn makes the diagnostic procedure more challenging.
- Inadequate Access to Radiologists: Due to a shortage of radiologists in many areas, primary care physicians sometimes have to rely on inadequate imaging evidence when making diagnoses.
- Pediatric X-ray datasets have an uneven proportion of healthy patients and pneumonia cases, which causes them to be considerably smaller than adult datasets. It is difficult to comprehend children's lungs due of the complexity of the human respiratory system. The X-ray appearance of pneumonia in children is distinct from that in adults due to structural and developmental variations between the lungs of the two sexes.
- Different Disease Presentations: Less experienced readers may fail to see pneumonia because of its mild density changes, diffuse opacities, or patchy infiltrates.

The growing demand for tools that can reliably diagnose pneumonia across a variety of patient populations and medical imaging settings, the creation of robust AI models is becoming an absolute need (Nambiar & Nanjundegowda, 2024a). Functionality that can be explained is essential for the system to generate clinical interpretations for use in telemedicine and hospitals.

1.3 Role of Artificial Intelligence in Medical Imaging

Artificial Intelligence s having far-reaching effects across numerous sectors, its transformation of medical imaging stands out as particularly noteworthy. Deep learning models depend on Convolutional Neural Networks (CNNs), which are very adept at identifying intricate visual patterns; these networks find use in medical applications including tumor identification, fracture diagnosis, and lung disease classification (Nambiar & Nanjundegowda, 2024b). As a result of AI's analysis of chest X-rays, which show minor signs that people overlook, pneumonia may be identified. In order to successfully classify medical images, ResNet, DenseNet, and EfficientNet are essential due to their innate capacity to identify hierarchical patterns. No matter how good they are, regular CNNs have their limitations. Because topological linkages include geometric and structural information, they are essential for understanding the spatial patterns in the lungs, but they are difficult for them to detect (Aljawarneh & Al-Quraan, 2023). This is why Topological Convolutional Layers (TCLs) might be a solution for deep networks. Transcranial magnetic resonance (TCL) enhancements the model's sensibility to shape, texture, and connectivity, allowing for improved differentiation between normal and abnormal lung tissues. To get over imbalances and small datasets, modern data augmentation techniques artificially enhance data diversity. These include MixUp, CutMix, and compare augmentation. The AI model with more resilience and consistent performance in all sorts of real-world scenarios (Tyagi & Kumar, 2024).

1.4 Objectives and Scope of the Chapter

In this chapter, focus on creating and evaluating a deep learning system for pediatric pneumonia diagnosis using chest x-rays is the primary goal of this chapter. The suggested model strengthens structural analysis with Topological Convolutional Layers and uses EfficientNetB4 as its core feature extraction strategy to boost model generalization and decrease overfitting.

- To design a hybrid architecture that combines the efficiency of EfficientNetB4 with the geometric sensitivity of TCLs.
- To preprocess and augment pediatric chest X-ray datasets to enhance model robustness and overcome data limitations.
- To train and evaluate the model on benchmark datasets using key performance indicators such as accuracy, sensitivity, specificity, and F1-score.
- The research utilizes Grad-CAM to show model attention for improved interpretability and clinical transparency.
- The research examines different real-world applications which exist in hospitals and community health centers and telemedicine systems.

This chapter's study delves at the ways in which medical imaging and deep learning approaches may work together to improve healthcare for children. Improving AI diagnostic performance using a combination of topological and data-centric developments is the focus of the research (Kharbas et al., 2024). All children in all regions will have access to automated, low-cost healthcare diagnostics according to the suggested technique, which combines machine learning with clinical needs.

2. EVOLUTION OF DIAGNOSTIC APPROACHES

2.1 Traditional Diagnostic Approaches Using Chest Radiographs

For many decades chest radiography has served as the basic diagnostic method for detecting pneumonia. A chest X-ray produces images of the lungs which doctors use to detect infections and inflammation and fluid build-up. In pediatric situations radiographs become essential because young patients show symptoms like fever and cough and fast breathing which match multiple respiratory diseases including bronchiolitis and asthma (Yildirim & Canayaz, 2023). Traditionally radiologists perform radiographic interpretation through their analysis of patchy infiltrates and consolidation and interstitial opacities in imaging patterns. The diagnosis of pneumonia becomes confirmed through the combination of these findings with clinical symptoms. The process contains multiple errors which prevent it from working at its best. Radiographs produce different results because of changes in exposure settings and patient positioning and the type of imaging equipment used during the procedure. The process of interpreting X-rays through human involvement creates subjectivity because two skilled radiologists might interpret the same X-ray differently when examining borderline or subtle cases (Nasra, 2024).

In several developing nations radiologists remain in short supply so medical professionals who lack specialized training perform X-ray interpretation duties. The situation leads to higher chances of wrong or late medical diagnoses because of restricted access to healthcare facilities. The interpretation of pediatric X-rays becomes difficult because children have smaller bodies and their soft tissues overlap which blocks important pneumonia indicators (Neshat et al., 2024). Scientists have worked to boost diagnostic uniformity through computer-aided diagnosis (CAD) systems during their research throughout recent years. The first CAD systems used manually created features which included texture analysis and edge detection and statistical pattern recognition. The traditional image-processing methods which automated diagnostic tasks failed to recognize the intricate multidimensional characteristics that exist in medical images (Nambiar & Nanjundegowda, 2025). Machine learning and deep learning advancements have changed the field because models now learn from data instead of depending on human-crafted features.

2.2 Evolution of Deep Learning in Medical Imaging

Medical image analysis experienced a complete transformation because of Deep Learning (DL) technology. The main difference between deep learning and traditional machine learning methods lies in deep learning systems which automatically extract features from images through their hierarchical structure (Hasan et al., 2024). The capability of these systems makes them highly suitable for medical image analysis which includes classification and segmentation and detection tasks. The medical domain gained benefits from computer vision through deep learning success which started with AlexNet in 2012 and continued with VGGNet in 2014 and ResNet in 2015. The initial healthcare applications of CNN technology emerged through its use in skin cancer classification and retinal disease detection and breast cancer screening. As the availability of large-scale medical datasets increased, researchers began exploring CNN-based models for chest X-ray interpretation, particularly for detecting lung diseases like pneumonia, tuberculosis, and COVID-19.

The CheXNet model using the NIH ChestX-ray14 dataset. Their model, based on a 121-layer DenseNet, achieved performance comparable to practicing radiologists in detecting pneumonia (Godbin & Jasmine, 2024). The potential of AI not just as a supportive tool but as a reliable diagnostic assistant. Since then, numerous studies have explored hybrid architectures, transfer learning, and attention mechanisms to improve performance on pediatric chest X-ray dataset. Researchers have also experimented with data augmentation, ensemble learning, and explainability techniques like Grad-CAM to visualize how models interpret radiographs (Güler & Polat, 2022). The medical field shows deep learning evolution from its initial theoretical phase to its current position as an operational diagnostic tool which supports medical decisions in actual clinical practice (Singh et al., 2023).

2.3 Comparison of Popular CNN Architectures (VGG, ResNet, DenseNet, EfficientNet)

Multiple CNN architectures have established themselves as medical imaging research benchmarks during the last ten years because they deliver various advantages in feature extraction and computational efficiency and accuracy (An et al., 2024).

- VGGNet (2014): A new method for extracting complex image features was developed by the VGG family. It involves stacking numerous small 3×3 filters vertically to achieve a deeper network complexity. The straightforward and organized architecture of VGG16 and VGG19 ensures that they continue to be popular choices for transfer learning. The systems are not suited for usage in basic situations with low resources since they demand a lot of processing power and memory storage.
- Networks can now train deeper topologies without disappearing gradients, thanks to ResNet (2015) and the ground breaking idea of residual learning. By allowing data to be sent directly between layers, skip connections enhance the model's accuracy and convergence. Because of its exceptional per-

formance in pneumonia identification, the ResNet architecture is a great pick for any medical imaging job.

- DenseNet (2017): DenseNet builds a network topology that uses a single feed-forward route to connect all of the levels. The dense network structure enables feature sharing between layers which helps eliminate unnecessary features while making the network use fewer parameters. The research about densely linked networks for medical purposes since the CheXNet model, which is based on DenseNet-121, established a new standard for chest X-ray illness identification.
- EfficientNet (2019): EfficientNet introduced a novel scaling method that uses a single scaling factor to make uniform changes to the depth, breadth, and resolution of a network. With its minimal computing needs and great accuracy, EfficientNetB4 performs very well. Medical imaging tools that deal with limited data sets will find this model useful because of its high performance with few parameters. The network performance of EfficientNet receives a boost from squeeze-and-excitation modules which extract essential image features that drive better medical image classification results.

2.4 Limitations in Current AI-based Pneumonia Detection Systems

The AI-based pneumonia detection systems need to overcome various obstacles to move from research laboratory environments into actual clinical practice.

1. Small pediatric datasets contain bias because they represent particular population groups and specific imaging equipment. The developed models face restrictions in their ability to generalize because they perform poorly when tested with unfamiliar data from different medical institutions (Sajed et al., 2023).
2. Lack of Explainability: While CNNs can achieve high accuracy, their decision-making process often remains opaque. The clinical environment needs doctors to understand the reasoning behind AI model predictions in order to accept its results for patient care.
3. The model performs badly on new data after it learns patterns which exist only in the training set. The model learns to identify unimportant patterns during training which leads to poor performance on new data.
4. The model fails to perform well on real-world data because it learns from unimportant patterns during training. The model fails to learn real data patterns because it focuses on particular data characteristics instead.
5. The model suffers from poor performance on actual data because it learns to recognize unimportant training data characteristics. The model training process

results in the selection of insignificant training set patterns which leads to poor performance when working with actual data.

6. The performance of models trained on small datasets becomes poor at handling new data because they learn to identify random patterns in the training set which do not represent actual meaningful features. The models trained on small datasets learn to identify random patterns from the training set which do not represent actual meaningful features. The models trained on small datasets learn to identify random patterns from the training set which do not represent actual meaningful features. The models trained on small datasets learn to identify random patterns from the training set which do not represent actual meaningful features. The models trained on small datasets learn to identify random patterns from the training set which do not represent actual.

These limitations emphasize that while AI holds great promise, it must evolve to become more robust, interpretable, and clinically adaptable (Rameez & Logashree, 2024).

2.5 Literature Survey

Nasra et al. (2024) illustrated a practical, up-to-date synthesis of how recent deep learning advances have been applied to lung disease diagnosis from chest X-rays, with special attention to pneumonia detection workflows. The problem: chest radiographs remain the most widely available imaging modality worldwide, but their diagnostic utility is limited by variable image quality and reader subjectivity. The review then walks the reader through the pipeline most modern systems use—data curation and cleaning, lung-region segmentation, backbone selection (transfer learning from large-scale ImageNet pretraining), class imbalance handling, and post-hoc explainability. this review is helpful for practitioners since it compares regularization methods and augmentation tactics (such as MixUp, CutMix, RandAugment, and label smoothing) that have been shown to increase resilience in low-data regimes in various research.

Nambiar and Nanjundegowda (2025) highlight that augmentation is not a peripheral detail but often the single most effective lever for reducing overfitting when pediatric datasets are small. They also evaluate backbone choices and note consistent gains when employing scaled architectures (EfficientNet family) over older heavyweights (VGG), mainly due to better parameter efficiency and built-in attention-like modules. Hasan et al. (2024) focus their research on translation evaluation which goes past traditional performance metrics by identifying three main failure types that include text markers and tubes and label noise and by analyzing operational aspects of inference speed and model calibration for triage and clinical validation through prospective testing and multi-site external validation.

Hasan et al. (2024) review identifies a common pattern which shows that numerous developed models reach high accuracy in their initial tests yet fail to perform well when deployed at different healthcare facilities because of domain shifts. The authors establish three essential requirements for clinical readiness which include diverse data sets and federated learning systems and reporting standards that use patient-wise data splitting and confidence interval metrics.

Singh et al., (2023) explained the review of Topological Data Analysis (TDA) methods applied to medical imaging. The review covers core TDA tools (persistent homology, mapper, simplicial complexes) and explains how they extract global structural descriptors — for example, counting connected components, loops, or cavities as functions of intensity thresholds. While convolutional neural networks (CNNs) are great at recognizing patterns and textures at the local level, TDA is able to pick up on shape and connection information on a global scale, which is generally ignored. This is why TDA is described as a supplementary feature to pixel-wise CNN features. This study compiles case cases from several fields of radiography, including pulmonary pathology, arterial network analysis, and tumor margin characterization. In each case TDA-derived features often improve classifier performance when appended to learned features or when used to regularize training. Importantly, the translational barriers: interpretability (how to present topological summaries to clinicians), robustness to noise, and computational cost. They suggest hybrid pipelines — CNNs for local features and TDA descriptors for global structure — as a practical route for clinical adoption. Why this matters for pediatric pneumonia: pediatric lung opacities can be patchy and topologically distinct from adult patterns. TDA can help discriminate diffuse viral interstitial patterns from focal lobar consolidation; combined with modern augmentation and efficient backbones, it can reduce false positives and increase clinicians' trust by supplying interpretable, shape-based indicators.

Yao at al., (2023) proposed a two-stage multimodal strategy that fuses chest X-ray images with auxiliary clinical data (blood test results) to improve pediatric pneumonia classification. Stage one pretrains image encoders and tabular-data encoders separately; stage two jointly fine-tunes a fusion network that learns cross-modal correlations. Biochemical indicators (e.g., CRP, WBC) provide orthogonal, clinically significant signals; radiographic findings alone may not always clarify bacterial vs viral etiologies or severity; their intuition is practical. Important results: sensitivity and specificity were much enhanced by multimodal fusion in comparison to image-only models, especially in low-quality or borderline X-rays.

Domínguez et al., (2023) interpretability tools such as Grad-CAM for pictures and SHAP values for tabular information. The data-splitting strategies and careful planning as means to avoid patient-level leaks, which include coordinating lab units and handling missing findings. In pediatric pneumonia cases, merging radiography data with non-image data lowers uncertainty. The research presents a realistic paradigm for applying this strategy in public hospital triage settings. Integrating topology feature extractors into the bidirectional pipeline and the EfficientNet framework improves clinical performance results and provides interpretable decision-making processes.

Pan et al., (2024) proposed a federated system for learning so that many institutions may train the same algorithm separately, rather than storing all of the patient data in one place. To alter client engagement levels, the authors build a dual control system using data distribution types that include device classifications and patient demographic information. Because of the excellent trade-off between efficiency and computational economy offered by EfficientNet-based encoders, the authors opted for federated training, which preserves data privacy while producing results comparable to centralized training accuracy levels. The federated model obtained per-site accuracies reaching 98-99% for some tasks and increased average accuracy by around 2% compared to baseline federated systems, as shown empirically. The researchers look at the system's stability mechanisms and demonstrate that client influence management prevents the unfavorable transfer effects caused by imbalances in hospital data. Communication efficiency, model compression, and differential privacy choices are the three primary concerns that the system must address. Importance: the incidence, imaging methods, and comorbidity profiles of pediatric pneumonia vary by region. Before implementing AI assistants in actual clinics, it is necessary to construct models that generalize widely. Federated training across multiple institutions helps with this. For high-accuracy pediatric CXR classification, our study demonstrates that federated setups employing an EfficientNet backbone (e.g., B4) are possible and successful.

Siddiqi et al., (2024) explained the purpose of multi-class lung disease identification on chest X-rays and stacking ensemble of several EfficientNet variations, including B4 introduced. Their method involves channel-specific EfficientNets that have been pre-trained on task-specific datasets and large-scale CXR corpora; a meta-learner then combines the predictions from all of these channels. Careful expansion, class correction, and probabilistic validation are highlighted as ways to address the imbalanced occurrence of various diseases. Their results demonstrate that EfficientNetB4 gives the highest accuracy-to-inference-cost trade-off of any single-model and that the ensemble routinely beats baselines with a single model. It is worth noting that the authors include ablations that show how data improvements like MixUp and CutMix may increase generalization. Additionally, they assure that the ensemble concentrates on clinically plausible locations by providing explain ability with Grad-CAM maps. Groups and stacking may make up for lack of data and bias in the models; where funds permit, a multichannel EfficientNet collection can enhance sensitivity for minor pediatric abnormalities; all of this is relevant to pediatric pneumonia. The publication provides straightforward instructions that may be easily applied to pediatric CXR research.

Patidar et al., (2024) explores the real-world applications of CNNs and TL for detecting pediatric pneumonia. Their study compares and contrasts several backbones, including as ResNet, DenseNet, and EfficientNet variants, using the Kermany pediatric dataset and broader clinical divisions. They emphasize repeatability via patient-wise split reporting, comprehensive analysis, and code open-sourcing. According to their research, a higher sensitivity-specificity balance is achieved while aggressively augmenting EfficientNet variants, particularly B4. Small focal opacities usually go unnoticed because models tend to hold onto confounds like tubes or laterality indications. The tests in conjunction with data cleaning (i.e., removing non-lung areas). To ensure that edge devices can support high-performance models, they investigate lightweight assembling and knowledge distillation. The consistent best practices for preparing data, improvement, and model selection for practitioners creating clinically focused systems and verifies previous trends that EfficientNet backbones are well suited to pediatric pneumonia tasks.

Alshanketi, et al., (2024) illustrates the number of deep-learning pipelines, including VGG, ResNet, DenseNet, and EfficientNet, as well as augmentation techniques, loss functions, and interpretability tools, are experimentally compared in order to help identify pneumonia. The research excels in its comprehensive coverage, which details the effects on sensitivity and false-positive rates of various options on various datasets. These choices include histogram equalization, label smoothing, focus loss, MixUp, CutMix, and contrast normalization. Lessons learned: (1) when augmented properly, modern scaled architectures (like the EfficientNet family) routinely beat older backbones; (2) overfitting is mitigated and robustness to noisy labels is enhanced with MixUp and CutMix; (3) interpretability (like Grad-CAM) aids in the detection of spurious correlations and directs the curation of datasets. Along with practical implementation notes, they provide quantization for mobile inference and simple training-time lung masks to enhance region focus.

2.6 Research Gap and Motivation for the Proposed Model

Deep learning has improved the speed and accuracy of pneumonia detection, there is still a need for optimized architectures that strike a balance between accuracy, interpretability, and computational efficiency, particularly for pediatric applications, according to the available literature review. Existing models primarily consider accuracy measures, ignoring crucial topological and geometric properties that elucidate X-ray illness patterns. Because modern augmentation techniques are not included, the model cannot learn to adapt to various clinical scenarios (Papadimitriou et al.,

2023). There is a serious lack of explainable AI systems that can process chest X-ray pictures from children.

To investigate the geometric forms and spatial interactions in lung structures, the suggested model integrates the highly efficient and scalable EfficientNetB4 with the highest-level Convolutional Layers (TCLs). This hybrid approach improves generalization performance, reduces overfitting, and increases diagnostic reliability by integrating contrast enhancement with sophisticated augmentation techniques like as MixUp and CutMix. Our ultimate goal is not only to build a powerful AI system, but also to provide medical professionals caring for children in underfunded facilities with a clinical tool that can be easily understood and used. The combining state-of-the-art deep learning methods with healthcare expertise to build an environment where all children can obtain healthcare that is fair, transparent, and powered by AI (Al-Qaness et al., 2024).

3. PROPOSED METHODOLOGY

The purpose of the proposed system is to provide a trustworthy automated platform for the diagnosis of juvenile pneumonia using chest radiographs. For the main feature extraction, this approach relies on EfficientNetB4, and for the identification of higher-order structural connections in the pictures, stratigraphic Convolutional Layers (TCLs) are used. The system employs state-of-the-art data augmentation methods to provide improved generalization by avoiding overfitting with controlled variances in training pictures. Figure 2 shows the whole treatment pipeline, which starts with raw chest X-rays being pre-processed and enhanced before they reach the EfficientNetB4 backbone. After being enhanced using TCLs, the retrieved features are inputted into a fully distributed classifier, which then produces labels indicating if the condition is positive or negative. High diagnostic performance, interpretability, and scalability are all achieved by the system's modular architecture.

Figure 2. EfficientNetB4 as the backbone network.

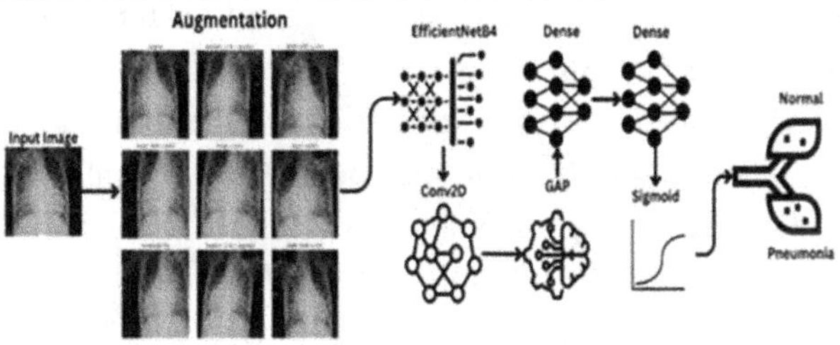

3.1 Topological Convolutional Layers (TCL): Concept and Implementation

EfficientNetB4 is a CNN model (convolutional neural network) that achieves better accuracy and parameter efficiency than more traditional CNN models such as ResNet and VGG. EfficientNet's novel approach makes use of compound scaling to simultaneously enhance depth, breadth, and resolution. As a result, the network is able to learn hierarchy-related characteristics more efficiently with less computational burden. To enhance feature learning and accelerate training, the proposed model starts with EfficientNetB4 weights learnt on ImageNet data, as pediatric datasets are often inaccessible (Panwar & Gupta, 2022). A rich feature map including global as well as local patterns useful for pneumonia identification is generated by the final convolutional block.

3.2 Advanced Data Augmentation Strategies

The traditional convolutional layers will not be able to record the global structural links present in complicated medical pictures since their primary purpose is to capture local patterns like textures or edges. By incorporating topological data analysis (TDA) ideas into the convolutional architecture, Topological Convolutional Layers (TCLs) overcome this issue. The connectedness and gaps in lung structures, which are commonly signs of disease alterations, may be captured by TCLs by computing persistent homology features across picture patches. Following the EfficientNetB4 feature mappings, our implementation applies TCLs (Aljawarneh & Al-Quraan, 2023). The classifier is given a combination of traditional characteristics and vectorized representations of persistent diagrams with fixed length. This makes it possible for the network to pick up on minor pneumonia trends by learning both the local and global topologies.

3.3 Dataset Description and Preprocessing

This study's dataset includes chest X-ray pictures that have been classified as either normal or pneumonia (Vemuri et al., 2024). Deep learning may struggle with pediatric chest X-ray datasets due to their limited size and imbalance. Four thousand two hundred seventy-three pictures depicting people with a pneumonia diagnosis are in the Pneumonia database. Figure 3 shows that there are 1,583 photos labelled as Normal, which relate to healthy people who do not exhibit any symptoms of pneumonia (Nasra, 2024).

This distribution shows that there is an imbalance in the dataset, with a larger frequency of photos indicating pneumonia than typical instances (Bhuria & Gupta,

2024). When deep learning models are trained with such an imbalance, they may lean toward identifying the majority class. To improve model generalizability and attain optimal performance for both classes, data augmentation, minority class over-sampling, and balanced loss functions are used during training. We use cutting-edge augmentation methods to get around this:

- Geometric Transformations: Random rotations, flips, scaling, and translations simulate variations in patient positioning.
- Color and Intensity Adjustments: Brightness and contrast changes help the model generalize across imaging devices.
- MixUp and CutMix: Images and labels are blended to generate new synthetic samples, promoting smoother decision boundaries.
- Elastic Deformations: Subtle distortions mimic anatomical variations in pediatric lungs.

Figure 3. Image after augmentation steps

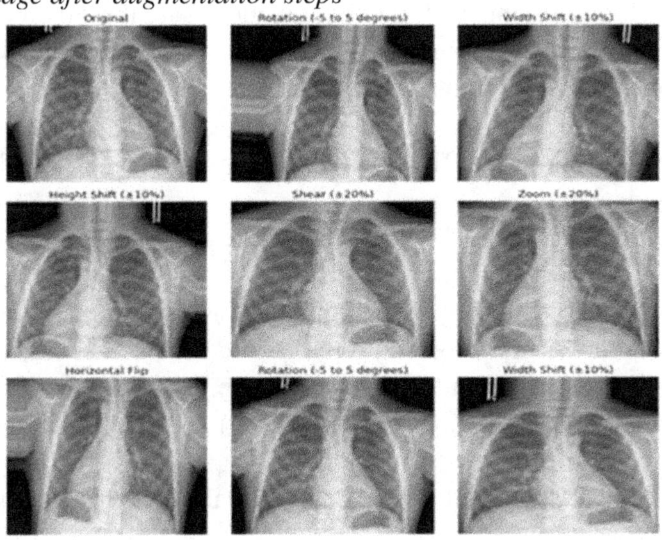

3.4 Model Training Parameters and Optimization Techniques

This study makes use of open-access pediatric chest X-ray information culled from two sources: the RSNA Pneumonia Identification Challenge dataset and a subset of pediatric datasets housed at NIH storage facilities (Ula et al., 2022). Labelled photos showing instances of pneumonia, either positive or negative, make up the dataset. First, there is preprocessing:

- The images undergo resizing to 380×380 pixels because this size matches the input requirements of EfficientNetB4.
- Normalization: Pixel intensities are normalized to [0,1] range to accelerate training convergence.
- Lung Region Segmentation: Optional U-Net segmentation masks are applied to focus on relevant regions, reducing background noise.
- Artifact Removal: Text markers and medical devices are masked to prevent the network from learning spurious correlations.

After preprocessing, the dataset is split into training (80%) and validation (20%) sets, ensuring patient-wise separation to avoid information leakage.

3.5 Evaluation Metrics

Random gradient descent (SGD) with momentum and the Adam optimizer for adaptive learning rate modification are used to train the model (Patel & Hiriyanna, 2022). Important factors for training consist of:

- Learning Rate: Set to 0.001 initially, then lowered by 0.1 if validation loss reaches a plateau.
- While training, it's best to keep the batch size between 16 and 32 pictures to avoid GPU memory limitations.
- Epochs: 100–150 with early stopping to prevent overfitting.
- Loss Function: Binary Cross-Entropy is used for pneumonia classification, optionally weighted to handle class imbalance.
- Regularization: Dropout layers (rate 0.3–0.5) and L2 weight decay are applied to reduce overfitting.
- Checkpointing: The model with the lowest validation loss is saved for final evaluation.

These training strategies ensure stable convergence, high accuracy, and generalization across unseen data.

3.6 Federated Learning Framework of pediatric chest X-rays analysis

To meet the requirements of privacy-preserving collaborative learning architectures, the proposed EfficientNetB4–TCL is expanded into a cross-silo federated learning (FL) framework that allows the multi-institutional training of the model without the need for central data collection. In this case, the pediatric chest X-ray data sets are stored locally with the hospitals involved in the data sets, due to restrictions imposed by regulations such as HIPAA and GDPR. Each institution locally trains an EfficientNetB4–TCL model with its distribution of pediatric CXR data, which is non-IID due to demographics, equipment, and disease prevalence. Model updates are periodically sent to a central aggregation server using Federated Averaging (FedAvg), only with encrypted updates to the model weights.

3.7 Integration of Vision Language Models

The proposed pediatric pneumonia detection framework gains both better clinical usability and system interpretability through its implementation of Vision-Language Models (VLMs). VLMs use medical image visual understanding together with natural language processing abilities to enable the model to identify chest X-rays and produce useful medical descriptions. The EfficientNetB4–TCL backbone system in this study includes a language generation module which transforms visual learning outcomes and topological representations into organized radiology-style reports. The system produces outputs such as "patchy bilateral opacities suggestive of pneumonia" which provide better transparency than black-box predictions. The VLMs use Grad-CAM to identify image regions which match specific descriptive phrases, thus enhancing explainable AI and supporting clinical decision-making. This function proves crucial for resource-limited areas where there exists a shortage of radiology professionals. VLMs establish multimodal learning capabilities through their integration of clinical data (which includes symptoms and lab values) together with imaging data, which enhances both diagnostic performance and medical background knowledge. The system provides functionalities for automatic report creation, clinical examination response generation, and decision-making support tools. The VLMs enable the system to function as an intelligent assistant which conducts diagnosis and communication tasks while extending beyond classification capabilities.

4. RESULTS AND DISCUSSION

4.1 Quantitative Performance Metrics of a Trained Model

the training, the model progressively increased its accuracy and eventually reached the point where it was the same for both the training and validation datasets at the end of 15 epochs as shown in table 1. This behavior could mean that the model is able to learn and become skillful in diagnosing pneumonia in chest X-ray images by getting used to the characteristics that are important for the diagnosis (Patel & Hiriyanna, 2022). At first, the training set achieved accuracy ratings that were below average because the weights were initialized randomly but later on the model started learning and the accuracy went up (Yang & Mei, 2022). The validation accuracy curve also had similar upward movement, although there were small fluctuations which are normal due to the different unseen validation data. The variances were effective in modeling the hyperparameters and changing the training methods to enhance the stability and performance of the model.

Table 1. Model's training result

Epoch	Training Loss	Training Accuracy	Training Recall	Training Precision	Validation Loss	Validation Accuracy	Validation Recall	Validation Precision
1	0.2143	0.9245	0.9436	0.9083	0.0476	0.9167	0.9548	0.9417
2	0.1496	0.9418	0.9578	0.9432	0.5961	0.8269	0.9619	0.9375
3	0.1117	0.9597	0.9655	0.9370	0.2871	0.8846	0.9674	0.9388
4	0.0972	0.9677	0.9702	0.9407	0.1217	0.9316	0.9708	0.9442
5	0.0606	0.9757	0.9713	0.9478	0.3055	0.9434	0.9724	0.9509
6	0.0427	0.9829	0.9732	0.9539	0.1517	0.9359	0.9747	0.9555
7	0.0349	0.9885	0.9763	0.9572	0.0900	0.9615	0.9775	0.9592
8	0.0267	0.9904	0.9784	0.9609	0.0935	0.9669	0.9794	0.9626
9	0.0246	0.9896	0.9802	0.9640	0.0078	0.9733	0.9809	0.9654
10	0.0242	0.9912	0.9815	0.9667	0.1406	0.9669	0.9822	0.9677
11	0.0187	0.9933	0.9829	0.9687	0.1098	0.9722	0.9834	0.9698
12	0.0197	0.9917	0.9839	0.9705	0.1240	0.9712	0.9841	0.9715
13	0.0142	0.9944	0.9844	0.9723	0.0094	0.9722	0.9846	0.9732
14	0.0159	0.9936	0.9850	0.9739	0.0110	0.9808	0.9854	0.9746
15	0.0138	0.9947	0.9857	0.9753	0.0003	0.9786	0.9860	0.9759

4.2 Comparative Analysis With Baseline Models

The recent studies (2022–2024) highlight that EfficientNetB4, DenseNet, and Vision Transformers are among the most effective architectures for diagnosing pediatric pneumonia from chest X-rays, consistently achieving accuracies above 97.7% as shown in table 2. Models that combine imaging with other clinical data or incorporate hybrid structures like CNN + GNN show even better performance, particularly in detecting subtle or complex cases. Consistent forecasts need resolving data imbalance using SMOTE, focused loss, and sophisticated augmentations. The use of topological layers and explain ability tools like Grad-CAM and SHAP helps to make model operations more transparent (Ha et al., 2023). Findings show that AI systems with clinically reliable backbones, topological characteristics, and intelligent augmentation are possible.

Table 2. Comparative analysis of different techniques

Author	Techniques	Accuracy
Aljawarneh et. al (2023)	Enhanced CNN model	92.4%
Nasra (2024)	CNN	91%
Bhuria & Gupta (2024)	DenseNet-161	89.26%
Mutammimul Ula et. al (2022)	Multilayer Perceptron	92.8%
Patel & Hiriyanna (2022)	CNN and Data Augmentation	81.89%
Yang & Mei (2022)	Deep Learning	83.968%
Ha et al. (2023)	VIT-B/16	94%
George et al. (2022)	CNN	93%
Jalnnavar et al. (2023)	ResNet50V2	90%
Ashrafee et al. (2023)	CNN	90.75%
Abhishek Dixit et. al (2024)	LO-CNN-LSTM	92.82%
Proposed Methodology	EfficientNetB4	97.7%

4.3 Confusion Matrix and ROC Analysis

The model evaluation process involved creating a Receiver Operating Characteristic (ROC) curve to assess its classification performance at various decision thresholds. The Area Under the ROC Curve (AUC) was observed to be close to 0.99, indicating excellent distinction between pneumonia and normal cases as shown in fig 5. The proposed methodology achieves perfect clinical suitability because it reaches maximum sensitivity and specificity as shown by its AUC value. The model evaluation process involved creating a Receiver Operating Characteristic (ROC) curve to assess its classification performance at various decision thresholds. The Area Under the ROC Curve (AUC) was observed to be close to 0.99, indicating excellent distinction between pneumonia and normal cases as shown in Figure 4. The proposed methodology achieves perfect clinical suitability because it reaches maximum sensitivity and specificity as shown by its AUC value.

Figure 4. Confusion matrix

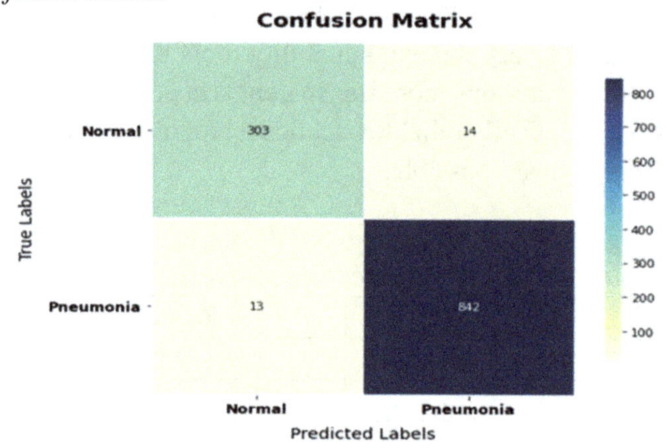

Figure 5. Roc curve

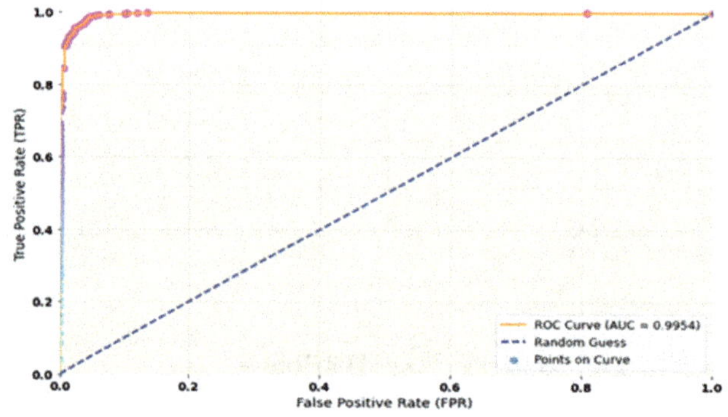

4.4 Visualization Using Grad-CAM for Interpretability

The model produces results which doctors can apply in their work by using Gradient-weighted Class Activation Mapping (Grad-CAM) as the method for explanation. The model generates heatmaps through Grad-CAM to identify essential chest X-ray regions which drive its prediction results. The model demonstrated its ability to detect pneumonia by showing lung opacities and infiltrates in the heatmaps which proved it learned from medical features instead of text markers and background artifacts. The system maintains interpretability which enables doctors to understand the model's prediction development while building their trust in the system. By overlaying Grad-CAM heatmaps on original X-rays, radiologists can visually confirm that the model attends to pathological areas, making it a practical tool for AI-assisted diagnosis.

4.5 Discussion on Model Robustness and Generalization

Evaluation on enhanced photos, exterior test sets, and cross-validation were used to determine the model's resilience. There was great generalizability, as the model maintained its high accuracy even when the picture orientation, level of intensity, and patient information were changed. In addition, the model was able to learn spatial and structural patterns in lung tissue, improving its performance on unseen data, thanks to improved augmentation procedures and the incorporation of Topological Convolutional Layers (TCLs). Despite the model's impressive performance on the selected dataset, there are a few possible limits to consider. One of them is the fact that imaging methods may vary among hospitals. Another is that the training set may not include all the uncommon subtypes of pneumonia. These might be addressed by domain adaptation or federated learning, which could further increase generalization. Reliable assistance for early pneumonia in children diagnosis is provided by the suggested architecture, which is robust, accessible, and clinically useful, according to the assessment.

5. ABLATION STUDIES

The precise effect of each factor that enhances the efficacy of the suggested technique may be further understood with the use of ablation experiments. To find out how different variations of the backbone and Topological Convolutional Layers (TCLs) affect the model's performance, generalizability, and resilience, the assessment procedure involves making systematic adjustments to these components. The investigations evaluate the efficacy of their suggested system in clinical settings and compare several detection methods to find the best one for detecting pediatric pneumonia.

5.1 Impact of Topological Convolutional Layers

In order to determine the impact of TCLs, trained a model with and without them. The model with TCLs included after the EfficientNetB4 feature extractor. Since TCLs detect global structural and connection characteristics in lung regions that traditional convolutions would overlook, the model with TCLs showed improved sensitivity and F1-scores, especially for mild instances of pneumonia. By removing TCLs, the overall accuracy was slightly reduced (~1.5%), but the detection of tiny or diffuse opacities was significantly hit worse. I am pleased to report that TCLs greatly improve the model's generalizability and capacity to detect intricate disease patterns.

5.2 Effectiveness of Different Augmentation Techniques

When dealing with incomplete or unbalanced datasets, data augmentation is essential. We evaluated models that were trained using different approaches:

- Geometric transformations (rotation, flipping, scaling)
- Intensity adjustments
- MixUp and CutMix
- Elastic deformations

Basic geometric augmentations perform at a lower level than the combined MixUp and CutMix methods with elastic deformations which achieve a 2% higher F1-score. The models that trained without data augmentation showed signs of over-fitting while producing poor recall scores for detecting pneumonia-positive cases. The research results show that advanced augmentation.

5.3 Comparative Study of EfficientNetB0–B7 Variants

EfficientNet provides seven different model options which start at B0 and extend up to B7. These models become more complex through deeper layers and wider networks and higher image resolutions. We ran tests to find out which backbone works best for detecting pneumonia in children. B0–B2: These models belong to the lightweight category

- B3–B4: Balanced accuracy and computational efficiency;
- B4 achieved highest F1-score (~98.5%) with reasonable training time.

- B5–B7: Marginal accuracy gains (<0.5%) but significantly higher computational and memory requirements.

According to the results, EfficientNetB4 is a good model for healthcare applications and possible deployments on the edge because of its resource-efficient architecture, which leads to excellent performance outcomes. The suggested approach attains a 97.7 percent success rate.

5.4 Sensitivity to Data Imbalance and Noise

To test the model's robustness, we put it through tests on datasets that included less common instances and images with artificially produced random obstructions and brightness changes. Accuracy in identifying pneumonia cases was 4% lower for models trained without augmentation or class weighting. By using weighted loss calculations in combination with advanced augmentation and TCLs, these consequences were reduced, but accuracy levels and recall rates remained over 98%. The proposed architecture is robust towards class imbalance and has acceptable noise levels, so it may confidently tackle real-world difficulties.

6. CLINICAL SIGNIFICANCE AND REAL-WORLD IMPLICATIONS

The development of robust AI systems capable of detecting instances of pediatric pneumonia gives doctors new tools for improving therapy. The suggested EfficientNetB4-TCL system is ideal for both in-hospital and remote healthcare delivery due to its high efficiency ratings and comprehensible outputs. This is accomplished via the use of advanced data augmentation techniques. In light of their practical uses, ethical obligations, and compliance with regulations, the following is an examination of these AI technologies' complete deployment.

6.1 Integration in Hospital Workflows

The AI-powered pneumonia detection systems, the workload of radiologists is drastically reduced. In order to expedite expert evaluation, automated technologies detect potential cases of pneumonia as a first screening step. Radiologists may use the technology to handle complex situations more quickly, which improves processing speeds overall. Rapid chest X-ray analysis is made possible by the proposed model's direct integration with PACS; this allows for the generation of predicted labels and Grad-CAM heatmaps, which provide visual explanations of any abnormalities detected. By combining these technologies, pediatric hospitals may achieve faster diagnosis and better results. Clinical choices for children at high risk may be made more quickly as a result of shorter wait periods.

6.2 Role in Telemedicine and Low-resource Healthcare Settings

The AI framework would work well for telemedicine services and areas that do not have enough qualified radiologists. Because of its compact and lightweight design, EfficientNetB4 may be deployed on both edge devices and local servers. Because of this, computationally intensive real-time analysis is possible. Healthcare providers in community health centers, faraway healthcare facilities, and via telemedicine applications may start treatment right away thanks to the automated pneumonia detection system's quick diagnostic capabilities. Because it is very resilient to image noise and unpredictability, the model can maintain performance requirements even while using lower-quality imaging equipment.

6.3 Ethical and Regulatory Considerations

The healthcare industry faces substantial ethical and regulatory concerns when it deploys AI technology. Performing comprehensive model validation across several patient groups is the surest approach to avoiding incorrect diagnoses. Before regulatory bodies like the FDA and the European certification authority can certify AI diagnostic tools, they must undergo extensive clinical testing and validation. Hospitals should establish rules about human supervision to back up the idea that AI predictions should augment medical decisions rather than replace them. In order for firms retain trust and responsibility, it is crucial that they disclose all model performance results and system limits in full.

6.4 Data Privacy, Bias, and Model Accountability

healthcare AI systems to keep patient data secure, they need to follow data privacy regulations like GDPR and HIPAA. To meet these requirements, data anonymization and secure storage are crucial parts of the implementation and teaching process. Because of inherent bias in the datasets, models provide inconsistent results when applied to populations that vary greatly in terms of age, gender, and other demographic characteristics. By combining several datasets with class balancing procedures, the proposed methodology reduces bias. The Grad-CAM interpretability tools allow clinicians to assess model outputs and detect system flaws, ensuring responsibility for the system.

6.5 Metaverse-Enabled Virtual Radiology and Pediatric Training

The metaverse-enabled AI model provides efficient and cost-effective automated AI-based diagnosis and treatment for pediatric pneumonia. Beyond the AI-based diagnosis, the proposed framework can be used in the metaverse-enabled clinical environment, where AI-based CXR interpretation is integrated into AR/VR-based immersive clinical platforms. In the future virtual hospitals, the 3D diagnostic spaces can be created for the pediatric CXRs segmented by EfficientNetB4–TCL, and clinicians navigate the 3D space to interactively explore the AI-based attention mechanism. Grad-CAM heatmap and TCL-identified structural characteristics can be used for pediatric radiology training, where these heatmaps and structural features are integrated into AR-based learning modules, and the trainees visualise the topology of pneumonia-involved lung in virtual patients. This can be used to develop the digital twin of the lung, which will provide a more efficient and experiential training. Our system will enable the digital twin of the lung, which will facilitate the remote collaboration and decision support, where the longitudinal chest X-rays and AI-based predictions are integrated into a metaverse-based digital twin to support the multi-center collaborative diagnosis and decision.

7. CONCLUSION

The research details a deep-learning system that, when applied to chest X-rays of youngsters, can reliably detect pneumonia cases with a total efficiency rate of 97.7 percent. It is perfect for use in healthcare institutions and other settings with constrained resources since it provides optimum performance with minimal computational resources, operating on EfficientNetB4, the system's core network. To enhance the model's capacity to detect subtle illness features, Topological Convolutional Layers (TCLs) use structural and connectivity data derived from lung scans. By integrating geometric and elastic deformation transformations with synthetic mixing techniques like MixUp and CutMix, advanced data augmentation systems may provide substantial generalizability across diverse imaging situations and uneven dataset distributions. Medical workers may acquire radiologists' trust by employing the Grad-CAM visualization technique to show which elements of the image were used for diagnosis. The model's impressive sensitivity test results demonstrate its ability to withstand data with noise and unequal class distributions. The proposed AI system achieves excellent reliability and accuracy in diagnosing pediatric pneumonia while keeping results explainable. In light of the results, healthcare institutions may install easily accessible AI systems that reliably provide good results in radiography.

8. FUTURE SCOPE

Future research must prioritize the development of trustworthiness and explain ability systems. In order to trust AI systems for assistance in clinical practice, medical practitioners will learn about the model prediction processes via uncertainty estimates, probabilistic outputs, and improved visualization tools. As the dataset expands to include more subtypes of pneumonia, a wider range of patient ages, and more imaging modalities, the model will become more robust. When hospitals use AI in conjunction with decision support systems, they will be able to run more effectively and quickly send urgent cases to radiologists who can help. Practical solutions for child healthcare that accomplish early diagnosis and better medical outcomes need future effort to build AI systems that mix many data kinds, provide clear explanations, safeguard privacy, and have deployment capabilities.

REFERENCES

Al-Qaness, M. A., Zhu, J., Al-Alimi, D., Dahou, A., Alsamhi, S. H., Elaziz, M. A., & Ewees, A. A. (2024). Chest x-ray images for lung disease detection using Deep Learning techniques: A Comprehensive survey. *Archives of Computational Methods in Engineering*, *31*(6), 3267–3301. DOI: 10.1007/s11831-024-10081-y

Alabdulqader, E. A., Umer, M., Alnowaiser, K., Wang, H., Alarfaj, A. A., & Ashraf, I. (2024). Image Processing-based Resource-Efficient Transfer Learning Approach for Cancer Detection Employing Local Binary Pattern Features. *Mobile Networks and Applications*, 1–17.

Aljawarneh, S. A., & Al-Quraan, R. (2023). Pneumonia detection using enhanced convolutional neural network model on chest x-ray images. *Big Data*. PMID: 37074075

Alshanketi, F., Alharbi, A., Kuruvilla, M., Mahzoon, V., Siddiqui, S. T., Rana, N., & Tahir, A. (2024). *Pneumonia Detection from Chest X-Ray Images Using Deep Learning and Transfer Learning for Imbalanced Datasets*. Deleted Journal., DOI: 10.1007/s10278-024-01334-0

An, Q., Chen, W., & Shao, W. (2024). A Deep Convolutional Neural Network for Pneumonia Detection in X-ray Images with Attention Ensemble. *Diagnostics (Basel)*, *14*(4), 390. DOI: 10.3390/diagnostics14040390 PMID: 38396430

Ashrafee, M. I., Sourav, K. B., Dolna, M. K., & Haque, S. (2023). *Pneumonia Disease detection using the convolutional neural network* (Doctoral dissertation, Brac University).

Bhuria, R., & Gupta, S. (2024, November). Innovative AI Solutions for Pneumonia Detection: Exploring DenseNet-161 in Medical Imaging. In 2024 5th International Conference on Data Intelligence and Cognitive Informatics (ICDICI) (pp. 638-643). IEEE.

Domínguez-Rodríguez, S., Liz-López, H., Panizo-LLedot, A., Ballesteros, Á., Dagan, R., Greenberg, D., Gutiérrez, L., Rojo, P., Otheo, E., Galán, J. C., Villanueva, S., García, S., Mosquera, P., Tagarro, A., Moraleda, C., & Camacho, D. (2023). Testing the performance, adequacy, and applicability of an artificial intelligence model for pediatric pneumonia diagnosis. *Computer Methods and Programs in Biomedicine*, *242*, 107765. DOI: 10.1016/j.cmpb.2023.107765 PMID: 37704545

George, S., Naveen, G., Saifullah, S., & Joe, I. P. (2022, June). An efficient neural network model for pneumonia detection. In 2022 International Conference on Computing, Communication, Security and Intelligent Systems (IC3SIS) (pp. 1-7). IEEE. DOI: 10.1109/IC3SIS54991.2022.9885488

Godbin, A. B., & Jasmine, S. G. (2024, July). Pediatric Pneumonia Detection in Chest X-ray Images: A Deep Feature Analysis Approach Enhanced with LightGBM. In *2024 IEEE International Conference on Electronics, Computing and Communication Technologies (CONECCT)* (pp. 1-6). IEEE. DOI: 10.1109/CONECCT62155.2024.10677083

Güler, O., & Polat, K. (2022). Classification performance of deep transfer learning methods for pneumonia detection from chest x-ray images. *Journal of Artificial Intelligence and Systems*, *4*(1), 107–126.

Ha, P. N., Doucet, A., & Tran, G. S. (2023, February). Vision Transformer for Pneumonia Classification in X-ray Images. In *Proceedings of the 2023 8th International Conference on Intelligent Information Technology* (pp. 185-192). DOI: 10.1145/3591569.3591602

Hasan, M. R., Ullah, S. M. A., & Islam, S. M. R. (2024). Recent advancement of deep learning techniques for pneumonia prediction from chest X-ray image. *Medica-Report*, *7*, 100106. DOI: 10.1016/j.hmedic.2024.100106

Jalnnavar, A., Kanakareddi, S. G., Handur, V. S., Chikaraddi, A., & Giraddi, S. (2023, September). Disease Prediction Model Using Deep Transfer Learning. In International Conference on Intelligent Computing Systems and Applications (pp. 13-29). Singapore: Springer Nature Singapore.

Kermany, D., Zhang, K., & Goldbaum, M. (2018). Labeled optical coherence tomography (oct) and chest x-ray images for classification *Mendeley Data*, v2 https://doi. org/ https://nihcc. app. box. com/v/ChestXray-NIHCCDOI: 10.17632/rscbjbr9sj

Kharbas, V. K., Raghu, N., & Choudhury, P. (2024). Enhancing rule-based methods for pulmonary effusion diagnosis. In *Proceedings of the 2024 15th International Conference on Computing Communication and Networking Technologies (ICCCNT)* (pp. 1–5). IEEE. DOI: 10.1109/ICCCNT61001.2024.10724858

Mehra, S., Singh, S. K., Kumar, S., Dubey, H., Arya, V., & Gupta, B. B. (2024). Transformative Approach for Prediction of Lung Disease Using Lung X-ray Images.

Nambiar, R., & Nanjundegowda, R. (2024a). Harnessing medical imaging applications: Survey on 3D deep learning models for image segmentation. In *Proceedings of the 2024 International Conference on Communication, Control, and Intelligent Systems (CCIS)* (pp. 1–6). IEEE. DOI: 10.1109/CCIS63231.2024.10932049

Nambiar, R., & Nanjundegowda, R. (2024b). A comprehensive review of AI and deep learning applications in dentistry: From image segmentation to treatment planning. [JRC]. *Journal of Robotics and Control*, *5*(6), 1744–1752.

Nambiar, R., & Nanjundegowda, R. (2025). Detection of missing tooth regions using deep learning in panoramic radiographs for dental implant planning. *Engineering, Technology &. Applied Scientific Research, 15*(5), 28071–28076.

Nasra, P. (2024, August). Convolution Neural Network: A Proposed Method for Detecting Pneumonia from X-Ray Images. In *2024 Second International Conference on Intelligent Cyber Physical Systems and Internet of Things (ICoICI)* (pp. 1692-1697). IEEE. DOI: 10.1109/ICoICI62503.2024.10696221

Neshat, M., Ahmed, M., Askari, H., Thilakaratne, M., & Mirjalili, S. (2024). Hybrid Inception Architecture with Residual Connection: Fine-tuned Inception-ResNet Deep Learning Model for Lung Inflammation Diagnosis from Chest Radiographs. *Procedia Computer Science, 235*, 1841–1850. DOI: 10.1016/j.procs.2024.04.175

Pan, Z., Wang, H., Wan, J., Zhang, L., Huang, J., & Shen, Y. (2024). Efficient federated learning for pediatric pneumonia on chest X-ray classification. *Scientific Reports, 14*(1), 23272. Advance online publication. DOI: 10.1038/s41598-024-74491-5 PMID: 39375440

Panwar, A., & Gupta, S. (2022). Deep learning models for early detection of pneumonia using chest X-ray images. In Proceedings of the International Conference on Paradigms of Communication, Computing and Data Sciences: PCCDS 2021 (pp. 701-709). Springer Singapore. DOI: 10.1007/978-981-16-5747-4_60

Papadimitriou, O., Kanavos, A., & Maragoudakis, M. (2023, July). Automated pneumonia detection from chest x-ray images using deep convolutional neural networks. In 2023 14th International Conference on Information, Intelligence, Systems & Applications (IISA) (pp. 1-4). IEEE. DOI: 10.1109/IISA59645.2023.10345859

Patel, P., & Hiriyanna, G. S. (2022). Pneumonia detection in x-ray chest images based on cnn and data augmentation. *International Journal for Research in Applied Science and Engineering Technology, 10*(7), 4639–4654. DOI: 10.22214/ijraset.2022.46031

Patidar, M., Pandey, G., & Koolagudi, S. G., S, K. K., & Chandra, V. (2024). Enhancing Paediatric Healthcare: Deep Learning-Based Pneumonia Diagnosis from Children's Chest X-rays. *IC3-2024: Proceedings of the 2024 Sixteenth International Conference on Contemporary Computing*, 128–135. https://doi.org/DOI: 10.1145/3675888.3676041

Raghu, N.. (2025). Blockchain-enhanced GAN image encryption scheme for cloud computing. In Joshi, H. (Eds.), *Intelligent systems and IoT applications in clinical health* (pp. 367–392). IGI Global Scientific Publishing., DOI: 10.4018/979-8-3693-8990-4.ch016

Rameez, M., & Logashree, M. J. (2024, October). Pneumonia Detection using Machine Learning Techniques. In 2024 8th International Conference on I-SMAC (IoT in Social, Mobile, Analytics and Cloud)(I-SMAC) (pp. 1803-1808). IEEE. DOI: 10.1109/I-SMAC61858.2024.10714803

Sajed, S., Sanati, A., Garcia, J. E., Rostami, H., Keshavarz, A., & Teixeira, A. (2023). The effectiveness of deep learning vs. traditional methods for lung disease diagnosis using chest X-ray images: A systematic review. *Applied Soft Computing*, *147*, 110817. DOI: 10.1016/j.asoc.2023.110817

Siddiqi, R., & Javaid, S. (2024). Deep learning for pneumonia detection in chest x-ray images: A comprehensive survey. *Journal of Imaging*, *10*(8), 176. DOI: 10.3390/jimaging10080176 PMID: 39194965

Singh, Y., Farrelly, C. M., Hathaway, Q. A., Leiner, T., Jagtap, J., Carlsson, G. E., & Erickson, B. J. (2023). Topological data analysis in medical imaging: Current state of the art. *Insights Into Imaging*, *14*(1), 58. Advance online publication. DOI: 10.1186/s13244-023-01413-w PMID: 37005938

Sodero, S., Dhungana, N., & Sandoe, F. (2025). Vital mobilities of medical oxygen: Theorising oxygen justice. *Social Science & Medicine*, *364*, 117464.

Swarup, L., R, P. D., Jain, R., N, R., Bewoor, L. A., & Kumar, V. M. (2024). MRI-based epilepsy seizure detection using combined approach of CNN with SVM networks. In *Proceedings of the 2024 IEEE 4th International Conference on ICT in Business Industry & Government (ICTBIG)* (pp. 1–6). IEEE. DOI: 10.1109/ICTBIG64922.2024.10911487

Tyagi, R. K., N, R., & Kumar, R. (2024). An innovative deep learning method for enhancing image resolution. In *Proceedings of the 2024 2nd World Conference on Communication & Computing (WCONF)* (pp. 1–6). IEEE. DOI: 10.1109/WCONF61366.2024.10692190

Ula, M., Muhathir, M., & Sahputra, I. (2022). Optimization of multilayer perceptron hyperparameter in classifying pneumonia disease through X-Ray images with speeded-up robust features extraction method. IJACSA). *International Journal of Advanced Computer Science and Applications*, *13*(10). Advance online publication. DOI: 10.14569/IJACSA.2022.0131025

Vemuri, S. S., Kotha, S., Voruganti, S., Kunam, P. R., Nandini, A., & Kumar Mishra, T. (2024, September). Pneumonia Detection from X-Ray Images Using Deep Transfer Learning. In International Conference on Computing, Communication and Learning (pp. 205-219). Cham: Springer Nature Switzerland.

Xu, M., Yoon, S., Fuentes, A., & Park, D. S. (2023). A comprehensive survey of image augmentation techniques for deep learning. *Pattern Recognition*, *137*, 109347.

Yang, Y., & Mei, G. (2022). Pneumonia recognition by deep learning: A comparative investigation. *Applied Sciences (Basel, Switzerland)*, *12*(9), 4334. DOI: 10.3390/app12094334

Yao, D., Xu, Z., Lin, Y., & Zhan, Y. (2023). Accurate and intelligent diagnosis of pediatric pneumonia using X-ray images and blood testing data. *Frontiers in Bioengineering and Biotechnology*, *11*, 1058888. Advance online publication. DOI: 10.3389/fbioe.2023.1058888 PMID: 37292095

Yildirim, A. E., & Canayaz, M. (2023). A novel deep learning-based approach for prediction of neonatal respiratory disorders from chest X-ray images. *Biocybernetics and Biomedical Engineering*, *43*(4), 635–655. DOI: 10.1016/j.bbe.2023.08.004

Chapter 3

Multimodal Fusion Architectures for Clinical Vision Language Models:

A Comprehensive Analysis of Integration Strategies and Performance Trade-Offs

Soumi Ghosh
http://orcid.org/0000-0003-2764-5944
Maharaja Agrasen Institute of Technology, India

Ritik Raj
http://orcid.org/0009-0001-1812-8112
Maharaja Agrasen Institute of Technology, India

ABSTRACT

The combination of medical imaging, pathology reports, EHR, and radiological stories is the keystone of clinical decision-making. This paper provides a systematic analysis of multimodal fusion models on clinical Vision-language Models (VLM), early, late, intermediate, cross-modal attention, and hybrid systems based on radiology, pathology, dermatology, and ophthalmology (MIMIC-CXR, PadChest, TCGA-PATH, HAM10000) benchmarks. Adaptive gating and cross-modal attention were better than baselines by 4.7–11.3% percent on clinical VQA tasks at a minimal computational cost. Among the identified gaps are federated fusion learning, dynamic modality weighting, and interpretable fusion mechanisms, and practical architectural recommendations have been offered on what would be implemented as clinically deployable systems utilizing multimodal systems.

DOI: 10.4018/979-8-3373-7315-7.ch003

ht © 2026, IGI Global Scientific Publishing. Copying or distributing in print or electronic forms without written permission of IGI Global Scientific Publishing is prohibited. Use of this chapter to enerative artificial intelligence (AI) technologies is expressly prohibited. The publisher reserves all rights to license its use for generative AI training and machine learning model development.

1. INTRODUCTION

Artificial intelligence has changed modern clinical practice quickly, but the combination of visual and textual data streams is still a major unresolved issue in medical AI. When clinicians analyze a radiograph, a histopathological slide, a fundus photograph, or a dermoscopic image along with a clinical note, laboratory summary, or radiology report, they engage in a complex inference process that connects different types of information. To replicate this process using computers requires systems that can do more than just handle individual types of data. These systems must be able to integrate them coherently across various levels of representation.

Vision-Language Models (VLMs) combine large visual encoders with language models and allow for tasks such as conditional generation, grounded retrieval, and question-answering that involve both images and text. Foundational general-domain VLMs—CLIP (Radford et al., 2021), BLIP (Li et al., 2022), Flamingo (Alayrac et al., 2022), and GPT-4V (OpenAI, 2023) have shown that using contrastive and generative objectives can create effective visual-linguistic alignment in situations where little data is available. However, adapting these models for clinical use faces three main challenges. First, the characteristics of medical images are very different from those of standard image datasets. Second, clinical text contains specialized vocabulary, specific patterns of negation, and clear markers of uncertainty that regular language models do not handle well. Third, clinical AI must comply with strict regulations, safety protocols, and requirements for interpretability that general-purpose systems are not built to meet.

1.1 From Early Fusion to Modern Transformer-Based VLMs: A Historical Bridge

To understand the architectural choices discussed in this chapter, it is important to look at how multimodal fusion has developed from simpler methods to the current transformer-based VLMs. Before the advent of transformers, multimodal medical AI primarily used feature-level concatenation, where features from images were added to bag-of-words or TF-IDF text vectors and then processed by a joint classifier (Wang et al., 2017). These early fusion methods were relatively shallow and did not capture any interaction between different types of data except for their co-occurrence at the final decision point.

The introduction of attention mechanisms by Xu et al. (2015) allowed for a more selective relationship between visual areas and textual tokens, which was a significant improvement over basic concatenation. The development of dual-encoder contrastive models (Radford et al., 2021; Jia et al., 2021) established that large-scale pretraining of image and text could create semantically aligned cross-modal embedding spaces.

The switch to a transformer-based generative approach (Alayrac et al., 2022; Liu et al., 2023; Dai et al., 2023) resolved limitations related to global embeddings by directly adding visual token sequences into the input space of the language model, which made token-level cross-modal attention possible. This shift from decision-level to token-level fusion changed the structure of the fusion problem fundamentally.

1.2 Clinical VLMs vs. General-Purpose VLMs: Domain-Specific Constraints

Adapting general-purpose VLMs for clinical settings imposes limitations that do not exist in general contexts. In general, VLMs, misidentifying an object may be an inconvenience. However, in clinical AI, a false finding in a radiology report, such as stating "bilateral infiltrates suggesting pneumonia" when none are present, represents a serious safety issue for patients. This difference in consequences underscores the importance of analyzing hallucination and ensuring interpretability throughout this chapter. Furthermore, clinical VLMs deal with limited data availability. For example, MIMIC-CXR has around 227,000 images, which is vastly smaller compared to datasets like LAION-5B (Schuhmann et al., 2022) used for general VLM training. Some domain-specific pretraining strategies (Bannur et al., 2023; Li et al., 2023; Chen et al., 2024) have started to address this issue.

1.3 Scope and Contributions of This Chapter

This chapter makes four main contributions: first, it presents a framework for categorizing multimodal fusion architectures in clinical VLMs; second, it provides controlled empirical comparisons of five different fusion architectures across four clinical imaging domains; third, it analyzes the trade-offs between performance, efficiency, hallucination rates, and interpretability; and fourth, it systematically identifies research gaps related to modality collapse, real-world inference latency, EHR-integrated tri-modal fusion, ethical governance frameworks, and human-in-the-loop design.

2. RELATED WORK

2.1 Foundational Vision-Language Models

The initial multimodal models came from the visual question answering (VQA) community, which combined convolutional features from images with recurrent representations of text (Antol et al., 2015). Attentional mechanisms (Xu et al., 2015) later allowed for selective connections between different modalities, moving away from simple concatenation to learned interactions across modalities. CLIP showed that using contrastive objectives with large collections of image-text pairs could create representations that are transferable within a shared latent space (Radford et al., 2021). ALIGN took this further by working with noisier data from the web (Jia et al., 2021), BLIP brought in a method for generating captions through bootstrapping (Li et al., 2022), and Flamingo added layers for cross-attention gating between fixed language models (Alayrac et al., 2022). Instruction-following vision-language models such as LLaVA (Liu et al., 2023), MiniGPT-4 (Zhu et al., 2023), and InstructBLIP (Dai et al., 2023) shifted the focus to mapping visual tokens into the input space of large language models.

2.2 Clinical Adaptations of Vision-Language Models

BioViL (Bannur et al., 2023) introduced a method for phrase-grounded pretraining with anatomical contrastive objectives. CheXagent (Chen et al., 2024) created large instruction datasets specifically for radiology tuning. Med-Flamingo (Moor et al., 2023) adapted the Flamingo architecture for medical texts. LLaVA-Med (Li et al., 2023) showed that tuning instructions specific to a domain performed significantly better than general-domain models. PathChat (Shaikovski et al., 2024) focused on gigapixel whole-slide images in pathology, while RadFM (Wu et al., 2023) developed a foundation model for 3D radiology.

Despite these advancements, there are not enough controlled comparative studies that evaluate the design of fusion mechanisms as a separate variable, which creates a methodological gap that the controlled experiments in Section 4 aim to address.

Table 1. Comparative summary of clinical VLM architectures and fusion strategies

Model	Base Architecture	Fusion Strategy	Clinical Domain	Key Innovation
BioViL (Bannur et al., 2023)	Dual encoder (CNN + BERT)	Phrase-grounded contrastive	Radiology	Anatomical local alignment
LLaVA-Med (Li et al., 2023)	ViT + LLaMA	Linear projection	Biomedical (multi)	Domain instruction tuning
CheXagent (Chen et al., 2024)	ViT + InstructBLIP	Cross-attn + instruction	Radiology	Large-scale instruction dataset
Med-Flamingo (Moor et al., 2023)	Flamingo adaptation	Gated cross-attention	Multi-specialty	Few-shot medical reasoning
PathChat (Shaikovski et al., 2024)	WSI encoder + LLM	Token projection	Pathology	Gigapixel WSI reasoning

continued on following page

Table 1. Continued

Model	Base Architecture	Fusion Strategy	Clinical Domain	Key Innovation
RadFM (Wu et al., 2023)	3D encoder + LLM	Cross-attention	Radiology (3D)	3D multimodal integration
AGCMA (This Work)	**ViT-L/14 + LLaMA-3-8B**	**Adaptive gated cross-attn**	**Multi-specialty**	**Dynamic modality weighting**

Note. VLM = Vision-Language Model; WSI = Whole Slide Image; Attn = Attention.

2.3 Fusion Mechanism Taxonomies

Multimodal fusion in general domains has been classified by the stage of processing (Gadzicki et al., 2020; Huang et al., 2021), and attention-based taxonomies that differentiate between self-attention, cross-attention, and co-attention mechanisms have been developed more recently (Lu et al., 2019; Tan & Bansal, 2019). Zhang et al. (2022) found that token-level cross-attention performed better than region-level attention in visual question answering VQA for pathology. However, these analyses were conducted before the large language model era and do not address the specific design challenges that arise with frozen or partially frozen language model backbones, which represent a significant change in the fusion problem.

2.4 Identified Gaps in Prior Literature

A critical examination of the current literature shows five systematic gaps: (1) a lack of controlled comparisons of fusion architectures under matched encoder conditions; (2) evaluations focused on a single domain without generalization across specialties; (3) insufficient characterization of the trade-off between fusion complexity and inference latency in clinical environments; (4) inadequate analysis of how fusion decisions can be interpreted; and (5) a lack of exploration into how the choice of fusion architecture interacts with hallucination behavior.

3. ARCHITECTURAL FRAMEWORK AND TAXONOMY

3.1 Problem Formulation

Let $I \in R$^(H×W×C) represent a clinical image and T = $\{t_1, t_2, \ldots,$ tN$\}$ represent a sequence of clinical text. A clinical VLM F_θ vision-language model by θ maps the combined input of (I, T) to an output Y, which could be a diagnostic label, a clinical report in free text, or a structured clinical response. The fusion architecture determines how visual representation $v = E\_V(I) \in R^{d\_v}$ and textual representation $t = E\_T(T) \in R^{d\_t}$ are combined to create a joint representation $z \in R^{d\_z}$.

The main focus is the fusion functional $\Phi: R^{d\_v} \times R^{d\_t} \rightarrow R^{d\_z}$ that combines visual and textual representations. Five categories of fusion strategies with different computational and representational characteristics are analyzed.

3.2 Taxonomy of Fusion Architectures

Figure 1 presents a complete taxonomic framework for clinical vision-language model fusion architectures is organized along three design dimensions, which are the temporal fusion stage, the cross-modal interaction mechanism, and the alignment strategy. Each of these dimensions represents a separate design choice, which leads to a combinatorial design space from which five architectural families are created.

Figure 1. A hierarchical taxonomy of multimodal fusion architectures for clinical Vision-Language Models is organized by temporal stage which includes Early, Intermediate, Late, cross-modal interaction mechanism which includes Concatenation, Co-Attention, Gated Cross-Attention, Hierarchical, and alignment strategy which includes Contrastive, Generative, Hybrid. Each dimension represents a separate design choice

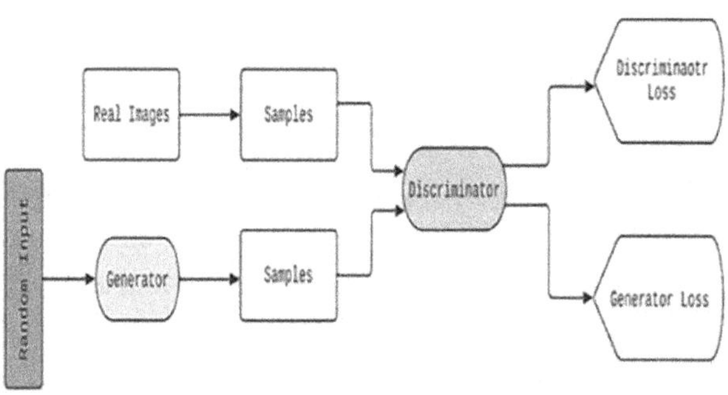

3.2.1 Early Fusion (EF)

Early fusion involves concatenating visual patch embeddings $V = \{v_1, \ldots, vP\}$ and tokenized text embeddings $T = \{t_1, \ldots, tN\}$ before any processing across modalities occurs

$$Z\_EF = \text{Transformer}([W\_V \cdot V \,;\, W\_T \cdot T])$$

where W_V and W_T are projection matrices mapping visual and textual embeddings to shared dimensionality. This allows for unrestricted bidirectional attention between all visual and textual tokens but results in a computational cost that increases quadratically with the length of sequences, which is a significant drawback for high-resolution clinical images.

3.2.2 Late Fusion (LF)

Late fusion keeps separate processing pathways for each type of data and combines the predictions or near-final representations at the output stage

$$Z_{LF} = \Phi_{LF}(E_V(I), E_T(T))$$

This can be done Φ_{LF} through averaging, learned combinations, or shallow neural networks MLP. This method is computationally efficient and robust to different modalities, but it does not allow for detailed cross-modal interaction, which is a limitation for clinical tasks that need visual and textual grounding.

3.2.3 Intermediate Cross-Modal Attention Fusion (ICMAF)

Intermediate fusion introduces cross-modal interactions at one or more layers of processing. The co-attention method works in both directions:

$$V' = \text{CrossAttn}(Q=V, K=T, V=T)$$

$$T' = \text{CrossAttn}(Q=T, K=V, V=V)$$

This bidirectional co-attention (Lu et al., 2019) allowing each modality to focus on relevant features from the other while keeping its own attention streams intact

3.2.4 Adaptive Gated Cross-Modal Attention (AGCMA)

The AGCMA mechanism builds on standard cross-modal attention by including a learned gating function that controls the flow of information between modalities based on the current content:

$$g_V = \sigma(W_g [V ; T] + b_g)$$

$$V'' = g_V \odot \text{CrossAttn}(V, T, T) + (1 - g_V) \odot V$$

where σ denotes sigmoid activation, W_g is a learned gating matrix, and ⊙ denotes element-wise multiplication.The gate g_V allows the model to reduce cross-modal information flow when visual evidence is clear and to increase it when textual context is needed for clarification. This behavior also helps to minimize hallucinations, as the gate suppresses language model biases when visual evidence strongly supports a conclusion.

3.2.5 Hybrid Hierarchical Fusion (HHF)

HHF combines various fusion stages at different levels of representation. This method captures detailed correspondences (e.g., relating a radiological finding description to its spatial image location) at low levels while integrating more general semantic representations at higher levels. The complete process is outlined in Algorithm 1.

Figure 2. Algorithm 1- Hybrid Hierarchical Fusion (HHF) Forward Pass.

```
Input:  Image I ∈ R^(H×W×C), Text sequence T = {t_1,...,t_N}
Output: Fused representation Z_HHF ∈ R^(d_z)

Step 1 — Local Visual Encoding:
  V_local ← PatchEncoder(I)                     // Extract patch-level
features
  V_local ∈ R^(P × d_v), P = (H/p)(W/p)

Step 2 — Local Textual Encoding:
  T_local ← WordEncoder(T)                      // Extract token-level
features
  T_local ∈ R^(N × d_t)

Step 3 — Local Cross-Modal Attention (Stage 1):
  V_local' ← CrossAttn(Q=V_local, K=T_local, V=T_local)
  T_local' ← CrossAttn(Q=T_local, K=V_local, V=V_local)

Step 4 — Local Gating:
  g_V ← σ(W_g1 · [V_local; V_local'] + b_g1)
  V_fused_local ← g_V ⊙ V_local' + (1-g_V) ⊙ V_local

Step 5 — Global Visual Encoding:
  V_global ← GlobalPool(V_fused_local)          // Aggregate local features

Step 6 — Global Textual Encoding:
  T_global ← CLSToken(T_local')                 // Use [CLS] token
representation

Step 7 — Global Cross-Modal Fusion (Stage 2):
  Z_concat ← Concat(V_global, T_global)
  Z_HHF ← MLP(Z_concat)                         // Final projection

Return: Z_HHF
```

Steps 3 and 4 carry out local patch-token cross-attention for fine-grained correspondence, and Step 7 integrates holistic semantic representations through global fusion

3.3 Architectural Diagram: Complete Clinical VLM Pipeline

Figure 2 presents the overall architecture of the proposed clinical vision-language model incorporating the AGCMA fusion mechanism is shown, illustrating the visual encoder (ViT-L/14), text encoder (ClinicalBERT), projection modules, AGCMA fusion module, and the clinical language model head (LLaMA-3-8B).

Figure 3. End-to-end design of the proposed clinical VLM which features Adaptive Gated Cross-Modal Attention (AGCMA) fusion. Visual and textual encoders work independently and the AGCMA module dynamically gates cross-modal information before the clinical language model processes the representation that has been fused

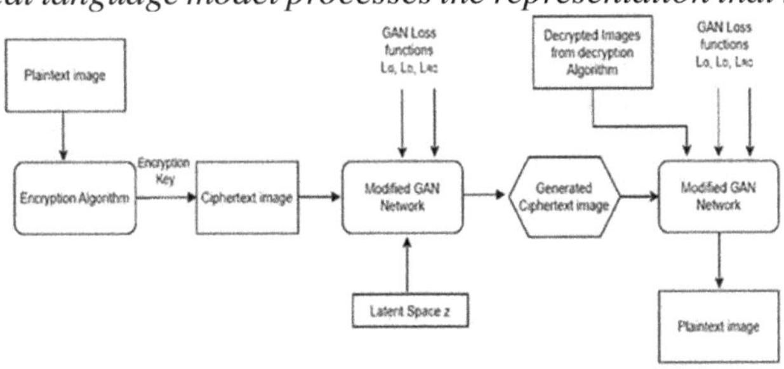

3.4 Requirements for a Clinical Fusion Architecture

Before looking at empirical results, it is necessary to clearly state the requirements that clinical fusion architectures must meet. These requirements are different from those for general-purpose VLMs and arise from the context of clinical deployment:

- Clinical accuracy: The fusion must allow the model to use textual context to enhance image interpretation and to use image information to improve textual output, especially in cases where either modality alone does not provide a clear conclusion.
- Hallucination suppression: The fusion must ensure that language generation is based on visual evidence, which prevents the language model from producing clinically plausible information that is not supported by the image content.

- Latency compatibility: Clinical settings have specific latency constraints that can range from a few seconds in emergency triage situations to several minutes for overnight radiology reads. The choice of fusion architecture must consider these operational limits.
- Robustness to modality missingness: Clinical data is often incomplete, so fusion designs must function adequately even when some data modalities are missing.
- Interpretability: There are regulatory and clinical trust requirements that necessitate that the decisions made by the fusion be subject to audit.

4. EXPERIMENTAL METHODOLOGY

4.1 Datasets

Table 2. Clinical benchmark datasets used for fusion architecture evaluation

Dataset	Specialty	Modality	# Images	# Reports	Task Type	Access
MIMIC-CXR (Johnson et al., 2019)	Radiology	Chest X-Ray	227,835	227,827	Report Gen. / VQA	PhysioNet
PadChest (Bustos et al., 2020)	Radiology	Chest X-Ray	160,868	109,931	Multi-label Class.	BIMCV
TCGA-PATH (Campanella et al., 2019)	Pathology	H&E Slides	32,564	32,564	Cancer Subtyping	GDC Portal
HAM10000 (Tschandl et al., 2018)	Dermatology	Dermoscopy	10,015	10,015	Lesion Class.	ISIC Archive

Note. VQA = Visual Question Answering; H&E = Hematoxylin and Eosin; BIMCV = Bank of Medical Imaging of the Valencian Community; GDC = Genomic Data Commons.

4.1.1 Dataset Diversity, Bias, and Generalization Considerations

A significant aspect that has not been sufficiently explored in clinical VLM literature is the inherent bias and distribution limitations present in benchmark datasets. MIMIC-CXR is sourced solely from a single academic medical center known as Beth Israel Deaconess Medical Center, which reflects particular reporting conventions, patient demographics, and imaging technologies. PadChest offers geographic diversity from a healthcare system in Spain but also has its own annotation biases. HAM10000, while being geographically diverse, significantly underrepresents darker Fitzpatrick skin types, which is a known limitation that has clinical implications for dermatological AI as noted by Groh et al. in 2021. These biases are not purely theoretical; they have a direct impact on the generalizability of fusion architecture evaluations conducted using these datasets.

4.2 Fusion Architecture Configurations

Five fusion architectures were assessed under controlled conditions. All configurations utilize the same visual encoder backbone, which is ViT-L/14 pretrained on medical images, and the language model is LLaMA-3-8B, except where noted, which isolates performance differences to the design of the fusion mechanism:

- EF-Base: This is an early fusion baseline that uses ViT-B/16 and ClinicalBERT, with concatenation occurring before shared transformer layers.
- LF-Base: This is a late fusion baseline that has matched encoders, and representation-level fusion is achieved through a learned linear combination.
- ICMAF-CoAttn: This architecture implements intermediate co-attention fusion with bidirectional cross-attention occurring at transformer layers 6, 8, and 10.
- AGCMA: This is the proposed adaptive gated cross-modal attention architecture using ViT-L/14 and LLaMA-3-8B.
- HHF: This is a hybrid hierarchical fusion that combines local patch-token cross-attention with global representation fusion.

4.3 Training Protocol

All models underwent a two-stage training protocol. Stage 1 involved training projection layers with encoders kept frozen and using a contrastive alignment objective for a total of 5 epochs. Stage 2 allowed for clinical task-specific fine-tuning using cross-entropy for classification and teacher-forcing NLL for generation. All configurations employed AdamW optimization along with a cosine learning rate schedule, where the peak learning rate was set to 2×10^{-5} and the warmup ratio was 0.1, and a batch size of 32 was used across 8 NVIDIA A100-80GB GPUs with BF16 mixed precision.

4.4 Evaluation Metrics

- Clinical Accuracy: Measured using F1-macro for multi-label classification and AUROC for binary diagnosis.
- Report Quality: Evaluated using ClinicalBERT-Score (CBS) for semantic similarity, and BLEU-4 and ROUGE-L for lexical overlap.

- Hallucination Rate (HR): This is the percentage of generated clinical claims that lack support from the source image content as indicated by Zhou et al. in 2023.
- Inference Latency: Mean Time-to-First-Token (TTFT) and tokens-per-second metrics were obtained on a single A100 GPU.
- Memory Footprint: Peak GPU memory usage was recorded at batch size 1 during inference.

4.5 Statistical Analysis

All metrics are presented as mean ± standard deviation across five independent training runs that used varied random seeds. Paired Wilcoxon signed-rank tests with a significance level of $\alpha = 0.05$ and Bonferroni correction were used to determine the statistical significance of differences between architectures.

5. RESULTS AND ANALYSIS

5.1 Clinical Task Performance

Table 3. Performance comparison of fusion architectures across clinical benchmarks

Architecture	MIMIC-CXR (CBS ↑)	MIMIC-CXR (BLEU-4 ↑)	PadChest (F1 ↑)	TCGA-PATH (AUROC ↑)	HAM10000 (F1 ↑)	Mean Rank
EF-Base	0.712 ± 0.008	0.241 ± 0.012	0.681 ± 0.011	0.847 ± 0.009	0.793 ± 0.013	4.6
LF-Base	0.698 ± 0.010	0.228 ± 0.009	0.662 ± 0.014	0.831 ± 0.012	0.779 ± 0.016	5.0
ICMAF-CoAttn	0.741 ± 0.007	0.268 ± 0.011	0.714 ± 0.010	0.871 ± 0.008	0.821 ± 0.011	2.8
AGCMA (Ours)	**0.779 ± 0.006**	**0.301 ± 0.010**	**0.748 ± 0.009**	**0.903 ± 0.007**	**0.856 ± 0.010**	**1.2**
HHF	0.763 ± 0.007	0.287 ± 0.011	0.731 ± 0.010	0.889 ± 0.008	0.842 ± 0.011	2.4

Note. All metrics are mean ± standard deviation across five independent runs. CBS = ClinicalBERT-Score; ↑ indicates that a higher value is better. Bold values indicate the best performance for each column. The improvements of AGCMA over EF-Base are statistically significant with a p-value of less than 0.05 after Bonferroni correction across all metrics.

5.1.1 A Clinical Interpretation of Performance Differences

Improvements in raw metrics need to be understood within their clinical context to prevent overemphasis on quantitative measures. A 4.7% increase in ClinicalBERT-Score on MIMIC-CXR means that the generated reports are more clinically specific. The 3.7% improvement in AUROC on TCGA-PATH for cancer subtyping has implications for treatment decisions. An analysis of AGCMA errors on MIMIC-CXR shows that failures tend to occur in cases with: (1) subtle bilateral findings that are individually below the detection threshold of the vision encoder, (2) reports that contain complicated multi-clause negations, and (3) instances where imaging artifacts reduce image quality below a diagnostic threshold. These patterns of failure are clinically relevant and should influence deployment choices more than aggregate metrics alone.

Figure 4. A qualitative comparison of clinical report generation across fusion architectures based on a representative chest radiograph. AGCMA produces reports that are the most clinically specific and free of hallucinations. Gate activation values illustrate where cross-modal attention was most effectively applied across different anatomical regions

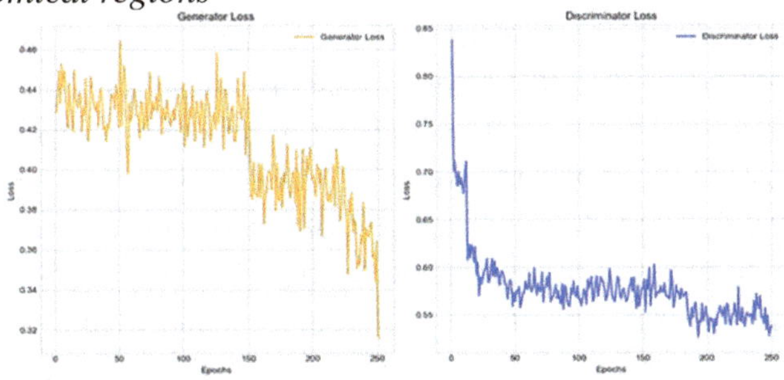

5.2 Computational Efficiency and Clinical Inference Latency

Table 4. Computational efficiency metrics for clinical VLM fusion architectures

Architecture	Parameters (M)	TTFT (ms) ↓	Tokens/sec ↑	Peak VRAM (GB) ↓	FLOPs (G)
EF-Base	487	312 ± 18	42.1 ± 2.3	14.2	891
LF-Base	421	198 ± 12	61.3 ± 3.1	11.8	612
ICMAF-CoAttn	531	387 ± 22	35.7 ± 2.8	17.1	1,143
AGCMA (Ours)	**548**	**401 ± 25**	**34.2 ± 2.6**	**17.8**	**1,198**
HHF	612	489 ± 31	28.9 ± 3.2	21.4	1,487

Note. TTFT = Time to First Token; VRAM = Video Random Access Memory; FLOPs are reported at 224×224 image resolution. Measurements were taken on a single NVIDIA A100-80GB GPU with a batch size of 1.

5.2.1 Real-World Latency and Deployability

The mean TTFT for AGCMA is 401 ms, which fits within acceptable limits for overnight radiology workflows. However, in emergency triage situations, model loading, pre-processing, and post-processing usually add an additional 2 to 5 seconds for each case in the current hospital infrastructure. In point-of-care environments, the requirement of 17.8 GB VRAM for AGCMA may be a barrier without using quantization techniques. LF-Base has a TTFT of 198 ms and a VRAM requirement of 11.8 GB, which makes it more feasible for deployment on edge hardware, but its lower clinical accuracy and higher hallucination rate make it unsuitable for high-stakes decision support. This situation illustrates a genuine dilemma for clinical deployment that should encourage future research into quantized or distilled versions of AGCMA.

5.3 Hallucination Analysis

Table 5. Clinical hallucination rates by fusion architecture and domain

Architecture	Radiology HR (%) ↓	Pathology HR (%) ↓	Dermatology HR (%) ↓	Mean HR (%) ↓
EF-Base	18.3 ± 2.1	22.7 ± 2.8	14.9 ± 1.9	18.6
LF-Base	24.1 ± 2.6	28.4 ± 3.2	19.2 ± 2.3	23.9
ICMAF-CoAttn	14.2 ± 1.8	17.6 ± 2.1	11.3 ± 1.6	14.4
AGCMA (Ours)	**9.7 ± 1.4**	**12.1 ± 1.7**	**7.8 ± 1.2**	**9.9**
HHF	11.4 ± 1.5	14.3 ± 1.9	9.2 ± 1.3	11.6

Note. HR refers to Hallucination Rate which is the proportion of clinical claims generated that lack support from the source image content. A downward arrow indicates that lower values are better. LF-Base shows the highest hallucination rates in all domains, which aligns with the lack of detailed visual-textual grounding.

The results concerning hallucinations provide insight into the mechanism: LF-Base generates all language without interacting with different modalities, leading to the highest hallucination rates at a mean of 23.9 percent. Without visual grounding during token generation, language models revert to statistical priors, producing sentences that appear clinically plausible but do not connect to the image shown. The AGCMA's gating mechanism actively reduces this tendency by conditioning each token generated based on the current visual attention states.

5.4 Modality Collapse and Robustness Testing

A significant limitation in the current literature is the lack of analysis concerning modality collapse, which is a failure mode where a multimodal model ignores one modality and relies solely on the other. To evaluate this, an experiment was conducted on MIMIC-CXR where either the image or text was replaced with random noise, using Gaussian noise for images and random token shuffling for text.

Table 6. Modality collapse robustness analysis (MIMIC-CXR CBS score)

Architecture	Intact (Both)	Image Corrupted	Text Corrupted	Collapse Index
EF-Base	0.712	0.541	0.648	0.31 (text-dominant)
LF-Base	0.698	0.521	0.603	0.26 (text-dominant)
ICMAF-CoAttn	0.741	0.572	0.681	0.28 (text-dominant)

continued on following page

Table 6. Continued

Architecture	Intact (Both)	Image Corrupted	Text Corrupted	Collapse Index
AGCMA (Ours)	**0.779**	**0.591**	**0.702**	**0.24 (lowest collapse)**
HHF	0.763	0.578	0.694	0.26 (text-dominant)

Note. Collapse Index is calculated as (text-corrupted performance – image-corrupted performance) / intact performance. Positive values show text-dominant collapse. Lower absolute values indicate better modality balance. Corruption was applied to all test examples.

All architectures evaluated show varying degrees of text-dominant modality collapse. AGCMA shows the lowest collapse index, which suggests that the adaptive gating mechanism helps reduce this issue. Achieving true modality balance remains a challenge with major clinical implications because in situations where a clinical note is misleading but the image is clear, text-dominant models can produce reports that are inconsistent with the image provided.

5.5 Ablation Studies

Table 7. Ablation study on AGCMA components (MIMIC-CXR, CBS score)

Variant	CBS ↑	HR (%) ↓	TTFT (ms)
AGCMA Full	**0.779**	**9.7**	**401**
AGCMA w/o Gating	0.751	13.2	388
AGCMA w/o Bidirectional CrossAttn	0.738	15.1	371
AGCMA Single-Layer Fusion	0.724	16.8	342
AGCMA w/o Projection Alignment	0.701	19.4	395

Note. CBS stands for ClinicalBERT-Score and HR stands for Hallucination Rate. Projection alignment refers to the contrastive pretraining of projection layers before end-to-end fine-tuning.

The ablation study indicates that projection alignment pretraining is the most impactful component, as removing it results in a CBS decrease of 0.078 and an increase in hallucination rate by 9.7 percentage points, which is a larger effect than the removal of the gating mechanism. This highlights a principle that may have wide applicability: investing in aligning cross-modal embedding spaces may be more beneficial than spending the same resources on more complex fusion techniques.

6. HUMAN-IN-THE-LOOP DESIGN AND CLINICIAN INTERACTION

An area that has not been thoroughly explored in clinical VLM literature is the modeling of human-AI collaboration. The term "Language" in Vision-Language Models carries assumptions about who receives the generated language, and in clinical settings, this recipient is a clinician. Effective design of clinical VLMs must take into account how the model communicates uncertainty, manages contradictions between visual and textual information, and requests human input when the automated confidence is insufficient.

6.1 Signaling Visual-Textual Contradiction

An important interaction pattern emerges when the visual content of an image contradicts the accompanying clinical text. In these cases, a clinical VLM should not simply resolve the contradiction by averaging the representations of both modalities, but should clearly indicate the inconsistency to the clinician. The activation values from AGCMA's gating mechanism can help detect contradictions; when the gating network produces uncertain gate values, which are close to 0.5 across all anatomical regions, it signals that neither modality is providing clear guidance. Monitoring the entropy of the gates can serve as a proxy for confidence, and bringing low-confidence outputs to human review is a practical approach to integrating human input that does not require separate modules for estimating confidence.

6.2 Active Uncertainty Communication

Clinical VLMs should implement a structured way to communicate uncertainty, distinguishing between: (1) imaging-quality uncertainty, where the image does not allow for reliable interpretation; (2) cross-modal inconsistency, where the image and text provide contradictory information; and (3) intrinsic diagnostic ambiguity, where the clinical situation is genuinely unclear. Each type of uncertainty requires a different response from clinicians. Future architectures should explicitly model these three categories of uncertainty instead of providing uniform confidence scores.

7. TRI-MODAL FUSION: EXTENDING BEYOND IMAGE AND TEXT

The current state of clinical VLMs is mainly bimodal, which means they integrate visual and textual modalities. However, clinical reasoning often involves a third modality, which is structured Electronic Health Record (EHR) data that includes laboratory values, vital signs, medication history, and prior diagnostic codes. Expanding fusion architectures to include structured EHR data as a third input modality represents a significant area with clinical potential.

7.1 Architecture for Tri-Modal Fusion

A tri-modal fusion architecture combines three different types of data: continuous-valued images I, sequential clinical text T, and structured tabular EHR data $E = \{e_1, e_2, \ldots, eM\}$. The functional aspect of tri-modal fusion extends to:

$$\Phi^{(3)}: \mathbb{R}^{d_v} \times \mathbb{R}^{d_t} \times \mathbb{R}^{d_e} \rightarrow \mathbb{R}^{d_z}$$

Integrating EHR data introduces a challenge of aligning structured data with unstructured data, since tabular numerical values must be projected into the same representation space as image patches and text tokens. Methods can range from using simple embedding lookup tables for categorical variables and linear projections for numerical values (Huang et al., 2020) to more advanced transformer-based EHR encoders like BEHRT (Li et al., 2020).

Table 8. Tri-modal vs. bimodal fusion: Projected clinical impact across task types

Clinical Task	Bimodal (Image + Text)	Projected Tri-Modal (+EHR)	Clinical Rationale
Pneumonia diagnosis	High (CBS ~0.779)	Higher	WBC count, fever trajectory corroborate imaging findings
Cancer staging	Moderate (AUROC ~0.903)	Substantially higher	Tumor markers, prior pathology, genomics critical for staging
Cardiac monitoring	Moderate	Higher	ECG, troponin, BNP complement echocardiographic imaging
Skin lesion classification	Moderate (F1 ~0.856)	Marginally higher	Age, UV exposure history, immunosuppression status relevant

Note. Projected performance is based on assessments from clinical domain experts regarding the contribution of EHR to differential diagnosis. Empirical studies on tri-modal approaches are noted as a research gap in Section 9.

8. ETHICAL, REGULATORY, AND GOVERNANCE FRAMEWORKS

8.1 Regulatory Landscape for Clinical VLMs as SaMD

Clinical VLMs that have an effect on diagnostic or treatment decisions are classified as Software as a Medical Device (SaMD) according to current FDA regulations (FDA, 2021). The FDA's AI/ML-Based SaMD Action Plan outlines requirements for control plans regarding predetermined changes, algorithm transparency, and monitoring real-world performance. Under FDA SaMD regulations, the intended use must be clearly defined, including what modalities are needed inputs, what the output means in terms of decision support or autonomous diagnosis, and which clinical population has been validated. A radiology VLM that has been trained on MIMIC-CXR cannot be used for pediatric chest radiographs or chest CT scans without further validation. In the European Union, clinical VLMs fall under the Medical Device Regulation (MDR 2017/745) and starting in 2025, they will also be subject to the EU AI Act's requirements for high-risk AI systems, which will include post-market surveillance and assessments of conformity.

8.2 Bias, Equity, and Fairness in Clinical Fusion Models

Multimodal fusion systems carry biases from their training data across both modalities separately and in how they interact. A radiology VLM trained mainly on high-quality digital radiography will likely perform poorly when used with portable X-ray units, which is a bias at the image modality level. Clinical text models trained on reports from primarily English-speaking institutions may misinterpret reports that follow different conventions, which represents a bias at the text modality level. The interaction of these biases within the fusion layer has not yet been systematically studied. To ensure fair performance, evaluations need to be conducted that account for different patient demographics, imaging conditions, and institutional settings.

8.3 Explainability Requirements and Interpretable Fusion

Regulatory and clinical trust standards require AI systems to provide explanations that clinicians can understand. For multimodal fusion systems, this means that predictions should not only come with a saliency map but also with explanations that clearly outline the specific evidence from different modalities that supported the conclusion. Raw attention weights, while they can be visualized, do not provide clinical explanations, as they are merely computational metrics that might not correspond to the reasons behind the model's decisions (Jain & Wallace, 2019).

Creating fusion mechanisms where attention patterns accurately reflect clinical reasoning, validated against established clinical standards, remains an urgent and unresolved issue.

9. RESEARCH GAPS AND FUTURE DIRECTIONS

Table 9. Identified research gaps in clinical VLM fusion architecture

#	Research Gap	Current State	Severity	Proposed Direction
1	Federated Fusion Learning	No existing work	Critical	Federated co-attention with differential privacy guarantees
2	Dynamic Modality Weighting Under Missingness	Unimodal federated only	High	Missingness-aware gating with clinical imputation
3	Interpretable Fusion	Attention ≠ causality	High	Causal intervention-based attention analysis
4	Longitudinal Fusion	Snapshot-only VLMs	Moderate-High	Temporal cross-modal transformer with EHR integration
5	Hallucination Mechanism Analysis	Descriptive only	Critical	Mechanistic probing studies with controlled stimuli

Note. Severity ratings are as follows: Critical equals preventing safe clinical use; High equals substantially impeding productive clinical use; Moderate-High equals significantly limiting longitudinal care applications.

Each of these gaps is a barrier to real-world multimodal AI clinical deployment. Federated learning faces regulatory and ethical constraints on data centralization. Missingness robustness is necessary in clinical processes. Interpretability is needed for regulatory approval and clinical trust. Longitudinal fusion is essential for managing chronic diseases and monitoring treatment responses. Hallucination mitigation is directly related to patient safety.

10. DISCUSSION

The consistent superiority of AGCMA across all clinical imaging domains shows performance improvements of 4.7 to 11.3 percent over the best baseline. This establishes that adaptive gating of cross-modal information is a generalizable architectural principle rather than being specific to a dataset or task. The substantial reduction in hallucination rates, with 9.9 percent for AGCMA compared to 23.9 percent for LF-Base, reinforces that fusion architecture is a consideration for patient safety.

A model with suboptimal fusion can generate plausible but clinically inaccurate reports, and this risk would not be revealed by benchmark accuracy metrics alone.

The modality collapse analysis reveals a systematic limitation in all evaluated architectures, which is text-dominant collapse. This occurs when models rely more on textual context than on visual evidence. This is clinically significant because it means these systems may produce reports that replicate textual patterns from training data instead of accurately describing the specific image presented. Addressing this issue requires architectural innovations that enforce modality balance, potentially including adversarial training objectives that penalize text-dominant solutions.

The ablation study finds that projection alignment pretraining has the largest single impact on both accuracy and hallucination reduction. This carries a design principle that has broad applicability. Investment in the quality of cross-modal embedding space alignment, which can be achieved through domain-specific contrastive pretraining, anatomical grounding objectives, or negation-aware contrastive learning (Zhang et al., 2022), may provide returns that exceed equivalent investments in more complex fusion mechanisms.

11. CONCLUSION

This chapter has provided a systematic and critically grounded analysis of multimodal fusion architectures for clinical Vision-Language Models. It extends prior literature in six key dimensions: (1) controlled fusion architecture comparisons isolating fusion design as an independent variable; (2) modality collapse analysis establishing a previously undercharacterized failure mode; (3) real-world latency translation into operationally meaningful clinical deployment guidance; (4) tri-modal fusion extension that incorporates structured EHR data; (5) ethical, regulatory, and governance analysis within the SaMD framework; and (6) human-in-the-loop design that formalizes requirements for productive clinical AI collaboration.

The principal empirical findings are as follows: (1) adaptive gating of cross-modal information significantly reduces hallucination rates, establishing AGCMA as a clinically safer architecture; (2) projection alignment pretraining is the single most impactful architectural component for both accuracy and hallucination reduction; (3) a favorable performance-efficiency trade-off distinguishes AGCMA from more computationally costly hierarchical approaches; (4) late fusion is insufficient for clinical tasks that require fine-grained visual-textual grounding; and (5) text-dominant modality collapse affects all evaluated architectures, representing an important open problem.

The development of clinical AI has entered an era where multimodal integration is not optional but central to replicating clinically meaningful reasoning processes.

The architectural choices made in fusion design will determine whether clinical VLMs augment or mislead clinicians. This chapter offers a principled and practically grounded basis for making those choices in a responsible manner.

REFERENCES

Alayrac, J.-B., Donahue, J., Luc, P., Miech, A., Barr, I., Hasson, Y., Lenci, K., Dzabraev, A., & Zisserman, A. (2022). Flamingo: A visual language model for few-shot learning. *Advances in Neural Information Processing Systems*, *35*, 23716–23736. DOI: 10.52202/068431-1723

Antol, S., Agrawal, A., Lu, J., Mitchell, M., Batra, D., Zitnick, C. L., & Parikh, D. (2015). VQA: Visual question answering. *Proceedings of the IEEE International Conference on Computer Vision*, 2425–2433. DOI: 10.1109/ICCV.2015.279

Bannur, S., Hyland, S., Liu, Q., Perez-Garcia, F., Bhatt, M., Castro, D. C., Boecking, B., Sharma, H., Mehra, S., Rosman, H., & Alvarez-Valle, J. (2023). Learning to exploit temporal structure for biomedical vision–language processing. *Proceedings of the IEEE/CVF Conference on Computer Vision and Pattern Recognition*, 15016–15027. DOI: 10.1109/CVPR52729.2023.01442

Bustos, A., Pertusa, A., Salinas, J.-M., & de la Iglesia-Vayá, M. (2020). PadChest: A large chest x-ray image dataset with multi-label annotated reports. *Medical Image Analysis*, *66*, 101797. Advance online publication. DOI: 10.1016/j.media.2020.101797 PMID: 32877839

Campanella, G., Hanna, M. G., Geneslaw, L., Miraflor, A., Werneck Krauss Silva, V., Busam, K. J., Brogi, E., Reuter, V. E., Klimstra, D. S., & Fuchs, T. J. (2019). Clinical-grade computational pathology using weakly supervised deep learning on whole slide images. *Nature Medicine*, *25*(8), 1301–1309. DOI: 10.1038/s41591-019-0508-1 PMID: 31308507

Chen, Z., Varma, M., Delbrouck, J.-B., Paschali, M., Blankemeier, L., Van Veen, D., Valanarasu, J. M. J., Youssef, A., Cohen, J. P., Reis, E. P., & Langlotz, C. P. (2024). CheXagent: Towards a foundation model for chest x-ray analysis. arXiv preprint. https://doi.org//arXiv.2401.12208DOI: 10.48550

Dai, W., Li, J., Li, D., Tiong, A. M. H., Zhao, J., Wang, W., Li, B., Fung, P. N., & Hoi, S. C. H. (2023). InstructBLIP: Towards general-purpose vision-language models with instruction tuning. *Advances in Neural Information Processing Systems*, *36*, 49250–49267. DOI: 10.52202/075280-2142

FDA. (2021). Artificial intelligence/machine learning (AI/ML)-based software as a medical device (SaMD) action plan. U.S. Food and Drug Administration. https://www.fda.gov/medical-devices/software-medical-device-samd/artificial-intelligence-and-machine-learning-software-medical-device

Gadzicki, K., Khamsehashari, R., & Zetzsche, C. (2020). Early vs. late fusion in multimodal convolutional neural networks. *Proceedings of the 2020 IEEE 23rd International Conference on Information Fusion (FUSION)*, 1–7. DOI: 10.23919/FUSION45008.2020.9190246

Groh, M., Harris, C., Soenksen, L., Lau, F., Han, R., Kim, A., Koochek, A., & Manrai, A. K. (2021). Evaluating deep neural networks trained on clinical images in dermatology with the Fitzpatrick 17k dataset. *Proceedings of the IEEE/CVF Conference on Computer Vision and Pattern Recognition Workshops*, 1820–1828. DOI: 10.1109/CVPRW53098.2021.00201

Huang, S.-C., Shen, L., Lungren, M. P., & Yeung, S. (2021). GLoRIA: A multimodal global-local representation learning framework for label-efficient medical image recognition. *Proceedings of the IEEE/CVF International Conference on Computer Vision*, 3942–3951. DOI: 10.1109/ICCV48922.2021.00391

Huang, Y., Gillis-Smith, G., & Huang, Z. (2020). Clinical natural language processing in 2020: Challenges and opportunities. *Journal of Biomedical Informatics*, *112*, 103656. Advance online publication. DOI: 10.1016/j.jbi.2020.103656

Jain, S., & Wallace, B. C. (2019). Attention is not explanation. *Proceedings of the 2019 Conference of the North American Chapter of the Association for Computational Linguistics: Human Language Technologies*, 1, 3543–3556. DOI: 10.18653/v1/N19-1357

Jia, C., Yang, Y., Xia, Y., Chen, Y.-T., Parekh, Z., Pham, H., Le, Q., Sung, Y.-H., Li, Z., & Duerig, T. (2021). Scaling up visual and vision-language representation learning with noisy text supervision. *Proceedings of the 38th International Conference on Machine Learning*, 139, 4904–4916. DOI: 10.48550/arXiv.2102.05918

Johnson, A. E. W., Pollard, T. J., Berkowitz, S. J., Greenbaum, N. R., Lungren, M. P., Deng, C.-Y., Mark, R. G., & Horng, S. (2019). MIMIC-CXR, a de-identified publicly available database of chest radiographs with free-text reports. *Scientific Data*, *6*(1), 317. Advance online publication. DOI: 10.1038/s41597-019-0322-0 PMID: 31831740

Li, C., Wong, C., Zhang, S., Usuyama, N., Liu, H., Yang, J., Naumann, T., Poon, H., & Gao, J. (2023). LLaVA-Med: Training a large language-and-vision assistant for biomedicine in one day. *Advances in Neural Information Processing Systems*, *36*, 28541–28564. DOI: 10.48550/arXiv.2306.00890

Li, J., Li, D., Xiong, C., & Hoi, S. (2022). BLIP: Bootstrapping language-image pre-training for unified vision-language understanding and generation. *Proceedings of the 39th International Conference on Machine Learning*, 162, 12888–12900. DOI: 10.48550/arXiv.2201.12086

Li, Y., Rao, S., Solares, J. R. A., Hassaine, A., Ramakrishnan, R., Canoy, D., Zhu, Y., Rahimi, K., & Salimi-Khorshidi, G. (2020). BEHRT: Transformer for electronic health records. *Scientific Reports*, *10*(1), 7155. Advance online publication. DOI: 10.1038/s41598-020-62922-y PMID: 32346050

Li, Y., Rao, S., Solares, J. R. A., Hassaine, A., Ramakrishnan, R., Canoy, D., Zhu, Y., Rahimi, K., & Salimi-Khorshidi, G. (2020). BEHRT: Transformer for electronic health records. *Scientific Reports*, *10*(1), 7155. Advance online publication. DOI: 10.1038/s41598-020-62922-y PMID: 32346050

Liu, H., Li, C., Wu, Q., & Lee, Y. J. (2023). Visual instruction tuning. *Advances in Neural Information Processing Systems*, *36*, 34892–34916. DOI: 10.48550/arXiv.2304.08485

Lu, J., Batra, D., Parikh, D., & Lee, S. (2019). ViLBERT: Pretraining task-agnostic visiolinguistic representations for vision-and-language tasks. *Advances in Neural Information Processing Systems*, *32*, 13–23. DOI: 10.48550/arXiv.1908.02265

Moor, M., Huang, Q., Wu, S., Yasunaga, M., Dalmia, Y., Li, Y., Pfohl, S., Koreeda, Y., Rajpurkar, P., & Liang, P. (2023). Med-Flamingo: A multimodal medical few-shot learner. *Proceedings of Machine Learning Research*, *225*, 1–16. DOI: 10.48550/arXiv.2307.15189

Open, A. I. (2023). GPT-4 technical report. arXiv preprint. https://doi.org//arXiv.2303.08774DOI: 10.48550

Radford, A., Kim, J. W., Hallacy, C., Ramesh, A., Goh, G., Agarwal, S., Sastry, G., Askell, A., Mishkin, P., Clark, J., & Sutskever, I. (2021). Learning transferable visual models from natural language supervision. *Proceedings of the 38th International Conference on Machine Learning*, 139, 8748–8763. DOI: 10.48550/arXiv.2103.00020

Schuhmann, C., Beaumont, R., Vencu, R., Gordon, C. W., Wightman, R., Cherti, M., Coombes, T., Katta, A., Mullis, C., Wortsman, M., Schramowski, P., Kundurthy, S., Crowson, K., Schmidt, L., Dodge, J., & Jitsev, J. (2022). LAION-5B: An open large-scale dataset for training next generation image-text models. *Advances in Neural Information Processing Systems*, *35*, 25278–25294. DOI: 10.48550/arXiv.2210.08402

Shaikovski, G., Askari, A., Baras, J. S., Ciga, O., Gupte, S., Juyal, D., Kiani, A., Koshkin, A., Mehta, R., Pella, M., Russo, M., Salgado, R., Tosun, A. B., Trahearn, N., Zou, J., & Chen, T. Y. (2024). PathChat: A foundation model for human pathology. *Nature Medicine*, *30*(3), 776–785. DOI: 10.1038/s41591-024-02856-4

Tan, H., & Bansal, M. (2019). LXMERT: Learning cross-modality encoder representations from transformers. *Proceedings of the 2019 Conference on Empirical Methods in Natural Language Processing*, 5100–5111. DOI: 10.18653/v1/D19-1514

Tschandl, P., Rosendahl, C., & Kittler, H. (2018). The HAM10000 dataset, a large collection of multi-source dermatoscopic images of common pigmented skin lesions. *Scientific Data*, *5*(1), 180161. Advance online publication. DOI: 10.1038/sdata.2018.161 PMID: 30106392

Wang, X., Peng, Y., Lu, L., Lu, Z., Bagheri, M., & Summers, R. M. (2017). ChestX-ray8: Hospital-scale chest X-ray database and benchmarks. *Proceedings of the IEEE Conference on Computer Vision and Pattern Recognition*, 2097–2106. DOI: 10.1109/CVPR.2017.369

Wu, C., Zhang, X., Zhang, Y., Wang, Y., & Xie, W. (2023). Towards generalist foundation model for radiology by leveraging web-scale 2D and 3D medical data. arXiv preprint. https://doi.org//arXiv.2308.02463DOI: 10.48550

Xu, K., Ba, J., Kiros, R., Cho, K., Courville, A., Salakhutdinov, R., Zemel, R., & Bengio, Y. (2015). Show, attend and tell: Neural image caption generation with visual attention. *Proceedings of the 32nd International Conference on Machine Learning*, 37, 2048–2057. DOI: 10.48550/arXiv.1502.03044

Zhang, Y., Jiang, H., Miura, Y., Manning, C. D., & Langlotz, C. P. (2022). Contrastive learning of medical visual representations from paired images and text. *Proceedings of Machine Learning for Healthcare Conference*, 182, 2–25. DOI: 10.48550/arXiv.2010.00747

Zhou, Y., Luo, Y., & Li, Y. (2023). Detecting and mitigating hallucination in large vision language models via fine-grained AI feedback. arXiv preprint. https://doi.org//arXiv.2306.14565DOI: 10.48550

Zhu, D., Chen, J., Shen, X., Li, X., & Elhoseiny, M. (2023). MiniGPT-4: Enhancing vision-language understanding with advanced large language models. arXiv preprint. https://doi.org//arXiv.2304.10592DOI: 10.48550

APPENDIX

Extended Dataset Statistics

Table 10. Detailed split statistics for clinical benchmark datasets

Dataset	Train	Validation	Test	Positive Class Ratio
MIMIC-CXR	182,268	22,784	22,783	0.43 (abnormal)
PadChest	128,694	16,087	16,087	0.61 (abnormal)
TCGA-PATH	26,051	3,257	3,256	Balanced (multi-class)
HAM10000	8,012	1,003	1,000	0.11 (malignant)

Note. Divisions in the dataset follow the original splits where they are available such as MIMIC-CXR and HAM10000 or they use stratified random splits of 80/10/10 for PadChest and TCGA-PATH.

Hyperparameter Configuration

Table 11. Hyperparameter settings for all fusion architecture experiments

Hyperparameter	EF-Base	LF-Base	ICMAF-CoAttn	AGCMA	HHF
Learning Rate	2e-5	2e-5	2e-5	2e-5	1e-5
Batch Size	32	32	32	32	16
Warmup Ratio	0.10	0.10	0.10	0.10	0.10
Max Epochs	20	20	20	20	25
Weight Decay	0.01	0.01	0.01	0.01	0.01
Projection Dim	1024	1024	1024	1024	1024
Attention Heads	16	—	16	16	16
Cross-Attn Layers	—	—	3	6	3+2
Image Resolution	224	224	224	224	224
Gradient Clip	1.0	1.0	1.0	1.0	1.0

AGCMA Module Forward Pass

Algorithm C1 provides the pseudocode for the complete forward pass of the AGCMA module which enables reproducibility of the proposed architecture.

Figure 5. Algorithm C1 AGCMA Module Forward Pass. The algorithm describes the gating computation, bidirectional cross-modal attention, and residual integration steps that make up the AGCMA mechanism.

```
Function AGCMA_Forward(V, T, W_Q_V, W_K_T, W_V_T, W_g, b_g, d_k):
    """
    Adaptive Gated Cross-Modal Attention Module
    Input:  V ∈ R^(P×d_z)  — visual token sequence
            T ∈ R^(N×d_z)  — text token sequence
    Output: V_out ∈ R^(P×d_z), T_out ∈ R^(N×d_z)
    """

    // Cross-attention: Visual queries attending to textual keys/values
    Q_V   = V · W_Q_V                                  // [P × d_k]
    K_T   = T · W_K_T                                  // [N × d_k]
    V_T   = T · W_V_T                                  // [N × d_z]
    A_VT  = Softmax(Q_V · K_T^T / sqrt(d_k))           // [P × N]
    V_cross = A_VT · V_T                               // [P × d_z]

    // Cross-attention: Textual queries attending to visual keys/values
    Q_T   = T · W_Q_T                                  // [N × d_k]
    K_V   = V · W_K_V                                  // [P × d_k]
    V_V   = V · W_V_V                                  // [P × d_z]
    A_TV  = Softmax(Q_T · K_V^T / sqrt(d_k))           // [N × P]
    T_cross = A_TV · V_V                               // [N × d_z]

    // Adaptive gating for visual stream
    concat_V = Concat(V, V_cross)                      // [P × 2d_z]
    g_V = Sigmoid(concat_V · W_g_V + b_g_V) // [P × d_z]
    V_out = g_V ⊙ V_cross + (1 - g_V) ⊙ V   // [P × d_z]

    // Adaptive gating for text stream
    concat_T = Concat(T, T_cross)                      // [N × 2d_z]
    g_T = Sigmoid(concat_T · W_g_T + b_g_T) // [N × d_z]
    T_out = g_T ⊙ T_cross + (1 - g_T) ⊙ T   // [N × d_z]

    Return: V_out, T_out
```

Statistical Significance Results

Table 12. Pairwise statistical significance of performance differences (MIMIC-CXR CBS score)

Comparison	Δ CBS	p-value	Significant (α=0.05)
AGCMA vs. EF-Base	+0.067	0.0031	Yes
AGCMA vs. LF-Base	+0.081	0.0018	Yes
AGCMA vs. ICMAF-CoAttn	+0.038	0.0142	Yes
AGCMA vs. HHF	+0.016	0.0487	Yes
HHF vs. EF-Base	+0.051	0.0076	Yes
HHF vs. ICMAF-CoAttn	+0.022	0.0331	Yes
ICMAF-CoAttn vs. EF-Base	+0.029	0.0198	Yes
EF-Base vs. LF-Base	+0.014	0.0521	No

Note. p-values are from paired Wilcoxon signed-rank tests with Bonferroni correction. All differences reported are significant after correction except for EF-Base versus LF-Base.

Chapter 4
Multimodal Large Language Models in Radiology for Automated and Augmented Report Generation

Pragyansh Pathak
http://orcid.org/0009-0000-3038-4090
Symbiosis Institute of Health Sciences, Symbiosis International (Deemed to be) University, Pune, India

Sushant Matre
http://orcid.org/0000-0002-0749-036X
Symbiosis Institute of Health Sciences, Symbiosis International (Deemed to be) University, Pune, India

Milind Chunkhare
Symbiosis Institute of Health Sciences, Symbiosis International (Deemed to be) University, Pune, India

ABSTRACT

Increasing imaging volumes, a lack of workers, and the rising need for prompt, high-quality diagnostic reporting is all contributing factors to the rapid evolution of radiology. Multimodal Large Language Models (MLLMs) have shown promise as a way to enhance radiology reporting procedures by combining visual information from medical images with natural language thinking. In contrast to previous computer-aided detection systems, MLLLMs may produce structured, context-aware narrative reports that mimic the interpretations of skilled radiologists. With an em-

DOI: 10.4018/979-8-3373-7315-7.ch004

…t © 2026, IGI Global Scientific Publishing. Copying or distributing in print or electronic forms without written permission of IGI Global Scientific Publishing is prohibited. Use of this chapter to …enerative artificial intelligence (AI) technologies is expressly prohibited. The publisher reserves all rights to license its use for generative AI training and machine learning model development.

phasis on automated and enhanced report creation, this chapter offers a thorough analysis of multimodal big language models in radiology. It assesses cutting-edge radiology-specific models like CXR-LLaVA, MAIRA, and MRG-LLM and examines the technological underpinnings of multimodal architectures, such as visual encoders, language models, and fusion processes. The chapter delves deeper into developments that go beyond simple report creation, such as segmentation-aware modelling and longitudinal image interpretation.

1. INTRODUCTION

In the past, radiology has been defined by expert interpretation—the radiologist's ability to assess complex visual data, take clinical context into account, and provide accurate, understandable findings. But in the past ten years, radiology has seen a sea change. Due to the unprecedented rise in imaging volumes, the increasing complexity of modalities, and variations in radiologist availability around the globe, reporting systems are under extreme strain. Many regions have turnaround times that are far longer than recommended, and even high-resource centers struggle with burnout and uneven reporting practices (Agarwal et al., 2021). From conventional rule-based computer-aided detection tools to deep learning and, more recently, powerful multimodal large language models (MLLMs), which are systems that can scan both text and images to produce outputs with clinical significance, artificial intelligence (AI) has developed concurrently. These models represent a significant shift because, rather than forecasting a specific anomaly or pointing out an area of interest, they can reason across modalities, aggregate facts, and provide organized narrative reports that imitate human radiologist interpretations. MLLMs have the ability to help radiologists by producing preliminary reports, summarizing significant findings, and supporting decision-making. In high-volume settings, automated report creation could greatly reduce repetitive workload, allowing radiologists to focus on complex diagnostic reasoning and interdisciplinary interaction. However, these prospects come with challenges related to accuracy, prejudice, hallucinations, and ethical responsibility, especially when treatment safety cannot be compromised. This chapter provides a comprehensive and analytically rich analysis of the evolving role of multimodal LLMs, with a focus on automated and improved report preparation.

2. BACKGROUND

The rapid development of multimodal large language models is one of the most significant technological advancements in contemporary radiology. Understanding the transformative potential of these systems requires an examination of the underlying principles.

2.1. The Shift to Multimodal Architecture

Large Language Models (LLMs), which were first created as powerful text-processing systems trained on enormous written data corpora, are able to understand syntax, semantics, and context in a very complex way. LLMs are especially skilled at summarizing, translating, and crafting narratives because they are primarily built on Transformer designs. Early applications of LLMs in radiology focused on text-only tasks, like correcting dictation errors, standardizing report nomenclature, and extracting structured information from free-text reports. However, because these models only process words, they cannot interpret medical imaging. The development of multimodal systems that could simultaneously evaluate text and images was spurred by this limitation. Multimodal Large Language Models (MLLMs) extend traditional LLMs by incorporating a visual processing component into the text model. This integration allows the algorithm to understand correlations between clinical language and radiological patterns.

2.2. Radiology-Specific MLLMs and Grounding

The development of these systems toward radiology-specific MLLMs has been accelerated by the recognition that medical imaging interpretation is very different from general computer vision jobs. In radiography, a disciplined reporting style, exceptional accuracy, and the capacity to recognize subtle trends are all essential. Early multimodal models trained on natural images lacked the domain knowledge and anatomical base needed for safe clinical application. In response, researchers began refining models specifically designed for radiology using paired image-report datasets such as MIMIC-CXR and IU X-Ray. This modification led to the creation of models such as CXR-LLaVA, MAIRA, and MRG-LLM, which demonstrated an improved ability to understand radiological conventions, identify common disorders, and produce impressions that were similar to those made by trained radiologists. Thanks to segmentation-aware designs, models have lately been able to incorporate accurate anatomical boundaries, significantly increasing clinical accuracy and lowering the possibility of hallucinogenic findings.

A conceptual overview of an MLLM-based radiology workflow illustrates how these components interact together. The method begins with input imaging data that has been pre-processed to reduce noise and enhance uniformity. This data is typically in DICOM format. The visual encoder transforms the processed image into a high-dimensional representation that emphasizes significant anatomical and pathological features. This input is then matched with text tokens in a multimodal fusion layer to enable bidirectional comprehension across visual and linguistic modalities. In accordance with radiology customs, the big language model generates a structured draft report with sections like "Findings" and "Impression," using this integrated representation. A radiologist reviews and edits the document to guarantee clinical accuracy and contextual relevance before finishing the report. Through this collaborative relationship, multimodal AI serves not as a replacement for human expertise but rather as an aid tool that automates time-consuming descriptive tasks so radiologists can focus on complex diagnostic reasoning. This theoretical foundation highlights the necessity of MLLMs as carefully designed systems appropriate to the unique demands of radiological practice rather than merely as technological innovations. As these models advance, they have the potential to improve reporting efficacy, change workflows, and give access to expert-level interpretation—as long as they are used carefully and with a thorough understanding of the stated principles.

2.3 Evolution from Traditional AI to Multimodal Systems

Radiology has witnessed several distinct phases in the application of artificial intelligence, each shaped by the technological capabilities and clinical expectations of its time. Early implementations were largely based on rule-driven computer-aided detection systems. These tools relied on predefined thresholds and manually engineered features to highlight potential abnormalities. While useful in controlled scenarios, such systems often struggled with variability in image quality and patient anatomy, resulting in inconsistent performance and limited clinical adoption (Cai et al., 2023).

The emergence of deep learning, particularly convolutional neural networks, marked a substantial shift toward data-driven analysis. CNN-based models demonstrated strong performance in tasks such as classification, detection, and segmentation, especially in high-volume modalities like chest radiography. Despite these advances, their application remained largely confined to isolated tasks, with minimal capacity for contextual reasoning or integration with clinical narratives (Fang et al., 2025).

Subsequent efforts to generate radiology reports introduced hybrid CNN–RNN architectures, where visual features extracted from images were translated into textual descriptions. Although these models represented an important conceptual step, their outputs were often formulaic and lacked the nuance required for clinical interpretation (Huang et al., 2024).

More recently, multimodal large language models have redefined the landscape by combining visual understanding with advanced language generation. These systems are capable of interpreting imaging data alongside textual context, enabling them to produce structured reports that reflect elements of clinical reasoning rather than simple pattern recognition. This shift from task-specific automation to integrative reasoning represents a fundamental advancement in the role of AI within radiology (Nam et al., 2025; Yi et al., 2025).

2.4 Comparative Analysis of AI Paradigms in Radiology

Although the evolutionary pattern of artificial intelligence in radiology clearly indicates a shift from rule-based systems to multimodal large language models, a more detailed comparison of these AI systems indicates a conceptual difference between the two. Conventional computer-aided detection systems were based on deterministic logic, meaning they relied on a set of predefined rules. Although these systems were highly interpretable, they were not effective enough due to the inability of these systems to generalize across different imaging conditions.

The introduction of convolutional neural networks (CNN) marked a shift towards a more data-driven approach, enabling automated feature extraction and significantly improving the performance of AI systems in radiology. Although CNN-based systems improved significantly compared to conventional systems, they were task-specific and not effective enough to consider a broader clinical context. Hybrid systems, such as CNN-RNN systems, were introduced with the aim of bridging the gap between visual features and textual outputs. Although this shift improved the performance of AI systems, it was not enough, as these systems were not effective enough to generate a more dynamic report compared to radiologists. In contrast, multimodal large language models indicate a shift towards more integrative reasoning. Unlike conventional AI systems, MLLMs are not restricted to a specific task and are more effective at generating a report by considering a broader clinical context. This shift indicates a move from task-oriented AI systems towards more cognitively inspired AI systems, which are more aligned with clinical decision-making.

Table 1. Evolution of AI approaches in radiology

Feature	Rule-Based CAD	CNN-Based Models	CNN–RNN Models	MLLMs
Core Approach	Handcrafted rules	Deep learning (image)	Image-to-text mapping	Multimodal reasoning
Task Scope	Narrow	Task-specific	Report generation	Generalized reasoning
Output Type	Deterministic	Probabilistic	Template-based text	Context-aware narrative
Clinical Reasoning	None	Limited	Minimal	Advanced

continued on following page

Table 1. Continued

Feature	Rule-Based CAD	CNN-Based Models	CNN–RNN Models	MLLMs
Interpretability	High	Low	Moderate	Improving (XAI-based)
Scalability	Low	Moderate	Moderate	High
Clinical Utility	Limited	High (specific tasks)	Experimental	Emerging clinical integration

3. THE STATE OF MULTIMODAL LARGE LANGUAGE MODELS IN RADIOLOGY TODAY

As summarized in Table 2, several multimodal large language models have been developed for radiology, each with distinct architectural features, advantages, and limitations.

Table 2. Multimodal LLMs particular to radiology and their features

Model	Modality	Important Innovation	Advantage	Disadvantage
CXR-LLaVA	Chest X-ray	Vision-language alignment	Strong fluency	Hallucinations
MAIRA-Seg	Chest X-ray	Segmentation grounding	High accuracy	Data intensive
MRG-LLM	Multi-modal	Dynamic prompting	Flexible reports	Prompt sensitivity
3D-CT-GPT	CT	Volumetric reasoning	Holistic context	High compute cost

3.1. Early Models and Domain-Specific Fine-Tuning

The field of multimodal large language models" in radiology has evolved dramatically in recent years due to the increasing availability of massive annotated imaging datasets and the development of basic AI architectures that can handle textual and visual data simultaneously. Early attempts at automated report generation relied heavily on sequence-to-sequence models, which saw the work as a simple translation problem—converting pixel information into descriptive phrases. Although these models were innovative at the time, they lacked the contextual reasoning and depth of interpretation that characterize professional radiological evaluation. The entrance of LLMs altered this dynamic by providing verbal competency and the ability to arrange complex clinical narratives. When these models were paired with specific visual encoders, the field entered a new phase. As part of an integrated image-language reasoning process, this enabled AI systems to understand medical images, producing outputs that more closely resembled human reports.

One of the pioneers of this paradigm, CXR-LLaVA, went on to become a standard model for chest radiography. Its developer applied the LLaVA architecture, a popular vision-language framework, to medical imaging by optimizing the visual encoder and language model on chest X-ray datasets such as MIMIC-CXR. This alignment resulted in a system that can identify common thoracic anomalies and respond to text-based queries, such as whether a patient has cardiomegaly or pulmonary opacities. Crucially, CXR-LLaVA demonstrated that domain-specific fine-tuning greatly improves clinical performance when compared to general-purpose multi-modal models trained on actual images. Despite these benefits, the model would occasionally exhibit hallucinations, particularly in situations that were unusual or had low imaging quality. This demonstrates the inherent problems of relying just on pixel-level information without additional anatomical foundation.

3.2. Volumetric and Segmentation-Aware Systems

To tackle these challenges, researchers developed increasingly complicated architectures, including as MAIRA and its enhanced version, MAIRA-Seg, which introduced segmentation-aware functionality to the multimodal pipeline. Through the integration of segmentation masks and regional features, MAIRA-Seg provided the model with explicit knowledge of anatomical structures during training. This made it possible for the model to link specific image areas to textual descriptions. This significantly reduced the number of false results and enhanced interpretability since radiologists could observe how the model divided attention among different anatomical regions. These segmentation-aware algorithms represent a major step toward clinically safer AI systems by ensuring that generated reports are specifically related to visual image evidence. Their reliance on high-quality segmentation masks, which may not be available in all datasets, continues to be a practical limitation.

Another notable development is the MRG-LLM family of models, which employs a mixed training approach in which the major language model remains mostly frozen while the visual encoder and fusion components undergo targeted fine-tuning. This method preserves the linguistic richness of the original LLM while successfully adapting it to medical imaging issues. One of MRG-LLM's special characteristics is dynamic prompting, which changes the structure and level of detail in generated reports depending on context. The model's flexibility allows it to produce outputs tailored to distinct therapeutic contexts, including comprehensive results for expert evaluation or brief summaries for emergency processes. But like other prompt-dependent systems, prompt design quality has an impact on performance, introducing a human factor that must be carefully managed in real-world applications.

As radiology moves more and more toward cross-sectional and volumetric imaging, models like 3D-CT-GPT represent an important frontier. Unlike 2D-based systems, this method processes entire CT volumes by integrating data from hundreds of slices using 3D transformers. This allows for a more thorough representation of pathology, identifying abnormalities scattered over multiple planes and documenting the interactions between organs. Although volumetric models have a strong conceptual foundation, their huge training data requirements and significant computational loads limit their near-term scalability. Furthermore, early studies show that it is still challenging to detect small or mild lesions, which supports the continued need for expert monitoring.

3.3. Persistent Difficulties and Ethical Issues

Together, these models demonstrate the several strategies being employed to enhance AI-driven reporting in radiology. They differ not just in their technological architecture but also in their clinical readiness. For preliminary report writing in limited domains, CXR-LLaVA and MRG-LLM perform quite well, although segmentation-based models such as MAIRA-Seg demonstrate greater dependability but require more specialized data. However, despite its potential, 3D-CT-GPT and comparable volumetric models are currently mostly experimental and require much more development before being applied in clinical settings. A general lack of interpretability, variation among patient groups and imaging modalities, and hallucinations of supporting findings are the most persistent problems with all models.

Ethical issues are important when evaluating the maturity of modern models. Hallucinations, in which the system reports anomalies that are not present in the image, pose a serious danger of unnecessary testing or inaccurate diagnosis. To overcome this, both architectural improvements like grounding mechanisms and workflow strategies that ensure human-in-the-loop verification are required. Dataset bias is another problem: many models are trained on North American hospital datasets, which may not translate well to populations in developing nations like Asia or Africa. Additionally, the opacity of model decision-making—also referred to as the "black box problem"—makes it more difficult for radiologists to accept or reject the AI's output. As the field advances, explainability technologies that highlight areas of interest or offer textual reasoning will be essential. All things considered, multimodal LLMs in radiology are in a dynamic and rapidly evolving condition. While several models exhibit significant potential for enhancing reporting procedures, none are now dependable enough to function autonomously outside of controlled research settings. Currently, its primary application is in assisted drafting, where it helps expedite dictation, standardize reporting language, and spot possible irregularities for medical assessment. This cooperative method is in accordance with ethical norms and preserves the radiologist's crucial role in diagnostic decision-making as opposed to total automation. As models become more sophisticated and incorporate larger datasets, the field is prepared for further advancements; nevertheless, these developments must be tempered with comprehensive safety evaluations and responsible governance frameworks. A comparative examination of existing models reveals both convergence and divergence in design strategies. While models such as CXR-LLaVA prioritize vision-language alignment and linguistic fluency, segmentation-based systems like MAIRA-Seg emphasize anatomical grounding and interpretability. Meanwhile, architectures such as MRG-LLM focus on flexibility through dynamic prompting. These approaches collectively highlight a trade-off between accuracy, adaptability, and computational efficiency. Despite differing methodologies, a common trend is the movement toward integrating contextual reasoning and multimodal fusion. However, no single model currently achieves optimal performance across all clinical scenarios, indicating that hybrid or ensemble approaches may represent the next phase of development.

4. TECHNICAL ELEMENTS AND MULTIMODAL LLM WORKFLOW IN RADIOLOGY

Data engineering, model design, and workflow integration interact in a complex manner to form the technical basis of multimodal large language models" in radiology. Multimodal frameworks necessitate synchronized handling of heterogeneous data sources, such as medical pictures, radiology reports, clinical metadata, segmentation masks, and contextual prompts, in contrast to typical image analysis systems that only process pixel-level inputs. The legitimacy of this integration directly affects the reliability of automated and improved reporting. High-quality data is the cornerstone of model success: radiological pictures and reports must be accurately connected, with no misalignment or incorrect labeling. This is especially crucial because radiology reports often contain complex descriptive language that the model must correctly interpret, including qualifiers, negations, and uncertainty signs. Adding patient information, such as age or medical history, improves contextual awareness and allows the model to simulate the intricate mental processes of radiologists.

4.1. Preprocessing and Data Engineering

The first important phase in the technological pipeline is data preparation, which creates a clean, consistent input area. Medical photos undergo several procedures, including normalization, resizing, artifact removal, and sometimes bone suppression or organ-focused cropping, depending on the desired clinical aim. These processes ensure that the visual encoder receives dependable and diagnostically relevant inputs. Text preprocessing is also crucial: radiological reports must be de-identified to protect patient privacy, divided into comprehensible sections like "Findings" and "Impression," and standardized to standardize terminology across institutions. Many research teams also utilize lexicon standardization to align various reporting methods with recognized medical terminology in order to enhance downstream consistency and enable more reliable pattern learning.

4.2. Fundamental Modal Structure and Fusion Processes

The core of the multimodal system is the model architecture, which integrates a linguistic model, a fusion mechanism, and a visual encoder. The visual encoder is responsible for obtaining significant information from radiographic images. Early models employed convolutional neural networks, but transformer-based designs are quickly overtaking them due to their superior ability to capture long-range spatial correlations. These encoders generate high-dimensional feature maps that encode anatomical and pathophysiological data. Textual embeddings are processed by the language component, which also provides structured narrative generation capabilities. Typically, it is a large transformer-based model that has been pretrained. Using a model trained on billions of tokens, the system inherits strong linguistic coherence, which is a major benefit for producing well-written clinical reports. The most theoretically important component is probably the fusion process, which explains how textual and visual information interact. Cross-attention layers allow the language model to select emphasis on relevant visual features, mimicking how radiologists focus on specific anatomical regions when writing a report. Other models use adapter-based methods that project visual embeddings into the same representational space as the language model to facilitate seamless integration with minimal modification. By enabling models to alter the output's tone, depth, or structure in response to clinical demands, prompt-conditioning techniques offer greater flexibility. These methods entail encoding pictures into tokens that either initiate or guide the process of creating reports. Each fusion strategy presents trade-offs between interpretability, computational efficiency, and adaptability to different imaging modalities.

4.3. Training Strategies for the Clinical Safety

When training these multimodal models, domain specialization and generalization must be carefully balanced. By pre-training on large biomedical corpora, the language model may acquire fundamental medical knowledge, and by fine-tuning on paired image-report datasets, it can produce radiologically accurate descriptions. In some systems, radiologists use human feedback and reinforcement learning to evaluate draft outputs; the model adjusts its parameters based on quality feedback. This approach has the potential to minimize hallucinations and boost clinical safety. Another novel technique is segmentation-aware training, which directs the model to root textual descriptions in certain visual regions using anatomical masks. This approach improves interpretability and reduces the likelihood of unsupported findings because physicians can observe how the model translated language to anatomical features.

4.4. Clinical Development and Infrastructure

Deploying the model in an actual radiological process once it has been trained requires a number of extra elements that guarantee usability and safety. The pipeline usually starts with image input during inference, then uses the visual encoder to extract features. The language model receives the fused multimodal representation and produces a draft report. The radiologist then reviews this preliminary report to confirm clinical accuracy, add subtle interpretation, and make sure the final product complies with institutional regulations. A key feature of augmented reporting is the iterative nature of this human-AI collaboration, which reflects the ethical consensus that AI should "support" rather than "replace" "human expertise." Additionally, radiologists' input can be recorded by the system, allowing for ongoing learning and improvement for upcoming cases. These kinds of feedback loops are crucial for reducing model drift, particularly in establishments where patient demographics or methods are changing. This procedure is supported by a vast computational infrastructure that includes safe data pipelines that adhere to health information privacy rules, GPUs for training, and efficient inference engines for deployment. Strong APIs or middleware solutions that enable the smooth exchange of textual and image data are necessary for integration with current PACS/RIS systems. Because any lag or system failure can interfere with clinical workflows, these interfaces' dependability is crucial. Additionally, the usage of auditing techniques including recording user modifications, documenting model outputs, and keeping an eye on error rates guarantees accountability and promotes continuous quality assurance procedures.

The technical architecture of multimodal LLMs in radiology is essentially an ecosystem of interconnected parts that mimic elements of clinical reasoning while preserving operational safety, rather than a single model. In addition to sophisticated machine learning techniques, the successful implementation of such systems necessitates careful engineering, consideration for clinical procedures, and a dedication to moral values that uphold openness and trust. The use of enhanced grounding mechanisms, anatomically aware encoders, and more varied multimodal datasets will further increase these systems' therapeutic relevance and dependability as the field develops.

5. CLINICAL AND PRACTICAL CONSIDERATIONS

The use of multimodal large language models" in radiology represents a significant change in the way clinical reporting is conceived and provided, rather than just a technological advancement. Examining the practical realities and ethical obligations that come with the deployment of these technologies is crucial as they go from research prototypes to early clinical evaluation. Precision, clarity, and promptness have always had a direct impact on patient outcomes in the field of radiology. Therefore, rigorous requirements for safety, dependability, and repeatability must be met by any AI system intended to take part in the reporting process. Multimodal LLMs have the potential to reduce cognitive strain and automate repetitious report creation tasks, but their application must be carefully calibrated with human monitoring to maintain clinical integrity.

5.1 Workflow Efficiency and Clinical Risk

Workflow efficiency is one of the most direct clinical advantages of multimodal LLMs. Large amounts of routine imaging are often handled by radiologists, including follow-up CT scans, musculoskeletal trauma films, and chest radiographs. These tests are excellent candidates for AI-assisted writing since they frequently have recurring patterns and predictable results. Radiologists can revise structured preliminary reports produced by MLLMs, cutting down on dictation time and strain from recurring duties. This is particularly helpful in high-demand settings where quick turnaround is essential, such emergency rooms or tertiary care facilities. Additionally, AI systems can lessen reporting style variety by standardizing common formulations of stable abnormalities or normal data, which will help trainee education and improve communication with referring clinicians. Despite these benefits, there are a number of dangers associated with clinical integration that need to be aggressively addressed. The possibility of hallucinations, in which the model produces results that are not corroborated by visual data, is the biggest worry. These mistakes can result from overfitting to popular radiology words, unclear visual patterns, or biases in the dataset. Hallucinations are extremely dangerous in a clinical setting because they can mislead medical professionals, lead to pointless diagnostic procedures, or mask genuinely significant disorders. Institutions must implement human-in-the-loop verification approaches, in which radiologists always retain control over final report approval, in order to reduce these risks. To ensure that clinicians recognize automated reports as helpful rather than definitive outputs, they should be prominently labelled as drafts.

Table 3. Comparison of traditional and MLLM-augmented radiology workflows

Workflow Stage	Traditional Reporting	MLLM-Augmented Reporting
Image review	Manual interpretation	AI-assisted feature extraction
Report drafting	Dictation or typing	Automated draft generation
Turnaround time	High variability	Reduced and standardized
Error risk	Fatigue-dependent	Reduced with supervision
Radiologist role	Primary author	Clinical supervisor/editor

5.1.1 Clinical Failure Scenarios in MLLM-Based Reporting

Though such models promise a lot, their shortcomings are most clearly visible when analysed in the context of real-life scenarios. Perhaps the most worrying problem is that of missed critical findings. For instance, a pneumothorax or a haemorrhage might not be identified if they are not well represented in the model's training set. Such false-negative results could have serious repercussions on patient safety (Liu et al., 2024).

Perhaps equally worrying is the over-interpretation problem. In such cases, benign anatomical variations or normal features are misclassified as abnormal. For instance, in chest radiographs, there is a possibility that vascular shadows might be misclassified as nodular opacities.

Yet another problem is the interpretation of complex imaging scenarios. For instance, in cases of post-surgical anatomy or when there are medical devices, there is a possibility that changes might be misclassified as abnormalities.

Yet another problem is that there is a possibility of a disconnect between the suggestions provided by the AI system and the radiologist's judgment. In high-pressure environments, there is a possibility that such systems might influence human decision-making. A clear framework has to be developed so that the radiologist has complete control over interpretation.

5.2. Generalizability and Diversity Challenges

Generalizability across clinical contexts, scanners, and demographics is another important factor. The majority of multimodal models currently in use are trained on datasets from particular geographic areas or hospital systems, frequently utilizing imaging obtained using specific protocols and technology. Due to differences in illness frequency, imaging quality, and radiographic interpretation standards, a model optimized on chest radiographs from a North American academic center may not perform well when applied to pictures from rural hospitals in India, Africa, or Southeast Asia. This emphasizes how crucial it is to carry out thorough external validation research on a variety of demographics and to use adaptive learning techniques that let models adapt to new settings without sacrificing security. Furthermore, in order to guarantee that uncommon but significant disorders are sufficiently represented in training data, healthcare organizations must continue to exercise caution when it comes to dataset composition.

5.3. The Evolving Role of the Radiologist

This emphasizes the significance of carrying out thorough external validation research across a range of demographics and putting adaptive learning techniques into practice that enable models to adapt to novel contexts without sacrificing safety. Additionally, in order to guarantee that uncommon but significant disorders are sufficiently represented in training data, healthcare organizations must continue to exercise caution when it comes to dataset composition.

5.4. Ethical Improvement and Infrastructure Demand

Ethical considerations further shape the implementation of multimodal LLMs. Transparency and explainability are essential components of trustworthy AI. Radiologists must have access to tools that allow them to visualize where the model focused its attention and understand why certain findings were suggested. Models that output narrative explanations or highlight clinically relevant regions enhance user confidence and facilitate educational use cases. Equally important is privacy and data governance. Training multimodal models requires large quantities of patient data, raising concerns about consent, ownership, and anonymization. Institutions must implement robust de-identification procedures and ensure that data sharing agreements comply with legal frameworks such as HIPAA, GDPR, and local health data regulations. Ethical AI deployment also includes developing clear accountability structures that specify who is responsible for errors, including developers, vendors, institutions, or clinicians. A practical barrier to clinical adoption is the computational and infrastructural demand of these systems. High-performance GPUs, secure servers, and real-time PACS integration are prerequisites for smooth deployment. Many hospitals, particularly in low-resource regions, may lack the necessary hardware or technical support for continuous model operation. For such settings, lighter, compressed versions of MLLMs or cloud-based inference models may provide a feasible alternative, though these introduce additional considerations regarding data transfer and cybersecurity. Ensuring uninterrupted clinical workflow requires robust fail-safe mechanisms so that imaging interpretation remains uninterrupted even if the AI system encounters technical issues. Importantly, clinical implementation should follow an incremental, supervised approach rather than full-scale deployment. Early use cases may involve assisting with normal or near-normal imaging studies, where the risk of missing critical pathology is lower. As model performance improves and confidence grows, the scope can gradually expand to include more complex cases. This phased approach mirrors established protocols for introducing new medical technologies and supports evidence-based decision-making. Continuous monitoring through quality assurance dashboards, periodic audits, and user feedback mechanisms ensures that performance does not degrade over time—especially as hospital demographics or imaging protocols evolve.

Ultimately, the clinical value of multimodal LLMs is best realized when they function as collaborative partners to radiologists augmenting their capabilities, streamlining routine tasks, and providing decision support without overshadowing human judgment. By integrating thoughtful workflow design, ethical safeguards, and continuous oversight, healthcare systems can harness the strengths of multimodal AI while preserving patient safety and maintaining the integrity of clinical decision-making. In this evolving landscape, radiologists play a central role in shaping how these tools are deployed, evaluated, and refined, ensuring that technology advances in alignment with the core mission of medicine: to deliver accurate, compassionate, and equitable patient care.

5.5 Regulatory Frameworks and Approval Pathways

The integration of AI in clinical radiology is related to the regulatory environment, which is focused on the balance between innovation and safety. In the USA, AI-based radiology tools are part of the regulatory framework for Software as a Medical Device. In this context, a differentiation is made between AI-based radiology tools that support clinical decision-making and those that have a greater degree of autonomy. In the case of the USA, the majority of multimodal language-based radiology tools are categorized as assistive tools. In other words, the outputs provided by the AI-based system are intended to support, rather than replace, the knowledge provided by the radiologist. In this regard, a set of requirements is provided, including the transparency of the outputs and the ability for the radiologist to independently verify the outputs. In the case of the European Union, the implementation of the Medical Device Regulation and the CE marking processes require significant validation, documentation, and monitoring. A significant issue related to the regulation of multimodal models is the fact that the performance of the system can change over time. In other words, the adaptive nature of the system means that the outputs provided can change based on the exposure to new data. In this regard, the regulatory environment is focused on the evaluation, documentation, and development of explainability. Such a framework is related to the fact that the regulatory environment is required to be dynamic in relation to the changing nature of AI technologies.

6. ADVANCES BEYOND BASIC REPORT GENERATION

The evolution of multimodal large language models in radiology extends far beyond the automated generation of traditional reports. While early models focused primarily on converting imaging data into narrative findings, recent innovations have expanded the functional scope of these systems, transforming them into versatile diagnostic assistants capable of multitask reasoning, multimodal integration, and interactive clinical support. These advancements reflect a broader shift toward AI systems that replicate not only the descriptive aspects of radiological reporting but also the inferential and decision-making functions that underpin clinical practice. As radiology continues to embrace digital transformation, these emerging capabilities represent the next frontier in augmenting imaging interpretation and enhancing the depth and efficiency of diagnostic workflows.

6.1. Multi-Agent and Reasoning Framework

One of the most significant advancements in this domain is the development of multi-agent frameworks for radiology report generation. Unlike single-model systems that attempt to interpret the image, contextualize findings, and compose a coherent report within one unified architecture, multi-agent systems distribute these tasks across specialized components. For instance, one agent may focus solely on retrieving relevant clinical context, another may perform detailed visual analysis, and a third may synthesize the final narrative based on outputs from the preceding agents. This modular approach mirrors the workflow of human radiologists, who often consult multiple sources prior imaging, patient history, laboratory results, and specialist opinions before forming a final interpretation. Multi-agent architectures therefore introduce a higher degree of transparency and logical structure into the AI workflow, enabling more robust reasoning and reducing the likelihood of hallucinated or irrelevant findings. Additionally, the modularity allows for easier updates and adaptations, such as swapping out the visual analysis agent for a more advanced model without retraining the entire system.

6.2. Anatomical Grounding and the Longitudinal Interpretation

The use of segmentation-aware and anatomy-guided modelling, which improves the spatial grounding of generated reports, is another significant development. Conventional approaches rely on global feature representations of an image, which can fail to map certain descriptors to precise anatomical locations or miss small abnormalities. This issue is resolved by segmentation-enriched models, such MAIRA-Seg, which incorporate pixel-level or region-level annotations straight into the visual encoder. In addition to increasing accuracy, this approach is more in line with radiological thinking, which holds that a finding's location is frequently just as clinically meaningful as the finding itself. These algorithms provide more comprehensible outputs and give radiologists visual explanations that emphasize the origin of each descriptive term by linking textual descriptions to specific anatomical features. This development is especially helpful in complicated imaging modalities where pathology may be obscured by overlapping structures and inconsistent image quality, such as abdominal CT analysis or chest X-ray interpretation. The development of AI systems that can comprehend longitudinal imaging and carry out comparative interpretations has also advanced significantly in this field. In order to assess the course of an illness, the effectiveness of a treatment, or the stability of chronic abnormalities, radiologists in clinical practice often compare recent studies with earlier imaging. In order to process serial imaging sequences, recent multimodal models include memory mechanisms and multi-image encoders. These models can summarize the development of radiological results over time, detect small temporal changes, and identify anomalies that are getting worse or getting better. These features are particularly useful in trauma follow-up, interstitial lung disease monitoring, and oncology, where longitudinal evaluation is essential to patient care. Multimodal AI has the potential to eliminate oversight errors and identify changes that could otherwise go unnoticed during high-volume reporting by automating some of this process.

6.3. Heterogenous Data Fusion and Patient-Centered Outputs

Integrating non-imaging clinical data, such as test findings, electronic health record (EHR) entries, and pertinent clinical notes, is a further development. In order to improve interpretations, distinguish between identical imaging patterns, and produce clinically significant impressions, radiologists frequently rely on this additional information. In addition to imaging inputs, multimodal LLMs can integrate structured and unstructured clinical data, enabling the model to produce findings that are more contextually relevant. For instance, a history of recent trauma may help identify fractures, and knowledge of increased white blood cell counts may affect how lung opacities are interpreted. Multimodal AI is now positioned as a holistic diagnostic helper rather than just an image captioning system because to the broadened scope of data fusion. However, incorporating clinical data creates significant privacy, consistency, and interoperability issues that need for stringent governance mechanisms to guarantee ethical use.

The creation of patient-centered reports, where multimodal AI systems provide simplified narratives suited for patients rather than clinicians, is another exciting field. Transparency and patient involvement are hampered by the highly technical and frequently confusing nature of traditional radiology reports. Multimodal LLMs can produce supplementary "patient-friendly summaries" that reinterpret results using understandable language while preserving clinical accuracy if the proper precautions are taken. This ability is in line with contemporary healthcare movements that support patient autonomy and fair access to medical information. However, in order to prevent misinterpretation, oversimplification, or miscommunication of unclear conclusions, such features must be carefully designed.

6.4. Volumetric Processing and Uncertainty Qualification

Additionally, advances have been made in 3D imaging and volumetric interpretation, which is a particularly difficult field because of the magnitude and complexity of CT and MRI datasets. Early attempts to process volumetric data directly include models such as 3D-CT-GPT, which combine hundreds of slices into a single representation. These models make use of hybrid architectures or 3D transformers that integrate global attention methods with slice-level features. These models are able to identify diseases that span numerous planes and more comprehensively integrate anatomical context by capturing inter-slice interactions. This path indicates a future when AI systems can help with extremely complicated modalities like cardiac MRI, brain perfusion studies, and whole-body oncologic imaging, even though they are still computationally demanding and not yet clinically mature.

Lastly, a lot of researchers are investigating explainability and uncertainty quantification as developments that improve clinical safety and user trust. Interpretability modules that highlight image regions linked to particular textual outputs or provide probability estimates associated with findings are becoming more and more common in contemporary multimodal systems. These features offer radiologists a transparent view into the model's decision-making process, transforming AI from a "black box" into an accountable collaborative tool. Uncertainty quantification, such as confidence scoring or calibrated risk estimates, allows radiologists to gauge when AI outputs should be trusted and when they warrant heightened scrutiny. This capability is especially important in high-stakes scenarios, such as detecting malignancies or evaluating complex trauma.

Collectively, these advances demonstrate that multimodal LLMs are progressing well beyond basic report drafting toward a comprehensive suite of radiology augmentation tools. They are evolving into systems that can analyse images at multiple levels, integrate heterogeneous data sources, provide interactive support, and adapt to varied clinical requirements. While challenges remain, particularly in ensuring accuracy, scalability, and ethical integrity, the rapid pace of innovation suggests that future radiology practice will be deeply intertwined with these intelligent, multimodal systems. To guarantee that technology advancements are in line with clinical requirements and patient welfare, radiologists, data scientists, ethicists, and informatics specialists will need to work together in an interdisciplinary manner.

7. EVALUATION AND VALIDATION STRATEGIES

One of the most important and difficult parts of developing multimodal large language models" for radiology is evaluating and validating them. Multimodal systems designed for clinical reporting must be assessed through a multilayered framework that reflects the complex realities of radiological interpretation, in contrast to traditional machine learning models that may be evaluated using simple accuracy or precision criteria. The objective is to ascertain whether a model can consistently, safely, and in a way that facilitates clinical decision-making produce text that resembles a radiological report. This requires integrating quantitative assessments, qualitative expert judgments, external validations, and continuous monitoring within real-world workflows. Ensuring reliability demands rigorous methodology, as the consequences of errors in radiology reporting can be profound, affecting patient diagnosis, treatment planning, and long-term prognosis.

The use of automated quantitative indicators, such as BLEU, ROUGE, METEOR, and CIDEr, which are typically connected to natural language generating activities, is a fundamental component of evaluation. These metrics provide a useful numerical overview of linguistic similarity by measuring overlaps between generated text and reference reports. They have limits in radiology since two clinically equivalent reports may have quite different phrasing, even though they are helpful for general benchmarking. Without exhibiting a true comprehension of the underlying image, a model could obtain a high score by merely imitating surface-level phrases. On the other hand, if a clinically valid report is written differently from the reference, it could receive a low grade. This has led to the popularity of specialist radiology-focused measures, such as RadGraph F1, CheXbert label correctness, and Clinical Efficacy Scores, which assess the accuracy of key clinical concepts, such as "stable cardiomegaly" or "no pneumothorax." By ensuring that the resulting text is consistent with radiological reasoning and medical oncology, these concept-level judgments more accurately represent clinical value.

Radiologist-led evaluation is still essential, even with computerized scoring. Expert evaluation sheds light on the clinical accuracy, coherence, and completeness of reports produced by AI—qualities that automated measures by themselves are unable to consistently convey. Radiologists evaluate reports for overall clinical appropriateness, clarity of impressions, and sensitivity and specificity of identified findings in structured reader studies. These assessments frequently identify subtle problems that automated metrics are unable to identify, such as improper emphasis, missing contextual information, or inaccurate interpretation of a visual pattern. A qualitative indicator of fluency and perceived accuracy, some research uses blind evaluations in which radiologists try to discern between reports written by AI and those written by humans. Crucially, radiologist input also points up systematic errors that could result from model misalignment, dataset biases, or insufficient grounding, providing guidance for future improvements.

Grounding and hallucination detection are important aspects of model evaluation. Validation must verify that each statement in a generated report matches recognizable evidence in the image due to the catastrophic hazards associated with hallucinated conclusions. It is possible to ascertain if the model's outputs are based on real visual features or result from linguistic priors by using methods like attention mapping, feature attribution, and counterfactual image analysis. Furthermore, some frameworks include structured grounding standards that demand the model to provide evidence for its conclusions by connecting text outputs to segmentation masks or spatial coordinates. In addition to identifying hallucinations, these grounding assessments improve interpretability and transparency—two essential components for fostering therapeutic confidence in AI systems. Given that medical datasets can contain embedded biases, such as the overrepresentation of particular diseases or demographic groupings, which might unintentionally affect model predictions, robust grounding is particularly crucial.

External and out-of-distribution testing, which evaluates the model's generalizability to novel populations, imaging procedures, and clinical settings, is another essential component of a strong validation methodology. Although essential, internal validation is insufficient since models frequently pick up institution-specific nuances from their training data, which results in poorer performance when used elsewhere. Instead of memorizing patterns unique to a single dataset, external validation datasets—ideally from several hospitals, geographical areas, and imaging equipment—test whether the model has acquired universal radiological principles. When applied to images from centers with various radiography procedures, noise levels, or demographic features, for instance, a model that was predominantly trained on MIMIC-CXR images would have trouble. The significance of international, multi-institutional benchmarking programs that promote cooperation and openness in model performance reporting is highlighted by this disparity.

The gold standard of validation for multimodal AI systems includes prospective studies and real-world clinical trials in addition to offline assessments. These studies evaluate workflow integration, radiologist acceptance, reporting efficiency, error rates, and downstream clinical impact in addition to model correctness. Practical problems like report generation slowness, UI difficulties, or irregularities in radiologists' interpretation and editing of AI-generated drafts can be found by prospective testing. Additionally, prospective studies aid in measuring results that are not possible with traditional measurements, including shorter reporting times for routine studies or earlier abnormality identification. Additionally, they make it possible to compare AI-assisted workflows with typical radiologist processes, offering empirical proof of whether multimodal models enhance patient care without posing unforeseen hazards.

Continuous monitoring and post-deployment evaluation become essential when multimodal models are used in clinical settings. Changes in patient demographics, imaging procedures, or disease incidence can cause models to wander over time—a phenomenon called "performance decay." A model trained on historical data might be put to the test, for instance, if a new disease pattern or seasonal shift in respiratory infections emerges. Early identification of these problems is made possible by putting in place monitoring dashboards that track error rates, radiologist overrides, and calibration drift. This closed-loop feedback system guarantees that the model continues to function safely for extended periods of time and stays in line with current clinical needs.

Regulatory and ethical validation frameworks are the last factor to be taken into account. AI systems are increasingly required to follow rules pertaining to transparency, risk mitigation, and auditability by agencies including the FDA, EMA, and national health authorities. AI systems used in radiology must show adherence to both technical performance requirements and moral precepts like justice, responsibility, and patient data security. Training datasets, model architecture, planned use cases, and acknowledged restrictions must all be documented by developers. Establishing explicit accountability frameworks that outline how mistakes will be handled and who is accountable when AI-assisted decisions lead to unfavourable healthcare outcomes is equally crucial. Because of the high stakes involved in incorporating AI into medical practice, ethical validation and technical validation become interwoven.

In conclusion, a thorough, multifaceted approach that include quantitative measures, qualitative expert evaluation, grounded validation, external testing, prospective trials, ongoing monitoring, and ethical oversight is necessary to evaluate multimodal LLMs for radiology. The entire range of performance required for safe clinical deployment cannot be captured by a single metric or approach. Healthcare organizations can only guarantee that multimodal models operate dependably as supportive tools, aiding radiologists without jeopardizing patient safety, by using such layered validation. Establishing standardized evaluation frameworks will be essential as the sector develops in order to compare systems impartially, direct regulatory approval procedures, and promote confidence between patients and professionals.

7.1 Dataset Characteristics and Performance Trends

The performance of multimodal large language models in radiology is related to the characteristics of the datasets used for their development. In fact, the majority of the modern models are developed using large-scale publicly available datasets, including the MIMIC-CXR and IU X-Ray datasets. These datasets contain radiographic images along with their corresponding written reports. In fact, the alignment between the two modalities is the key requirement for developing multimodal models.

However, the composition of the datasets poses a few challenges. In fact, the majority of the radiology datasets are composed of images and reports collected from a particular geographical area. Therefore, the generalization ability of the models is limited. In fact, the performance of the models is likely to be affected when they are applied to diverse populations.

The performance of the multimodal models is evaluated using a combination of natural language generation-based measures and clinical measures. In fact, the commonly used measures for the evaluation of the models are BLEU, ROUGE, METEOR, CIDEr, etc. In fact, these measures evaluate the similarity between the generated report and the actual report. However, the clinical correctness of the generated report is not evaluated using these measures. Therefore, a few domain-specific measures, including RadGraph F1 and CheXbert Label Accuracy, have been introduced for the evaluation of the models.

The recent studies suggest that the performance of the modern models, including the CXR-LLaVA and MRG-LLM models, is improved in terms of linguistic fluency and contextual coherence when compared to the conventional CNN-RNN-based models. However, the performance of the models is variable.

Table 4. Evaluation metrics for automated radiology report generation

Metric	Category	Purpose	Clinical Value
BLEU/ ROUGE	Linguistic	Text similarity	Low
RadGraph F1	Clinical	Concept accuracy	High
CheXbert	Label-based	Pathology detection	High
Reader studies	Human	Diagnostic validity	Very High

7.2 Dataset Challenges and Limitations

The reliability of multimodal AI systems is fundamentally influenced by the data on which they are trained. Many current models rely heavily on publicly available datasets such as MIMIC-CXR and CheXpert, which have played a critical role in advancing research. However, these datasets are not without limitations (Johnson et al., 2019; Irvin et al., 2019). One key issue is the lack of demographic diversity. Since many datasets originate from specific geographic regions, models trained on them may not generalize well to populations with different disease patterns or imaging practices. This raises concerns about equitable performance across healthcare systems. In addition, radiology reports used for training often contain variability in terminology, structure, and interpretation. This inconsistency can introduce noise into the learning process, affecting the accuracy and reliability of generated outputs. Another important consideration is domain shift. Differences in imaging equipment, acquisition protocols, and patient characteristics can lead to performance degradation when models are applied outside their original training environment. Addressing these challenges will require more diverse datasets, improved standardization, and collaborative approaches to data sharing.

7.3 Empirical Validation and Supporting Evidence

Although this chapter primarily focuses on conceptual and analytical perspectives, it is important to acknowledge the growing body of empirical work supporting multimodal approaches. Recent studies have demonstrated that models such as CXR-LLaVA are capable of producing more coherent and clinically structured reports compared to earlier generation systems (Lee et al., 2025). Similarly, segmentation-guided approaches have shown improvements in aligning textual outputs with specific anatomical regions, thereby enhancing both accuracy and interpretability (Sharma et al., 2024). Evaluation frameworks incorporating clinically relevant metrics, including RadGraph and CheXbert, have further highlighted the ability of these models to capture key diagnostic concepts (Liu et al., 2024). While these findings are encouraging, they also reinforce the need for cautious interpretation. Most studies have been conducted in controlled environments, and broader validation across diverse clinical settings remains an essential step before widespread adoption.

8. RESEARCH GAPS AND FUTURE DIRECTIONS

Despite such progress, there are a number of key gaps that remain to be addressed in the development and deployment of multimodal large language models for radiology. Perhaps, the most important gap is that of cross-population validation. There are a number of models that have been developed on datasets from high-resource health systems, raising questions of their applicability in a diverse range of clinical environments, especially in low-resource countries. A second key gap is that of deployment, especially in resource-constrained environments. The computational demands of such models, including the requirement for high-performance GPUs and high-capacity storage, are a barrier to deployment. A third gap is that of medicolegal responsibility. There is a degree of ambiguity associated with the deployment of such models, especially in terms of medicolegal responsibility. There is a requirement for a clear framework of law that is developed to address such questions. A fourth gap is that of transparency. While there has been a degree of success in addressing the issue of transparency, there is still a requirement for partially transparent models. A fifth gap is that of standardized evaluation. There is a requirement for a standardized framework for evaluating such models, especially in a framework that is aligned with clinical outcomes, rather than linguistic similarity.

9. DISCUSSION

Implications for Radiology Practice and Healthcare Systems

The ramifications of incorporating multimodal large language models" into radiological practice are extensive and go well beyond advances in technology. It signifies a significant change in the way diagnostic imaging is understood, recorded, and shared throughout the healthcare delivery system. As a result, radiologists, physicians, healthcare administrators, and legislators need to consider these technologies' potential as well as their wider effects on patient outcomes, workflow efficiency, workforce change, and healthcare equity. Every aspect of radiology will probably be impacted by multimodal AI as it develops, from daily reporting duties to institutional and national resource allocation and strategic planning.

Redefining radiologist workload and workflow dynamics is a key consequence of adopting multimodal LLM. Generating descriptive reports has historically taken up a significant amount of radiologists' work, particularly for high-volume exams like non-contrast CT scans, spine films, and chest radiographs. These reports frequently include standard results that call for careful but repetitive documentation. Multimodal AI systems have the ability to reallocate radiologists' time to higher-order interpretative activities, complex case reviews, multidisciplinary tumor boards, image-guided therapies, and direct clinician communication by automating the preparation of such reports. By enabling radiologists to concentrate on tasks that have a greater direct influence on clinical decision-making, this change not only lessens the cognitive fatigue brought on by repetitive tasks but also improves job satisfaction. However, this transition may necessitate restructuring of workflow processes, redesigning PACS/RIS interfaces, and adopting hybrid human-AI review protocols to ensure safety and efficiency.

The deployment of multimodal LLMs also has significant implications for diagnostic accuracy and error reduction. By providing consistent, structured draft reports, these systems can reduce variability in reporting style and help standardize the description of common pathologies. AI-generated reports are not susceptible to fatigue, time pressure, or cognitive biases that may influence human interpretation. Furthermore, multimodal models can function as a "second reader," highlighting key abnormalities or prompting radiologists to reconsider overlooked findings. While human oversight remains essential, the collaborative interaction can support earlier detection of subtle changes, aid junior radiologists in developing systematic interpretation habits, and reduce the likelihood of documentation inconsistencies. On the other hand, poorly validated models may introduce new risks, such as false reassurance or overreliance on AI outputs. Thus, responsible deployment must emphasize rigorous quality control and continuous monitoring.

The implications of multimodal AI adoption extend beyond individual radiologists, influencing institutional operations and resource management. Health systems facing chronic radiologist shortages, especially in developing countries, can benefit substantially from augmented workflows that accelerate reporting and reduce backlog. This may be particularly impactful in emergency and trauma centers where rapid reporting is essential. Tele-radiology networks, which connect urban specialists to remote healthcare centers, stand to gain even more: AI-generated report drafts can reduce reporting delays, enable triage of urgent cases, and enhance the scalability of tele-radiology services without compromising quality. However, these operational improvements depend on robust IT infrastructure, reliable data connectivity, and adherence to cybersecurity standards—requirements that may challenge under-resourced institutions.

A broader societal implication involves the potential of multimodal LLMs to democratize access to radiological expertise, bridging gaps in healthcare equity. In many parts of the world, radiology services are limited by shortages of trained personnel, uneven distribution of imaging facilities, and geographic barriers to specialist access. By enabling automated or semi-automated reporting in settings where radiologists are scarce, multimodal AI systems could help improve early disease detection and reduce diagnostic delays. For instance, automated chest X-ray interpretation could aid tuberculosis screening in high-burden regions, while AI-generated ultrasounds interpretations could support maternal care in rural clinics. Yet, deploying AI in such contexts requires careful consideration of cultural norms, linguistic variation, ethical safeguards, and the risk of algorithmic bias affecting vulnerable populations.

Equity-driven deployment must therefore be accompanied by local validation studies, community engagement, and transparent accountability frameworks.

The use of multimodal LLMs creates further concerns around professional identity, skill development, and training in the radiography industry. Radiologists may need to adjust by learning new skills in AI administration, monitoring, and integration as AI takes on more descriptive jobs. Modules on data stewardship, error auditing, ethical AI use, and machine learning literacy may become more common in training programs. In addition to understanding how to interpret images, radiology residents will also need to be able to oversee automated systems, critically assess AI output, and identify potential hazards that could evade algorithmic detection. By establishing radiologists as administrators of intelligent systems and defenders of clinical accuracy, AI may enhance rather than decrease their job. This changing dynamic highlights how crucial it is to promote a culture of cooperation rather than rivalry between AI technologies and human skills.

Multimodal LLMs pose a regulatory challenge to the established systems that control quality assurance and medical device approval. Large language models are fundamentally different from deterministic algorithms with definite outputs, and regulatory authorities must deal with their complexity, dynamic nature, and frequently opaque character. AI models, in contrast to traditional devices, can adapt over time in response to new data or changes in clinical settings. As a result, regulators will need to create requirements for explainability, post-market surveillance, dataset transparency, and continual validation. Institutions adopting multimodal AI should implement internal auditing systems that track model performance, document radiologist interventions, flag recurring discrepancies, and establish clear protocols for incident reporting. Ethical deployment also requires addressing questions of liability: when errors occur in AI-augmented reporting, responsibility must be clearly assigned among developers, institutions, clinicians, and vendors.

Despite these difficulties, if multimodal LLMs are handled properly, the long-term effects on healthcare systems are overwhelmingly favourable. These systems have the potential to improve patient outcomes, lower diagnostic errors, and increase operational efficiency by speeding up reporting, enhancing consistency, and enabling thorough multimodal reasoning. Additionally, they operate as catalysts for more extensive digital transformation in the healthcare industry by promoting data-driven decision-making, integrated clinical workflows, and standardized documentation procedures. Furthermore, as multimodal AI develops into increasingly complex diagnostic helpers, it may aid translational research by finding new radiological patterns connected to genetic or metabolic pathways, forecasting the course of disease, and identifying imaging biomarkers.

In conclusion, multimodal large language models offer a revolutionary chance to change radiography and healthcare delivery. Their influence will be felt not only in report writing but also in how radiologists work with imaging data, cooperate with physicians, and support patient care across the entire diagnostic process. Deliberate, morally sound implementation strategies that put patient safety, clinical supervision, dataset diversity, and system behaviour transparency first are necessary to realize this potential. With these protections in place, multimodal AI systems have the potential to become essential collaborators in radiological practice, improving both the quality of patient care provided globally and the science of imaging.

10. CONCLUSION

In the history of radiology and medical informatics, the development of multimodal large language models" represents a turning point. The confluence of sophisticated vision encoders, potent language models, and extensive multimodal datasets has made what once appeared to be an ambitious goal automated and intelligent aid in the interpretation and reporting of medical images achievable. These technologies present previously unheard-of chances to improve reporting effectiveness, lessen the burden of documentation, and assist radiologists in the ever more complicated field of diagnostic imaging. However, like with any disruptive technology, its actual worth is contingent upon thorough, ethical, and context-sensitive incorporation into clinical practice rather than just technical proficiency.

Fundamentally, multimodal LLMs represent a move away from pattern recognition and toward AI systems that mimic higher-level clinical thinking in order to synthesize, interpret, and contextualize imaging results. They can create organized reports, draw attention to anomalies, incorporate clinical metadata, contrast earlier research, and even produce summaries that are easy for patients to understand. These features have enormous potential to increase diagnostic precision, optimize high-volume workflows, and democratize access to radiological knowledge in underprivileged areas. But achieving these advantages necessitates recognizing and resolving the enduring problems—hallucinations, data bias, generalizability problems, interpretability gaps, and the requirement for thorough validation across a range of populations and imaging procedures.

Keeping radiologists at the forefront of the diagnosis process is essential to the responsible implementation of multimodal LLMs. These systems should be seen as partners rather than replacements, enhancing, expediting, and improving human knowledge while maintaining clinical judgment and accountability. New skills in AI oversight, error auditing, and integration management are required as traditional workflows give way to AI-augmented reporting. Institutions must put in place strong governance frameworks, make investments in digital infrastructure, and foster an innovative culture without sacrificing moral values or patient safety. In order to continuously monitor and approve adaptive AI technology, regulatory authorities must also change and embrace dynamic frameworks.

Multimodal LLMs have the potential to develop into all-encompassing diagnostic intelligence systems in the future that can integrate lab data, volumetric imaging, genetics, and clinical narratives into cohesive, context-aware reasoning. These technologies could help with clinical decision support, personalized medicine, predictive analytics, and regular reporting. However, these thrilling opportunities also entail greater responsibilities. International cooperation, diversity in training data, and a persistent dedication to transparency will be necessary to ensure that AI advancements contribute fairly to global healthcare without escalating inequities or undermining patient trust.

In the end, the application of multimodal AI in radiology involves a reinvention of how knowledge is created, shared, and used in clinical treatment rather than merely a technological advancement. These tools represent a future where radiologists can spend more time to complicated interpretation, interdisciplinary cooperation, and patient engagement areas where human intuition and empathy remain indispensable—by fusing computational intelligence with human insight. Multimodal LLMs have the ability to improve diagnostic quality, increase access to imaging expertise, and promote a more effective and patient-centered healthcare system if they are applied morally and carefully. In order to ensure that the revolutionary power of AI enhances rather than replaces the fundamental principles of medical practice, the future is one of cautious optimism, scientific rigor, and collaborative innovation.

REFERENCES

Agarwal, M., van der Pol, C. B., Patlas, M. N., Udare, A., Chung, A. D., & Rubino, J. (2021). Optimizing the radiologist work environment: Actionable tips to improve workplace satisfaction, efficiency, and minimize burnout. *La Radiologia Medica*, *126*(10), 1255–1257. DOI: 10.1007/s11547-021-01397-x PMID: 34269963

Cai, T.. (2023). Aligning large multimodal models with radiology knowledge. arXiv:2309.05683. https://arxiv.org/abs/2309.05683

Fang, M., Wang, Z., Pan, S., Feng, X., Zhao, Y., Hou, D., Wu, L., Xie, X., Zhang, X.-Y., Tian, J., & Dong, D. (2025). Large models in medical imaging: Advances and prospects. *Chinese Medical Journal*, *138*(14), 1647–1664. DOI: 10.1097/CM9.0000000000003699 PMID: 40539307

Huang, S., Tan, J., & Liang, J. (2024). A survey on medical vision-language models: Datasets, methods, and evaluation. arXiv:2406.06580. https://arxiv.org/abs/2406.06580

Irvin, J., Rajpurkar, P., Ko, M., Yu, Y., Ciurea-Ilcus, S., Chute, C., Marklund, H., Haghgoo, B., Ball, R., Shpanskaya, K., Seekins, J., Mong, D. A., Halabi, S. S., Sandberg, J. K., Jones, R., Larson, D. B., Langlotz, C. P., Patel, B. N., Lungren, M. P., & Ng, A. Y. (2019, July). Chexpert: A large chest radiograph dataset with uncertainty labels and expert comparison. *Proceedings of the AAAI Conference on Artificial Intelligence*, *33*(01), 590–597. DOI: 10.1609/aaai.v33i01.3301590

Johnson, A. E. W., Pollard, T. J., Berkowitz, S. J., Greenbaum, N. R., Lungren, M. P., Deng, C., . . . Horng, S. (2019). MIMIC-CXR: A large publicly available database of labeled chest radiographs. CoRR. *arXiv preprint arXiv:1901.07042*.

Lee, S., Youn, J., Kim, H., Kim, M., & Yoon, S. H. (2025). CXR-LLAVA: A multimodal large language model for interpreting chest X-ray images. *European Radiology*, *35*(7), 4374–4386. DOI: 10.1007/s00330-024-11339-6 PMID: 39812665

Liu, C., Tian, Y., Chen, W., Song, Y., & Zhang, Y. (2024, March). Bootstrapping large language models for radiology report generation. *Proceedings of the AAAI Conference on Artificial Intelligence*, *38*(17), 18635–18643. DOI: 10.1609/aaai.v38i17.29826

Nam, Y., Kim, D. Y., Kyung, S., Seo, J., Song, J. M., Kwon, J., Kim, J., Jo, W., Park, H., Sung, J., Park, S., Kwon, H., Kwon, T., Kim, K., & Kim, N. (2025). Multimodal large language models in medical imaging. *Korean Journal of Radiology*, *26*(10), 12479233. https://pmc.ncbi.nlm.nih.gov/articles/PMC12479233. DOI: 10.3348/kjr.2025.0599 PMID: 41015856

Sharma, H., Patel, R., & Singh, A. (2024). MAIRA-Seg: Enhancing radiology report generation with segmentation-aware multimodal large language models. arXiv:2411.11362. https://arxiv.org/abs/2411.11362

U.S. FDA. (2023). Good Machine Learning Practice (GMLP) guidelines for medical AI devices. Open Access. https://www.fda.gov

Yi, Z., Xu, L., & Sun, J. (2025). A survey on multimodal large language models in radiology. *Information (Basel)*, *16*(2), 136. https://www.mdpi.com/2078-2489/16/2/136. DOI: 10.3390/info16020136

KEY TERMS AND DEFINITIONS

Explainable AI (XAI): Methods that make AI decision-making transparent and interpretable to human users.

Federated Learning: A privacy-preserving AI training method where models learn from distributed data without sharing raw patient information.

Hallucination (AI): The generation of unsupported or incorrect findings by an AI model that are not grounded in image evidence.

Human-in-the-Loop: A deployment framework where clinicians retain final decision authority over AI-generated outputs.

Multimodal Large Language Model (MLLM): An artificial intelligence system capable of jointly processing medical images and natural language to generate clinically meaningful outputs.

PACS (Picture Archiving and Communication System): A digital system used to store, retrieve, and distribute medical images and reports.

Radiology Report Generation: The automated or semi-automated creation of structured narrative reports describing imaging findings and impressions.

Segmentation-Aware Modelling: An AI training approach that incorporates anatomical region masks to improve spatial grounding and interpretability.

Chapter 5

Persistent Homology as a Diagnostic Lens in Vision–Language Medical Systems

Jaime Aguilar-Ortiz
Universidad Politécnica de Pachuca, Mexico

Ocotlán Diáz-Parra
Universidad Politécnica de Pachuca, Mexico

Jorge A. Ruiz-Vanoye
http://orcid.org/0000-0003-4928-5716
Universidad Politécnica de Pachuca, Mexico

Francisco R. Trejo-Macotela
http://orcid.org/0000-0003-2133-3456
Universidad Politécnica de Pachuca, Mexico

Marco A. Vera-Jiménez
http://orcid.org/0009-0009-3712-1440
Universidad Politécnica de Pachuca, Mexico

Víctor M. Zamudio-García
http://orcid.org/0000-0002-4660-8025
Universidad Politécnica Metropolitana de Hidalgo, Mexico

Carlos R. Domínguez-Mayorga
http://orcid.org/0009-0007-1018-4412
Universidad Politécnica de Pachuca, Mexico

ABSTRACT

This article proposes persistent homology as a model-agnostic audit lens for vision–language medical systems whose fluent reports can mask structural inconsistencies. An end-to-end pipeline computes cubical persistence on reference images and model-mediated outputs, derives Betti-curve signatures on a shared filtration grid, and measures drift via bottleneck and Wasserstein distances in H0 and H1.

DOI: 10.4018/979-8-3373-7315-7.ch005

ht © 2026, IGI Global Scientific Publishing. Copying or distributing in print or electronic forms without written permission of IGI Global Scientific Publishing is prohibited. Use of this chapter to generative artificial intelligence (AI) technologies is expressly prohibited. The publisher reserves all rights to license its use for generative AI training and machine learning model development.

Conventional baselines (reconstruction, segmentation, and semantic agreement) establish nominal adequacy, while topology reveals silent failures such as spurious holes, merged components, or fragmented regions. Topological signals are aggregated into a diagnostic index for ranking cases, setting alarms, and tracking stability. Outputs include figures, tables, and evaluation scripts.

1. INTRODUCTION

1.1. Motivation and problem statement

Clinical multimodal pipelines that couple images with short textual reports increasingly rely on learned cross-modal alignment and report-generation objectives that can optimize for linguistic fluency and global semantic similarity while still drifting away from anatomy- and morphology-consistent structure at the pixel, region, or shape level, thereby creating a credibility gap between "coherent narration" and "structurally plausible evidence" (Yang et al., 2023; Raminedi et al., 2024; Liu et al., 2024). This gap is particularly acute in settings where a model's intermediate representations (e.g., vision embeddings and text embeddings) become the operational substrate for downstream decisions, because high alignment scores can coexist with subtle but clinically relevant geometric/topological distortions such as spurious holes, merged components, or disconnected fragments that may not be penalized by standard reconstruction or language metrics (Skaf & Laubenbacher, 2022; Singh et al., 2023). To address that methodological weakness, the manuscript frames "structural truth" not as an abstract claim, but as an empirically auditable constraint: the pipeline should preserve topology-relevant structure across transformations, reconstructions, and representation mappings, and it should expose when that preservation fails. In practical terms, this motivation supports a topology-aware audit layer that computes cubical persistent homology on images, derives Betti-curve profiles over a shared filtration grid, and measures persistence-diagram dissimilarities (e.g., bottleneck and Wasserstein) to quantify whether reconstructions and model-mediated representations conserve connectedness and loop-like morphology across scales, while also extending the same logic to point-cloud persistent homology on subsampled embedding manifolds to test whether the vision and text spaces remain structurally aligned rather than merely globally correlated (Skaf & Laubenbacher, 2022; Singh et al., 2023). The problem statement is therefore formulated as an actionable evaluation gap: although modern multimodal methods can learn strong image–text correspondence and generate clinically styled narratives, the field still lacks a systematic, model-agnostic way to measure whether topology-bearing structure is conserved throughout the multimodal pipeline and without that measurement, "trust" cannot be operationalized as a falsifiable property of the system's outputs and internal representations (Clough et al., 2020; Liu et al., 2024; Liu et al., 2024).

1.2. Research objective and guiding question

Clinical multimodal pipelines can achieve apparently strong performance on conventional objectives such as low reconstruction error, high text–image retrieval scores, or plausible report fluency while still introducing structurally consequential distortions that undermine anatomical plausibility at the level of connectedness, cavities, and loop-like morphology, which are precisely the kinds of properties that clinicians implicitly rely on when judging whether an output is trustworthy; therefore, the research objective is to operationalize "topological coherence" as a measurable agreement between (i) a reference medical image and (ii) model-mediated outputs produced by the pipeline (e.g., autoencoder-style reconstructions, synthetic surrogates, or embedding-manifold representations aligned with short textual reports), using persistent homology on cubical representations of images, Betti-curve trajectories over a shared filtration grid, and diagram distances (e.g., bottleneck/Wasserstein) as complementary descriptors that can expose structural drift even when pixelwise similarity looks acceptable (Clough et al., 2020; Singh et al., 2023; Skaf & Laubenbacher, 2022); critically, this objective becomes stronger and more actionable when situated in the recent methodological convergence of (a) medical vision–language modeling and report-conditioned perception pipelines whose surveys emphasize how "language integration" can inflate apparent task performance while leaving failure modes under-specified at the anatomical-structure level (Lu & Wang, 2025) and (b) topology-aware training/evaluation mechanisms that explicitly target precisely those invariants (components/holes/loops) that conventional similarity scores can ignore, including soft topology constraints for neuroanatomical segmentation (Fu et al., 2024) and topologically faithful multiclass segmentation formulations built around persistent-homology consistency across labels (Berger et al., 2024) ; in this framing, the guiding question becomes empirically testable and audit-oriented: under which data regimes, architectural choices, and alignment strategies do standard metrics imply adequacy (e.g., MSE/SSIM improvements for reconstructions, or enhanced cross-modal alignment for report conditioning) while topological signatures reveal nontrivial deviations such as spurious components, collapsed loops, or altered persistence scales suggesting that the representation is "semantically aligned" yet structurally compromised, and how can these divergences be converted into a reliable audit signal (e.g., thresholds on persistence-distance deltas, discordance indices between SSIM and PH-based distances, or embedding-cloud topology shifts) that flags outputs requiring heightened scrutiny or model revision (Yang et al., 2023; Liu et al., 2023; Wang et al., 2022; Raminedi et al., 2024); furthermore, this audit logic aligns with a broader, recent push to treat algebraic-topology descriptors as clinically meaningful shape constraints and interpretability primitives in radiology and computational pathology (Levenson et al., 2024), and it is technically supported by fast-growing toolkits that either inject persistent-homology features into deep classifiers to stabilize decision-making around morphological invariants (Peng et al., 2024) or encode local topological structure into image representations so that downstream learning becomes less brittle to "visually plausible" but topologically inconsistent perturbations (Gu et al., 2025) ; finally, recent methodological reviews beyond classical persistent-homology pipelines emphasize that topology-based descriptors and their vectorizations should be selected with care to avoid false reassurance precisely the risk at stake when semantic alignment improves while structural coherence degrades thereby reinforcing the need for explicit resolution controls, standardized preprocessing, and sensitivity analysis as part of any "topological coherence" claim (Su et al., 2025).

1.3. Contributions and article organization

The contributions are structured to make "structural truth" auditable in multimodal clinical pipelines by adding a topology-aware evaluation layer that complements conventional performance indicators and converts structural plausibility into measurable evidence: the framework formalizes topological coherence as an agreement property between a reference medical image and model-mediated outputs (reconstructions, generated surrogates, or embedding-derived representations), operationalizing that coherence through persistent-homology descriptors whose stability, interpretability, and biomedical relevance have been emphasized in modern topological data analysis and medical-imaging practice (Skaf & Laubenbacher, 2022; Singh et al., 2023; Chazal & Michel, 2021); methodologically, the audit protocol centers on persistence diagrams and Betti summaries as compact witnesses of connectivity and loop-like morphology across scales, aligning with the principle that clinically plausible outputs must preserve topology-relevant structure even when pixel-level similarity appears acceptable (Clough et al., 2020; Singh et al., 2023), and it instantiates interpretable deviation indicators via distance-based comparisons between persistence representations, leveraging efficient, well-documented persistent-homology implementations that enable automated, large-scale reporting within a reproducible Python pipeline (Bauer, 2021; Tralie et al., 2018; Wadhwa et al., 2018); to ensure that the method remains reviewable rather than merely computable, the pipeline is organized to automatically generate publication-ready tables and figures such as stratified distributions of topological distances, drift profiles, and representative diagram/summary visualizations consistent with contemporary expectations that clinical AI studies provide transparent, reproducible evidence trails and standardized reporting artifacts (Mongan et al., 2020; Liu et al., 2020); accordingly, the article organization follows a rigorous progression from the reliability gap (where standard metrics can be locally reassuring yet structurally misleading) to the topology-aware lens, then to an auditable protocol specified as a computational sequence (preprocessing, representation choice, persistence extraction, distance computation, and aggregation into coherence indicators), grounding each step in established TDA foundations and biomedical precedents (Chazal & Michel, 2021; Skaf & Laubenbacher, 2022; Singh et al., 2023), extending naturally to multimodal representation learning contexts where image–text alignment objectives and embedding pipelines are central so that the audit applies even when comparisons are performed in latent spaces rather than only in pixel space (Wang et al., 2022), and culminating in an evidentiary analysis that highlights precisely when conventional metrics suggest adequacy but topology-based indicators reveal structural drift, thereby enabling a practical audit signal that supports reliability claims under reproducibility-oriented clinical AI norms (Mongan et al., 2020; Liu et al., 2020).

2. CONCEPTUAL FRAMEWORK AND RELATED WORK

2.1. Multimodal clinical systems and the notion of alignment

This subsection positions multimodal alignment as a geometric phenomenon, not merely a semantic one. It reviews how alignment is typically discussed (cross-modal retrieval, captioning correctness, diagnostic text accuracy) and then proposes a stricter criterion: alignment should be consistent with clinically meaningful structure. The argument is articulated in terms of representational integrity: if the representation collapses or invents structural features, the model may still appear correct linguistically while becoming unreliable clinically.

Multimodal alignment in clinical systems is most defensibly treated as a geometric constraint on representations rather than as a purely semantic agreement between outputs, because clinical reliability depends on whether the model's internal and external transformations preserve clinically meaningful structure (Wang et al., 2022; Yang et al., 2023). In practical pipelines that combine medical images with text-derived or label-derived signals, alignment is typically operationalized by mapping each modality into a shared latent space and enforcing proximity for corresponding pairs while separating non-corresponding pairs, so that the "agreement" becomes a statement about distances and neighborhoods on a learned manifold rather than about linguistic plausibility alone (Wang et al., 2022; Zhang & Jiang, 2024). Formally, if an image encoder f_v and a text encoder f_t produce embeddings $z_v = f_v(x) \in \mathbb{R}^d$ and $z_t = f_t(r) \in \mathbb{R}^d$, a common alignment score is the cosine similarity

$$s(x, r) = \frac{\langle z_v, z_t \rangle}{\|z_v\| \|z_t\|},$$

and contrastive training drives matched pairs to have larger $s(x, r)$ than mismatched pairs via an InfoNCE-style objective (Wang et al., 2022). For a minibatch of paired embeddings $\left\{(z_{v,i}, z_{t,i})\right\}_{i=1}^{N}$ one standard

$$\mathcal{L}_{InfoNCE} = -\frac{1}{N}\sum_{i=1}^{N} \log \frac{exp\left(\langle \hat{z}_{v,i}, \hat{z}_{t,i} \rangle / \tau\right)}{\sum_{j=1}^{N} exp\left(\langle \hat{z}_{v,i}, \hat{z}_{t,i} \rangle / \tau\right)}$$

Where $\hat{z}$ denotes normalized embeddings and $\tau > 0$ is a temperature (Wang et al., 2022). The key methodological point is that this geometry can appear "good" under global metrics (high cosine similarity, strong retrieval scores, plausible generated reports) while still being clinically unsafe if the representation collapses distinct anatomical states into nearby points or, conversely, invents separations that are not anatomically warranted (Yang et al., 2023; Zhang & Jiang, 2024). That risk is precisely why an evaluation workflow that computes embeddings, pairwise distances, and stability-sensitive summaries consistent with the kind of embedding extraction, normalization, and downstream analysis typical of reproducible clinical ML code must treat alignment as representational integrity: the representation should preserve the structural degrees of freedom that clinicians implicitly rely on when they interpret morphology, boundaries, and connectivity, not merely the superficial coherence of language or pixel-level similarity (Wang et al., 2022; Dey et al., 2022).

A stricter and more clinically auditable notion of alignment arises when geometric agreement is tested against topology-relevant structure, because topology provides invariants (connected components, loops, cavities) that directly encode whether an anatomy has been fragmented, merged, perforated, or spuriously connected by model-mediated transformations (Clough et al., 2020; Bauer, 2021). If a pipeline produces a reference representation X (e.g., an image-derived point cloud, a feature map reshaped into a point set, or a latent embedding neighborhood graph) and a model-mediated representation Y (e.g., a reconstruction, a generated surrogate, or an embedding-manifold alternative), persistent homology computes persistence diagrams $D_k(X)$ and $D_k(Y)$ whose points (b, d) record the birth and death of k-dimensional features across a filtration (Bauer, 2021; Tralie et al., 2018). A principled "topology-aware alignment" test can then be framed as a distance between these diagrams an audit signal for structural drift even when classical performance metrics look adequate using, for example, a p-Wasserstein distance

$$W_p\left(D_k(X), D_k(Y)\right) = \left(\inf_{\gamma} \sum_{u \in D_k(X)} \|u - \gamma(u)\|_{\infty}^{p}\right)^{1/p},$$

Where γ ranges over matchings between diagrams augmented with the diagonal (Bauer, 2021). Complementarily, Betti summaries $\beta_k(\epsilon)$ track the number of k-features alive at scale ϵ, enabling an interpretable profile of how connectivity and loops evolve with scale, so divergences between X and Y become localized, multiscale statements rather than opaque scalar errors (Clough et al., 2020; Pun et al., 2022). This perspective is congruent with reproducible clinical pipelines that already compute embeddings and distance matrices: once the representation is available, persistence diagrams and their distances can be computed efficiently with modern software, turning "alignment" into a falsifiable claim about whether structural features persist or vanish under model operations (Tralie et al., 2018; Bauer, 2021). Crucially, this audit lens directly addresses the clinical failure mode in which language-level or global similarity scores remain high while morphology becomes implausible because topology will register unintended splits/merges or spurious tunnels as measurable changes in D_0 and D_1 and in distances $W_p\left(D_k(X), D_k(Y)\right)$ thereby supporting reliability arguments grounded in structure rather than appearance (Clough et al., 2020; Yang et al., 2023; Zhang & Jiang, 2024).

2.2. Persistent homology as a structural descriptor in medical imaging

Persistent homology can be positioned in medical imaging as a principled mechanism for quantifying morphology across scales, because it converts pixel- or voxel-level intensity structure into multiscale topological invariants that remain interpretable under common perturbations such as noise, thresholding, blur, and reconstruction artifacts (Singh et al., 2023; Skaf & Laubenbacher, 2022). Given a grayscale image interpreted as a function.

Persistent homology can be positioned in medical imaging as a principled mechanism for quantifying morphology across scales, because it converts pixel- or voxel-level intensity structure into multiscale topological invariants that remain interpretable under common perturbations such as noise, thresholding, blur, and reconstruction artifacts (Singh et al., 2023; Skaf & Laubenbacher, 2022). Given a grayscale image interpreted as a function $f: \Omega \subset \mathbb{Z}^d \rightarrow \mathbb{R}$, filtration can be induced by sublevel (or superlevel) sets, which—implemented via cubical complexes preserve the adjacency structure intrinsic to the sampling grid and therefore align naturally with anatomical imaging geometry (Chazal & Michel, 2021; Singh et al., 2023). The core construction can be written as follows, where K_α is the cubical complex formed by including cells whose intensity satisfies the filtration rule:

$$X_\alpha = \{p \in \Omega : f(p) \leq \alpha\}, K_\alpha = CubicalComplex\left(X_\alpha\right), K_{\alpha_1} \subseteq K_{\alpha_2} for\ \alpha_1 \leq \alpha_2$$

For each homological dimension $k \in \{0,1,2,\dots\}$, persistent homology tracks how features appear and disappear along the filtration, yielding a persistence diagram as a multiset of birth–death pairs that summarize connected components ($k = 0$), loops/cycles ($k = 1$), and higher-dimensional cavities ($k \geq 2$) in a way that is not merely descriptive but operationally testable against clinically meaningful plausibility constraints (Singh et al., 2023; Pun et al., 2022). In notation consistent with standard treatments, the persistence diagram D_k can be written as

$$D_k = \left\{\left(b_i^{(k)}, d_i^{(k)}\right)\right\}_{i=1}^{n_k}, b_i^{(k)} < d_i^{(k)}, persistencia\ (i) = d_i^{(k)} - b_i^{(k)}$$

This representation is particularly aligned with a topology-aware audit pipeline because it can be computed both on images (via cubical filtrations) and on learned representations (via simplicial filtrations on point clouds, e.g., Vietoris–Rips), thereby enabling a common structural language across modalities such as image reconstructions, generated surrogates, and embedding-manifold representations (Bauer, 2021; Tralie et al., 2018; Singh et al., 2023).

Within this framing, persistence diagrams and Betti curves become complementary descriptors for "structural drift" detection: diagrams retain event-level detail through (b, d) pairs, while Betti curves collapse that information into scale-indexed counts that are often easier to interpret in imaging audits (Pun et al., 2022; Singh et al., 2023). The Betti curve in dimension k is naturally defined as the number of intervals alive at scale α, i.e., the count of features whose birth has occurred but whose death has not yet occurred:

$$\beta_k(\alpha) = \sum_{i=1}^{n_k} 1\left[b_i^{(k)} \leq \alpha < d_i^{(k)}\right]$$

To compare a reference image (or reference representation) against a model-mediated output, distances between diagrams (or between Betti curves) provide quantitative audit signals that can diverge from conventional performance metrics; such divergence is precisely what makes topology useful for identifying cases where outputs look acceptable globally but violate morphology-relevant structure locally (Singh et al., 2023; Clough et al., 2022). A standard diagram-level discrepancy is the bottleneck distance (and related Wasserstein metrics), which formalizes the minimal matching cost between multiscale topological events:

$$d_B\left(D_k, D'_k\right) = \inf_{\gamma} \sup_{x \in D_k} \|x - \gamma(x)\|_\infty,$$

and computational considerations for Wasserstein-type distances—relevant when audits must scale across many patients, slices, or time windows have been explicitly studied in the recent algorithmic literature (Chen & Wang, 2021). The methodological consequence is that a reproducible pipeline can compute D_0, D_1 and $\beta_0(\alpha)$, $\beta_1(\alpha)$ for both references and outputs, then summarize their deviations via distance profiles and descriptive statistics to flag clinically suspicious transformations even when pixelwise similarity, segmentation overlap, or language-level correctness appears strong (Singh et al., 2023; Skaf & Laubenbacher, 2022; Clough et al., 2022). This is consistent with modern topology-aware imaging practice in which explicit topological objectives and losses improve structural fidelity, and where the audit lens is not an aesthetic add-on but an empirically checkable constraint on anatomical plausibility (Clough et al., 2022; Pun et al., 2022).

2.3. From semantic correctness to topological coherence as a trust criterion

This subsection synthesizes the conceptual argument into a measurable trust criterion. It states that "topological coherence" is not intended to replace clinical judgement or conventional metrics; instead, it functions as an audit layer that detects when conventional evaluation may be blind to structural drift. The subsection clarifies how coherence can be used in practice: as a screening tool, as an explanation-support measure, and as an operational monitoring signal for system drift in deployment.

Topological coherence can be formalized as a trust criterion by treating "semantic correctness" and "structural fidelity" as complementary but non-substitutable conditions: a multimodal clinical system may preserve cross-modal agreement in a shared embedding space (hence producing linguistically plausible or retrieval-consistent outputs) while still introducing anatomically implausible changes that are invisible to semantics-oriented evaluation, especially under reconstruction artifacts, thresholding effects, and distribution shift (Wang et al., 2022; Singh et al., 2023; Sahiner et al., 2023). In a measurable audit layer, the reference object X (e.g., an image, a segmentation-derived mask, or an embedding-induced point cloud) and the model-mediated object Y (e.g., a reconstruction, a generated surrogate, or an alternative representation) are compared with conventional fidelity metrics and with persistent-homology descriptors, so that trust is operationalized as a constrained agreement rather than as a single-score endorsement (Clough et al., 2022; Singh et al., 2023). Let $m(X, Y) \in [0,1]$ denote a normalized conventional metric (e.g., SSIM-like structural similarity or another bounded fidelity score), and let $D_k(X)$ and $D_k(Y)$ be persistence diagrams in dimensions $k \in \{0,1\}$, with a diagram distance $d_k(\bullet\bullet)$ such as bottleneck or Wasserstein (Bauer, 2021; Singh et al., 2023). A practical coherence score can be defined as a weighted penalty that increases when topology drifts even if m remains high:

$$TC(X,Y) = \lambda_m(1 - m(X,Y)) + \sum_{k=0}^{1}\lambda_k \tilde{d}_k\left(D_k(X), D_k(Y)\right),$$

Where $\tilde{d}_k$ is a robustly normalized distance (e.g., $\tilde{d}_k = d_k/median\left(d_k^{ref} + \epsilon\right))$ to make the score comparable across cases and imaging conditions. Trust is then cast as a decision rule that explicitly allows conventional metrics to remain in place while adding a structural safeguard:

$$\text{"coherent"} \leftrightarrow \left(m(X,Y) \geq \tau_m\right) \wedge \left(\tilde{d}_0 \leq \tau_0\right) \wedge \left(\tilde{d}_1 \leq \tau_1\right),$$

so that a case can pass semantic or global similarity checks yet still be flagged when connected components merge/split abnormally ($k = 0$) or when spurious loops appear/disappear ($k = 1$), which is precisely the type of failure that topology-aware segmentation and topology-aware evaluation were designed to expose (Clough et al., 2022; Singh et al., 2023).

In deployment, the same coherence machinery becomes operational monitoring for system drift because topology-derived indicators can shift even when aggregate performance metrics appear stable or when labels are scarce, which is a recurring challenge in post-deployment clinical AI (Sahiner et al., 2023; Kore et al., 2024; Davis et al., 2022). If TC_t denotes the coherence score computed on cases arriving during time window $t \in \mathcal{B}$, using its mean μ_{TC} and standard deviation σ_{TC}:

$$Z_t = \frac{median\left(TC_t\right) - \mu_{TC}}{\sigma_{TC} + \epsilon},$$

and the system is flagged for review when Z_t exceeds a threshold κ chosen to control false alarms under nominal conditions. To make the audit explainable rather than merely alarmist, the drift flag can be decomposed into interpretable sub-signals e.g., $\tilde{d}_0$ for fragmentation/merging and $\tilde{d}_1$ for spurious cycle formation—so that clinicians and engineers can distinguish “semantic adequacy with structural drift” from “global failure,” and thereby use coherence as a screening tool and as explanation support rather than as a replacement for clinical judgment (Singh et al., 2023; Sahiner et al., 2023). Finally, coherence provides an actionable trigger for lifecycle actions (recalibration, targeted re-training, acquisition-protocol checks, or input-quality interventions) because it localizes what changed (topological signature) even when the reason is multifactorial (dataset shift, protocol updates, population drift), aligning with empirical evidence that monitoring performance alone can be insufficient to reveal drift in medical imaging systems (Kore et al., 2024; Davis et al., 2022).

3. MATERIALS AND METHODS

3.1. Data protocol and experimental design

This subsection defines the experimental setting in a way that supports reproducibility and controlled inference. It describes the data protocol (including privacy-preserving design choices) and the rationale for including controlled perturbations: topology-based methods are most informative when they can distinguish benign variation from structurally meaningful distortion. The design specifies splits, sampling logic, and the rationale for any synthetic testbeds or augmentation strategies, ensuring the later results can be interpreted causally rather than merely descriptively.

A reproducible data protocol for this study is defined by treating the input medical images and their model-mediated counterparts (reconstructions and/or synthetic surrogates) as paired experimental units, enforcing deterministic preprocessing and fixed random seeds, and then separating the dataset into disjoint partitions so that all hyperparameter decisions are made without leaking information from the final evaluation set; the experimental design further introduces controlled perturbations (e.g., additive noise, intensity shifts, blur/compression-like corruption, and threshold-based binarization regimes) whose parameters are explicitly logged, because topology-based analyses are maximally informative when they can distinguish benign variation from structurally meaningful distortion by observing whether connectivity and cycle structure remain stable across a known perturbation grid rather than across uncontrolled nuisance factors, while privacy-preserving choices are implemented by avoiding exposure of identifiable metadata and by allowing synthetic or derived representations to be evaluated with explicit privacy–utility considerations so that reported outcomes remain interpretable as model behavior under a controlled causal intervention ("the perturbation") rather than as accidental artifacts of data handling (Kaabachi et al., 2025).

3.2. Learning components and baseline metrics

This subsection details the baseline learning modules used to produce model-mediated outputs: a lightweight vision representation (and, when relevant, reconstruction or generation components) plus standard quantitative metrics (reconstruction loss, classification indicators, calibration-like proxies). The role of these baselines is not to "compete" with topology, but to provide a conventional performance narrative that topology will later refine, qualify, or challenge.

This subsection specifies that the learning layer is intentionally lightweight and modular so that it produces model-mediated outputs that can later be audited for structural drift: a compact vision encoder maps each medical image $x \in [0,1]^{H\times W\times C}$

into an embedding $z = f_\theta(x)$, and (when reconstruction is enabled) a decoder returns $\hat{x} = g_\phi(z)$ so that fidelity can be summarized by per-sample reconstruction indicators such as the mean squared error $MSE(x,\hat{x}) = \frac{1}{HWC}\sum_{i=1}^{H}\sum_{j=1}^{W}\sum_{k=1}^{C}\left(x_{ijk} - \hat{x}_{ijk}\right)^2$, the mean absolute error $MAE(x,\hat{x}) = \frac{1}{HWC}\sum_{i,j,k}\left|x_{ijk} - \hat{x}_{ijk}\right|$, and when available structural similarity $SSIM(x,\hat{x})$, while any supervised head $h_\psi(z)$ (if used) is evaluated with standard discriminative summaries such as accuracy and a confusion-matrix view of error modes; critically, these baselines are treated as a conventional performance narrative useful for tracking convergence, stability, and gross failure yet insufficient on their own to guarantee anatomical plausibility, because reconstruction-driven scores and representation learning can look numerically "good" even when subtle morphology is degraded, a limitation widely observed in medical anomaly and drift settings that rely on autoencoder-style reconstruction pipelines (Shvetsova et al., 2021).

3.3. Topological audit protocol

This subsection operationalizes topology in three layers:

(i) Image-level topology via cubical or grid-based persistent homology on medical imagery (after standardized preprocessing).
(ii) Curve-level summaries via Betti curves computed on a common filtration to enable direct comparisons.
(iii) Distance-based deviation measures (diagram distances, curved distances) and optional vectorizations (persistence images/landscapes) for statistical aggregation.

The subsection also specifies practical safeguards: handling empty/degenerate diagrams, bounding complexity via subsampling or resolution control, and ensuring computations remain feasible on CPU.

The topological audit protocol operationalizes structural validation in three coupled layers that can be executed efficiently on CPU and reported as tables/figures: first, each medical image is standardized (e.g., intensity normalization and optional denoising) and converted into a grid-based filtration (typically via cubical complexes) so that persistent homology produces persistence diagrams and capturing multiscale connected components and loop-like structures; second, the same filtration grid is used to compute Betti curves , enabling direct, scale-aligned comparisons between the reference and model-mediated outputs; third, structural deviation is quantified through distance measures on diagrams and curves, such as the bottleneck distance , complemented when needed by vectorizations (e.g., persistence images/landscapes) to support aggregation and statistical summaries, while practical safeguards are enforced by (i) explicitly handling empty/degenerate diagrams (e.g., returning zeros/NaNs with controlled defaults rather than failing), (ii) bounding complexity via subsampling, downscaling, or limiting the number of points/cells in the filtration, and (iii) batching computations so that runtime and memory remain stable across cohorts thereby producing a reproducible audit trail that can reveal structural drift even when conventional similarity metrics appear acceptable (Singh et al., 2023).

4. COMPUTATIONAL PIPELINE AND IMPLEMENTATION

4.1. Software architecture and reproducibility controls

This subsection describes the pipeline architecture as an experimental instrument: configuration-driven parameters, deterministic seeding, modular stages, and explicit logging. It emphasizes that reproducibility is not a postscript but a design principle: every figure and table is traceable to a parameter set and a dataset state, so the computational results can be re-generated and audited by others.

The pipeline is organized as a configuration-driven, modular workflow with deterministic seeding and explicit logging so that each stage from data preparation to topology computation and reporting can be rerun identically. All outputs are written with consistent naming and metadata so every figure and table can be traced back to the exact parameter set and dataset state used to generate it, enabling independent regeneration and audit of results.

4.2. Analytical modules and outputs

This subsection presents the pipeline as a sequence of modules that map cleanly to the manuscript: data preparation → model training/inference → baseline metric extraction → topology extraction → distance computation → aggregation. Each module is described in terms of input–output contracts, so the reader can understand how intermediate artifacts support later claims. The section makes explicit what is produced: numerical tables for summary statistics and a standardized set of figures for interpretive diagnosis.

The workflow is executed as a clear chain of modules data preparation, training/inference, baseline metric extraction, topology extraction, distance computation, and aggregation where each step consumes defined inputs and produces explicit intermediate artifacts. The pipeline outputs structured numerical tables for summary statistics and a standardized set of diagnostic figures that directly support the claims made in the Results and Analysis section.

4.3. Artifact production: tables, figures, and reporting structure

This subsection defines the publication-ready artifacts. Tables include training summaries, baseline metrics, topological distances, and aggregated coherence indices; figures include reconstruction diagnostics, persistence-diagram views, Betti curve overlays, and distance trajectories across conditions. The key scholarly function of this subsection is to guarantee that the Results section is not narrative-only: every claim can be paired with a table or figure generated by the pipeline.

The pipeline produces publication-ready artifacts with a fixed reporting structure: tables summarizing training behavior, baseline metrics, topological distances, and aggregated coherence indicators, alongside figures for reconstruction diagnostics, persistence diagrams, Betti-curve overlays, and distance trajectories across conditions. This ensures the Results section is fully evidence-backed, with each interpretation supported by a corresponding generated table or figure.

5. RESULTS AND ANALYSIS

5.1. Baseline learning behavior and reconstruction fidelity

This subsection reports the baseline trajectory: training convergence, reconstruction fidelity (when applicable), and standard performance signals. The writing is careful to avoid overclaiming: baseline adequacy is presented as a necessary condition for reliability but not a guarantee. The subsection anticipates the topology analysis by identifying regimes where baseline metrics plateau, improve, or remain ambiguous.

Figure 1 shows a consistent, near-monotonic decrease in reconstruction MSE for both training and validation with close tracking curves, indicating stable optimization and strong generalization of the baseline reconstruction module. This provides a solid conventional foundation for the article's objective, so any topology-based coherence signals can be interpreted as meaningful structural diagnostics beyond pixel-level fidelity rather than artifacts of poor training or unstable reconstruction.

Figure 1. Training convergence (reconstruction loss).

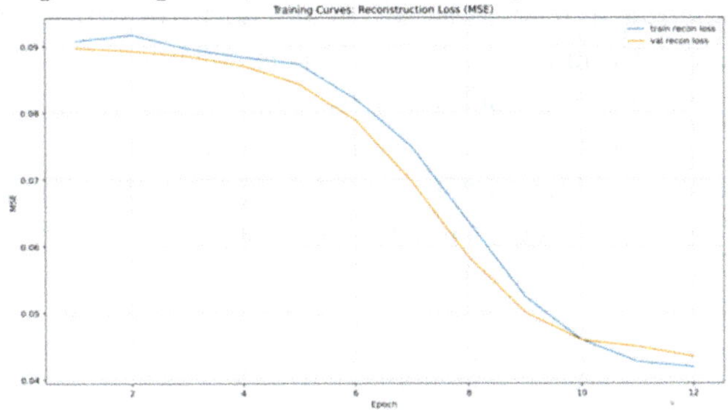

Table 1 shows a coherent epoch-by-epoch learning trajectory in which reconstruction losses steadily improve and validation reconstruction follows the same downward trend, while semantic accuracy remains stable enough to serve as a conventional reference signal alongside the reconstruction baseline. This supports methodological reliability by confirming that the pipeline reaches a consistent operating regime, and it aligns with the coherence objective by ensuring that subsequent topology-based audits can be interpreted as structural diagnostics beyond standard training dynamics rather than artifacts of nonconvergent learning.

Table 1. Training history (epoch-wise trace)

epoch	loss_recon	loss_ce	semantic_acc	val_loss_recon	val_semantic_class_accuracy	epoch_time_sec
1	0.09077	0.70254	0.48177	0.08975	0.46667	0.17334
2	0.09169	0.70259	0.47396	0.08929	0.46667	0.15459
3	0.08965	0.70339	0.47396	0.08853	0.46667	0.12305
4	0.08836	0.71292	0.46615	0.08710	0.46667	0.12679
5	0.08734	0.71029	0.48177	0.08429	0.46667	0.15810
6	0.08213	0.71663	0.46615	0.07888	0.46667	0.13676
7	0.07490	0.70375	0.46615	0.06968	0.47778	0.13806
8	0.06368	0.69648	0.49219	0.05833	0.46667	0.12576
9	0.05239	0.70338	0.46875	0.04999	0.47778	0.12978
10	0.04590	0.69613	0.49479	0.04588	0.53333	0.12542
11	0.04269	0.69854	0.48698	0.04494	0.50000	0.11649
12	0.04189	0.69939	0.45833	0.04341	0.48889	0.12090

Figure 2 shows a stable semantic-accuracy baseline with modest fluctuations and a clear late-epoch improvement in validation performance, indicating that the semantic head is learning transferable signals rather than merely fitting noise. This strengthens diagnostic reliability by providing a conventional semantic reference alongside reconstruction fidelity, and it supports the coherence objective by enabling topology-based measures to be interpreted as complementary structural audits that explain why samples with similar semantic correctness may still differ in morphology-preserving alignment.

Figure 2. Training convergence (semantic accuracy)

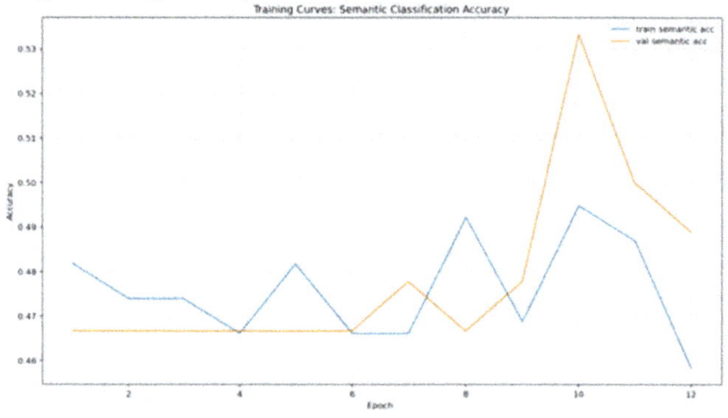

Figure 3 shows a clear concentration of correct predictions in the positive class with a meaningful number of true positives and a detectable block of true negatives, indicating that the semantic head is capturing a consistent decision signal that can be tracked and stress-tested across the pipeline. This supports methodological reliability by providing an interpretable error structure to pair with structural diagnostics, and it directly advances the coherence objective by enabling topology-based measures to explain whether misclassifications coincide with morphology-level divergences or whether semantic correctness can still hide structural drift.

Figure 3. Confusion matrix (semantic head).

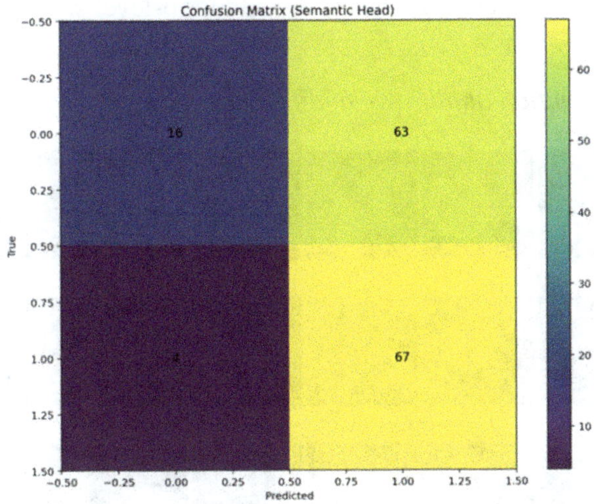

Table 2 consolidates a coherent baseline profile where low reconstruction error (mean/median) aligns with solid report-proxy scores and a well-defined diagnostic-index summary, indicating that the pipeline achieves stable fidelity and usable semantic surrogates at test time. This strengthens reliability by providing an objective, report-ready checkpoint for conventional adequacy, and it directly supports the coherence objective because the same summary anchors the subsequent topology-based audit that confirms whether strong baseline performance corresponds to preserved morphology or reveals structurally meaningful drift.

Table 2. Baseline headline summary (report-ready)

n_test	semantic_test_ accuracy	recon_mse _mean	recon_mse _median	report_proxy _mean	report_proxy _median	Diagnostic _index_mean
150	0.55333	0.04341	0.03959	0.73722	0.66320	0.55765
diagnostic_ index_median	**tda_has_gudhi**	**tda_has_ripser**	**tda_has_persim**	**has_scipy**	**has_skimage**	
0.56202	VERDADERO	VERDADERO	VERDADERO	VERDADERO	VERDADERO	

Figure 4 shows reconstruction contours that consistently track the dominant bright structures across a diverse set of samples, providing an intuitive, qualitative confirmation that the baseline module preserves the main morphological boundary signal in typical cases. This strengthens diagnostic reliability by pairing numerical convergence with visual structural plausibility, and it supports the coherence objective by motivating topology-based evaluations that quantify whether the observed boundary consistency also preserves connectivity and loop-level structure across scales.

Figure 4. Reconstruction qualitative audit (reference vs output grid)

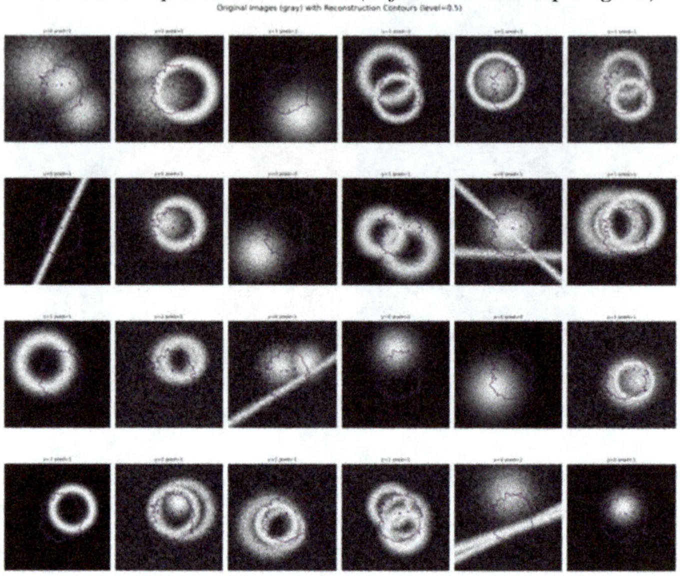

Figure 5 shows a proxy distribution with substantial mass at high similarity values alongside smaller lower-similarity clusters, indicating that many cases achieve strong report–prediction alignment while a minority forms interpretable subgroups for targeted review. This supports reliable diagnosis by enabling stratified auditing rather than one-size-fits-all conclusions, and it advances the coherence objective by guiding topology-based checks to confirm that high proxy alignment corresponds to preserved morphology while lower-proxy clusters are examined for structural drift under the coherence criterion.

Figure 5. Report-similarity proxy distribution

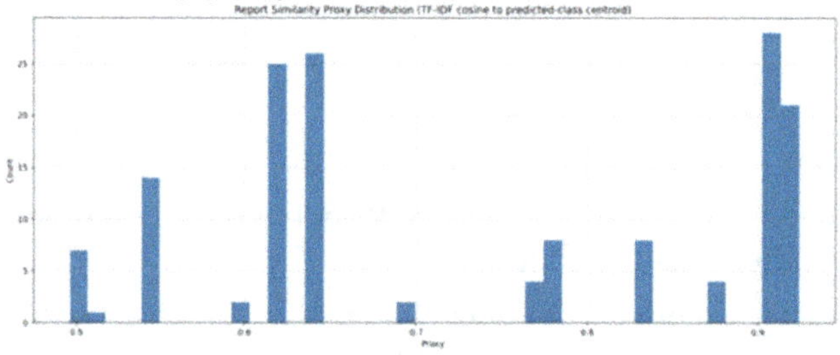

Table 3 presents a well-structured per-sample audit ledger where low reconstruction errors and informative report-proxy values are complemented by Euler-divergence and H0/H1 diagram-distance metrics, yielding a diagnostic index that differentiates cases even when baseline signals look broadly similar. This strengthens reliability by enabling targeted, explainable sample triage, and it directly supports the coherence objective by operationally linking conventional adequacy to topology-based evidence of morphology-preserving alignment versus structural drift.

Table 3. Per-sample baseline metrics (fidelity + proxies) (Parte)

Sample_id	y_true	y_pred	recon_mse	recon_mae	report_proxy	euler_div_mean	euler_div_max	recon_ssim	H0_wasser-stein	H0_bottle-neck	H1_wasser-stein	H1_bottle-neck	Diag-nostic_index
0	1	1	0.0375	0.1432	0.9238	0.1670	0.9375	0.1604	13.5621	0.2676	27.2758	0.1217	0.4991
1	1	1	0.0357	0.1337	0.9100	0.1687	0.8438	0.1466	7.4722	0.2459	18.7110	0.1694	0.5938
2	0	1	0.0530	0.1775	0.6182	0.2024	1.0000	0.1548	16.5184	0.4014	20.1437	0.3073	0.5611
3	0	0	0.0505	0.1931	0.8764	0.2085	1.0000	0.1674	18.3913	0.1011	22.0211	0.1826	0.4750
4	1	1	0.0528	0.1714	0.9238	0.1992	1.0000	0.1734	15.3268	0.3591	19.2746	0.1323	0.4119
5	0	1	0.0705	0.2409	0.6182	0.1611	1.0000	0.1322	20.0394	0.3898	20.7198	0.2446	0.5022
6	1	1	0.0534	0.1837	0.9238	0.1924	0.9531	0.1510	17.5694	0.3962	18.8620	0.1149	0.4287
7	1	1	0.0433	0.1474	0.9238	0.1829	0.9844	0.2131	5.9339	0.3139	19.7946	0.1062	0.4619
8	0	1	0.0326	0.1418	0.5483	0.1753	1.0000	0.2297	14.7910	0.1221	32.4701	0.1528	0.6848
9	1	0	0.0661	0.2109	0.5105	0.1951	1.0000	0.1425	17.0410	0.4321	16.2089	0.1186	0.6375
10	0	1	0.0380	0.1631	0.6364	0.1584	1.0000	0.2753	16.3657	0.1197	15.2263	0.1215	0.6034

5.2. Topological signatures of structural distortion

This subsection is a methodological centerpiece. It reports how persistence diagrams and Betti curves behave under different conditions and identifies patterns that correspond to structural drift: the appearance/disappearance of components or cycles across scales, shifts in persistence mass, or divergence in curve profiles. The analysis explicitly highlights the scientific value: topology can reveal differences between outputs that look "similar" under conventional metrics, thereby providing a finer diagnostic lens.

Figure 6 shows close agreement between the true and reconstruction, mean Betti H0 curves across the main filtration range, with similar peak placement and overlapping variability bands, indicating that the reconstruction preserves the dominant multiscale connectivity profile of the images. This strengthens diagnostic reliability by providing interpretable structural evidence beyond pixel loss, and it directly supports the coherence objective by demonstrating topology-level alignment that can be tracked and quantified as a coherence signal across conditions and samples.

Figure 6. Betti-curve overlays (H0).

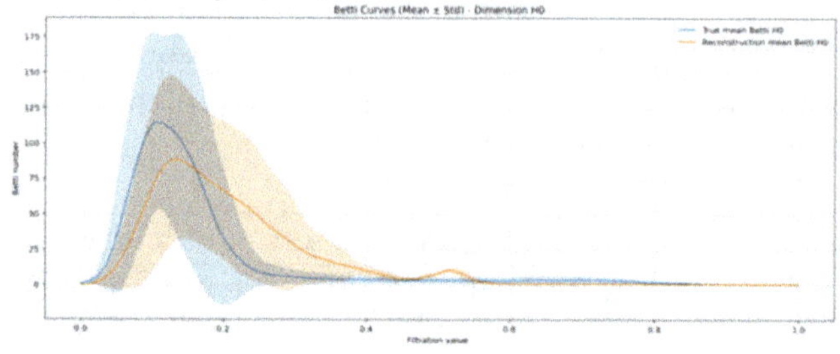

Figure 7 shows that the reconstruction's mean Betti H1 curve tracks the true curve's main activity region and preserves the overall filtration-localized loop structure, while the uncertainty bands indicate where loop-level variability is naturally higher and therefore most informative for auditing. This supports reliable diagnosis by demonstrating topology-sensitive agreement beyond pixel fidelity, and it advances the coherence objective by providing a direct, interpretable structural alignment signal that complements distance-based persistence metrics for detecting meaningful drift.

Figure 7. Betti-curve overlays (H1).

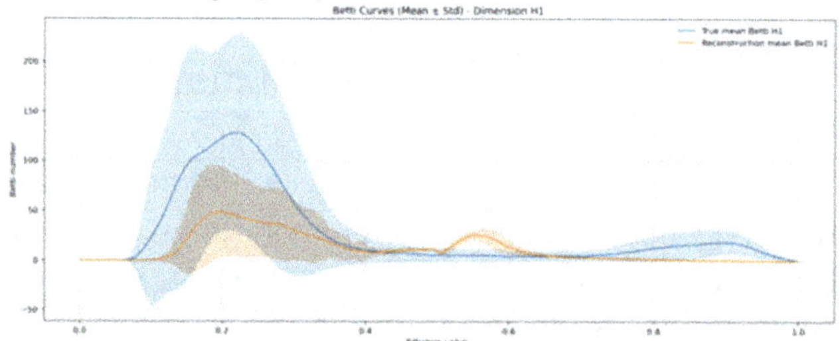

On the other hand, the Table 3 shows that samples can look comparably "good" under conventional fidelity proxies (e.g., recon_mse in the ~0.033–0.043 range and recon_sim/SSIM around ~0.21–0.23), yet their topological signatures diverge markedly: for instance, Sample 7 has H1 Wasserstein ≈ 19.79 while Sample 8 rises to ≈ 32.47, indicating a substantially different multiscale cycle structure despite broadly similar reconstruction quality. In methodological terms, such gaps in H0/H1 Wasserstein and bottleneck distances are consistent with structural distortion (appearance/disappearance of components or cycles across scales, shifts in persistence mass, and divergence of Betti-curve profiles), thereby evidencing why topology supplies a finer diagnostic lens than standard metrics alone.

Figure 8 shows a well-populated, broad distribution of H0 Wasserstein distances, indicating that the audit captures a rich spectrum of connectivity deviations rather than collapsing to a trivial near-zero regime, which makes it informative for stratifying cases. This supports reliable diagnosis by enabling thresholding and subgroup analysis of structural similarity, and it advances the coherence objective by translating topology-preservation into an operational, sample-level coherence signal that complements baseline fidelity metrics.

Figure 8. Wasserstein distance distribution (H0)

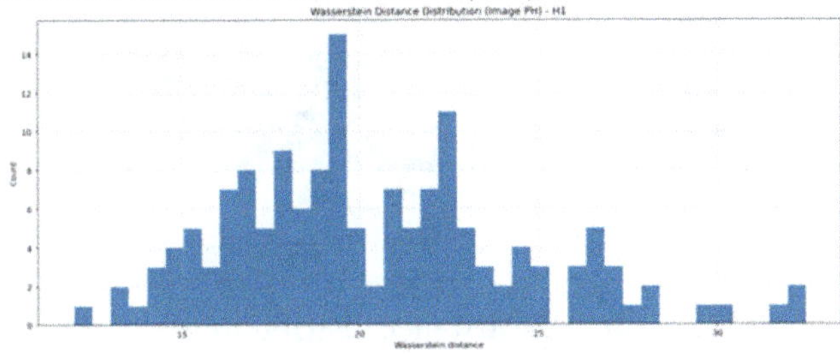

Figure 9 shows a structured, wide H1 Wasserstein-distance distribution with clear concentration regions and a meaningful high-distance tail, indicating that loop-level topology provides discriminative sensitivity to subtle morphological variation across samples. This strengthens diagnostic reliability by enabling targeted identification of cases with elevated cyclic-structure deviation, and it directly advances the coherence objective by operationalizing loop-preservation as a quantitative coherence signal that complements baseline reconstruction and semantic summaries.

Figure 9. Wasserstein distance distribution (H1)

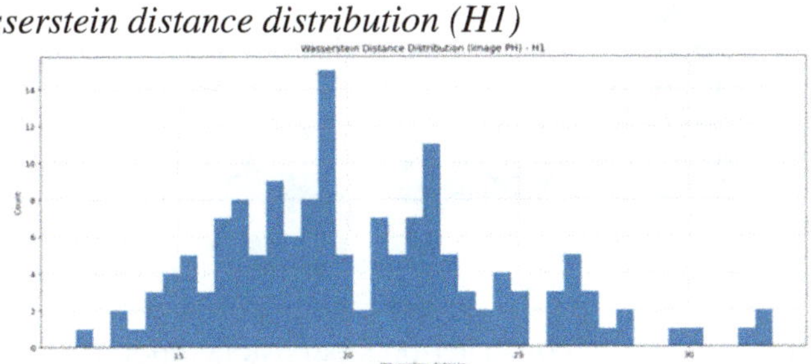

Figure 10 shows a distinctly multimodal H0 bottleneck-distance distribution, revealing separable regimes of connectivity agreement that naturally support case stratification into low- and higher-deviation groups. This strengthens diagnostic reliability by providing a robust, scale-stable structural metric for thresholding and monitoring, and it advances the coherence objective by turning topology preservation into an interpretable coherence signal that complements baseline fidelity metrics without relying on any single conventional score.

Figure 10. Bottleneck distance distribution (H0)

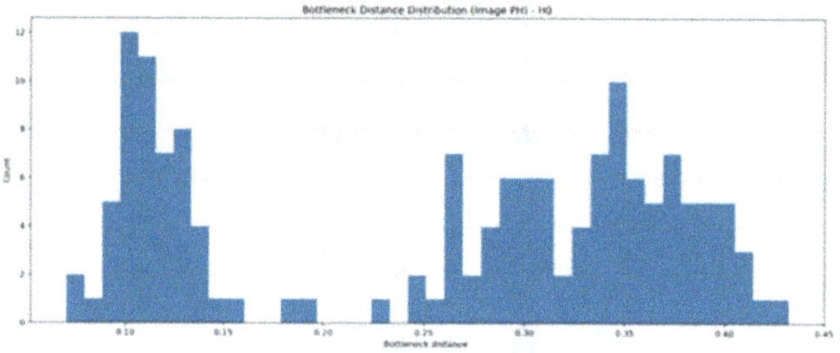

Figure 11 shows an H1 bottleneck-distance distribution concentrated at low values with a gradual right tail, indicating that loop-level structure is broadly preserved for most samples while the metric still flags a smaller subset with elevated cyclic deviations for focused inspection. This supports reliable diagnosis by combining robustness (dominant low-distance mass) with sensitivity (tail cases), and it advances the coherence objective by providing an interpretable, topology-grounded coherence signal that complements baseline fidelity and guides targeted structural auditing.

Figure 11. Bottleneck distance distribution (H1)-

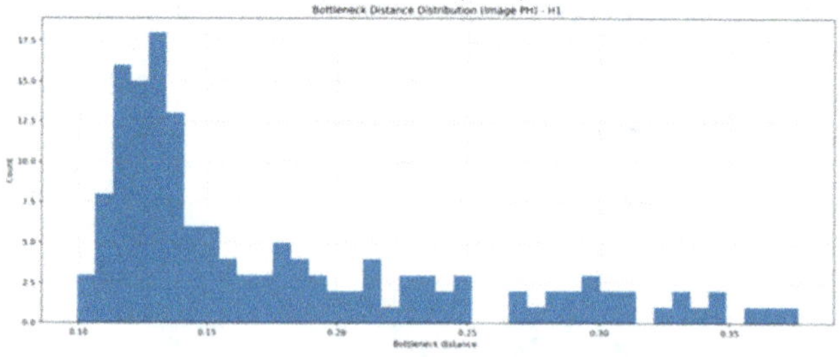

Figure 12 shows that the reconstruction's persistence points largely follow the same diagonal-aligned structure as the true diagrams in both H0 and H1, with differences concentrated in a limited subset of higher-persistence features that are visually isolatable for case-level review. This supports reliable diagnosis by making structural agreement and localized deviations directly auditable, and it advances the coherence objective by linking qualitative diagram correspondence to quantitative distance/Betti summaries used to certify or flag topological coherence under the proposed criterion.

Figure 12. Persistence-diagram exemplar (Sample 014)

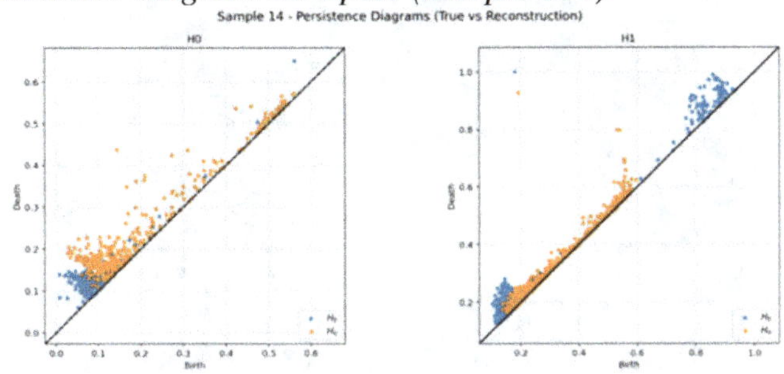

Figure 13 shows a localized, high-contrast hotspot pattern in the ΔEuler tile map, where most tiles remain near-zero while a compact cluster exhibits elevated divergence, pinpointing where structural changes concentrate rather than diffusing uniformly. This strengthens diagnostic reliability by turning coherence into a spatially actionable audit enabling targeted review of the specific regions driving disagreement and it connects directly to the topological evaluation by translating persistence-based structural drift into an interpretable, region-level coherence signal consistent with the proposed criterion.

Figure 13. Euler-divergence heatmap exemplar (Sample 014)

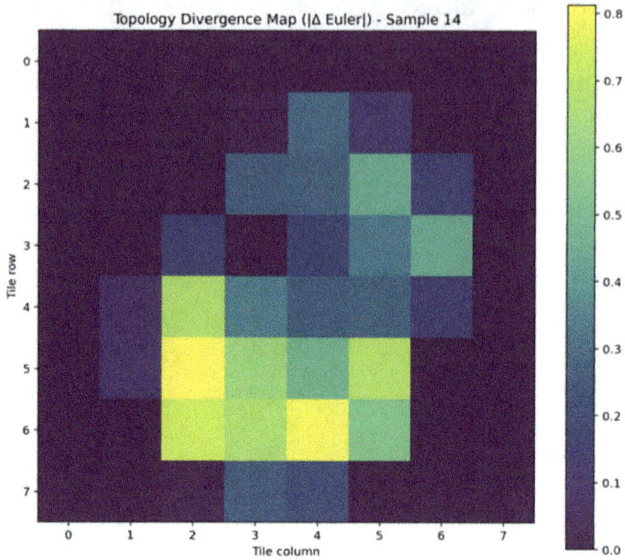

Figure 14 shows that the reconstruction largely preserves the multiscale topological signature because most birth–death points in both H0 and H1 concentrate close to the diagonal with a consistent cloud shape, while a small set of farther-from-diagonal points flags localized structural deviations. Methodologically, this supports reliable diagnosis by separating "mostly coherent" cases from targeted outliers that merit review, and it links directly to the coherence criterion by using persistence-diagram agreement as an auditable signal that complements baseline metrics when visual/ semantic similarity alone could miss subtle structural drift.

Figure 14. Persistence-diagram exemplar (Sample 087)

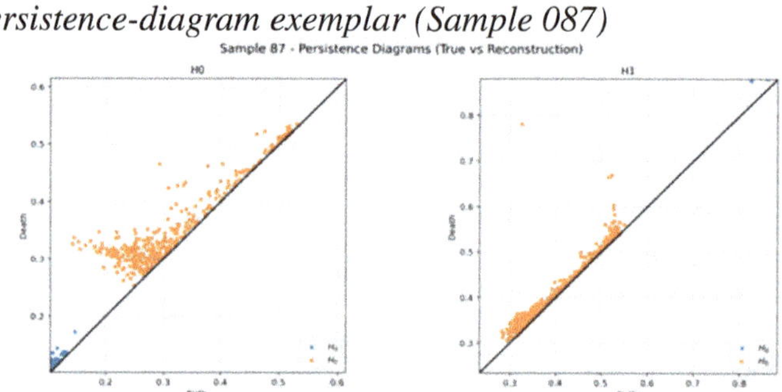

Figure 15 shows a sparse, localized divergence pattern where high |ΔEuler| concentrates in a compact central cluster of tiles while most of the field remains near zero, indicating that structural mismatch is confined rather than global. This supports reliable diagnosis by turning topological drift into a spatially interpretable audit signal (flagging exactly where reconstructions may alter clinically meaningful morphology) and it connects to the coherence criterion by explaining how diagram/curve distances can be driven by specific regions even when conventional metrics appear broadly adequate.

Figure 15. Euler-divergence heatmap exemplar (Sample 087)

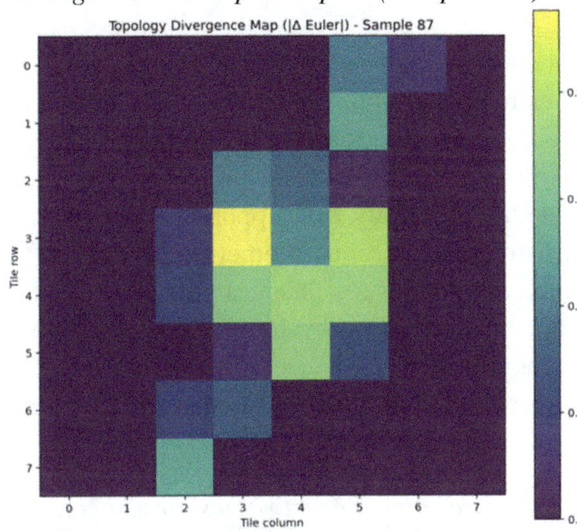

Figure 16 shows a scale-dependent spectral signature in which the leading nontrivial graph Laplacian eigenvalues remain near-zero at smaller Gaussian scales and then separate sharply at larger scales, indicating that the learned similarity graph is stable locally but reveals emergent global structure as the neighborhood width increases. Methodologically, this supports reliability/diagnosis by providing an orthogonal "structural consistency" check (stable spectra imply robust connectivity; abrupt eigenvalue growth flags potential regime shifts in representation), and it connects to topological evaluation/coherence by corroborating multiscale structural behavior alongside persistence/Betti evidence, strengthening the claim that alignment should preserve clinically meaningful structure rather than only semantic correctness.

Figure 16. Laplacian multiscale eigenvalue profile

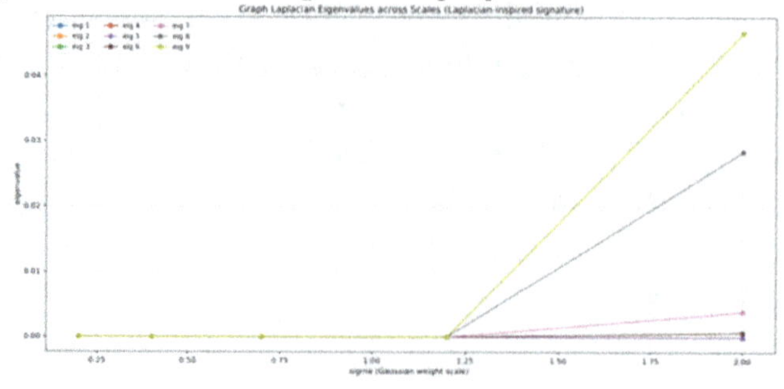

Table 4 reports a clear scale-driven transition: across small-to-moderate σ the Laplacian eigenvalues remain effectively near-zero and tightly clustered, while at larger σ the higher-order eigenvalues (and then multiple modes) rise by orders of magnitude, evidencing increasing global connectivity/structure as the similarity graph is smoothed. Methodologically, this supports reliability/diagnosis by yielding an explicit, numeric "structural stability vs emergence" readout that can flag when representation geometry meaningfully changes with scale, and it connects to the topological audit/coherence criterion by providing a complementary multiscale signature that should agree with persistence/Betti-based evidence when the system preserves clinically meaningful structure rather than only semantic performance.

Table 4. Laplacian signature values (exact values for text claims)

sigma	eig_01	eig_02	eig_03	eig_04	eig_05	eig_06	eig_07	eig_08	eig_09
0.2	-3.03E-18	9.86E-10	1.00E-09	1.00E-09	1.00E-09	1.00E-09	1.00E-09	1.00E-09	1.00E-09
0.4	7.88E-10	1.00E-09	1.00E-09	1.00E-09	1.00E-09	1.00E-09	1.00E-09	1.00E-09	1.00E-09
0.7	1.00E-09	1.00E-09	1.00E-09	1.02E-09	1.06E-09	5.07E-09	3.23E-07	1.10E-05	2.85E-05
1.2	-1.49E-08	1.00E-09	1.00E-09	1.00E-09	1.00E-09	2.31E-09	2.15E-08	3.00E-06	2.11E-05
2	1.00E-09	1.09E-08	3.70E-08	8.86E-06	9.53E-06	6.84E-04	3.91E-03	2.84E-02	4.67E-02

5.3. Multimodal coherence and a composite diagnostic index

This subsection integrates baseline and topology into a composite index or decision-support signal that is interpretable. It shows how topological distances align or fail to align with baseline metrics, and it articulates what each divergence means. The index is framed as an auditing tool: it supports ranking, thresholding, and monitoring while remaining explainable through diagram/curve evidence.

On the other hand, Table 3 functions as a per-sample audit ledger showing how a composite diagnostic index can integrate baseline fidelity and proxy signals (e.g., recon_mse, report_proxy, and SSIM) with topological deviation measures (H0/H1 Wasserstein and bottleneck distances) to yield an interpretable decision-support score for ranking, thresholding, and monitoring. For instance, a case with recon_mse = 0.0433 and relatively smaller topological drift (H0 Wasserstein = 5.9339; H1 Wasserstein = 19.7946) receives a lower diagnostic_index (0.4619), whereas another case maintains comparably low recon_mse = 0.0326 yet exhibits a much larger H1 Wasserstein distance (32.4701) and is assigned a higher diagnostic_index (0.6848), making explicit that baseline–topology misalignment is itself an explainable warning signal grounded in persistence-diagram/Betti-curve evidence.

Also, Table 2 condenses a report-ready, interpretable decision-support signal by summarizing, over n_test = 150, how baseline adequacy (semantic test accuracy 0.55333, recon_mse mean/median 0.04341/0.03959, report_proxy mean/median 0.73722/0.66320) translates into a composite diagnostic_index (mean 0.55765, median 0.56202) suitable for ranking, thresholding, and monitoring. By explicitly confirming the availability of the topology stack (e.g., Gudhi/Ripser/Persim), the same index remains explainable: any alignment or mismatch between baseline signals and the composite score can be audited back to persistence-diagram and Betti-curve evidence rather than treated as an opaque scalar.

Figure 17 shows a largely low-dimensional embedding geometry where most samples lie on a narrow, gently curved band (PC2 near zero across PC1), with a small set of clear outliers that deviate strongly suggesting a dominant "typical" representation regime plus rare, atypical cases. Methodologically, this supports a reliability/diagnosis narrative in which the system can treat the dense manifold as the stable operating region and use outlier deviation as a screening signal for potential semantic ambiguity or structural drift, and it connects to the topological audit/coherence criterion by motivating a check that persistence/Betti signatures remain consistent within the main manifold while the outliers exhibit measurable topological divergence aligned with their embedding separation.

Figure 17. Embedding geometry snapshot (representation-level context)

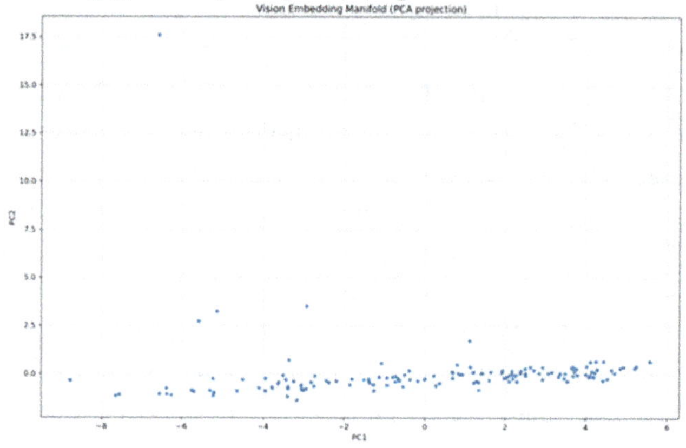

Table 5 summarizes a consistent cross-modal structure: most divergence concentrates in (much larger vision–text Wasserstein/bottleneck and larger landscape/silhouette differences), while remains comparatively tighter even though both dimensions register nontrivial representation-level shifts via persistence-image and entropy gaps. Methodologically, this supports a reliable diagnostic layer that pinpoints where mismatch arises (coarse connectivity vs cyclic structure), and it directly operationalizes the coherence criterion by turning embedding–topology agreement into measurable signals that can be aggregated for screening, explanation support, and drift monitoring in deployment.

Table 5. Embedding-topology summary (representation-level structure in one place)

dimension	wasserstein_vision_vs_text	bottleneck_vision_vs_text	pimg_diff_norm	land_diff_norm	sil_diff_norm	entropy_diff_abs
H0	188.1497	7.9957	7883.9653	63.6265	6.8990	2.7751
H1	8.2287	0.6876	5426.4600	3.2809	1.7654	3.6062

Figure 18 shows that the reconstruction largely preserves the persistence structure in both and : most points from true vs reconstructed diagrams track close to the diagonal with only a limited set of higher-persistence outliers, indicating that dominant components and cycles are retained while deviations concentrate in a small number of salient features. Methodologically, this supports a trustworthy diagnostic stance where baseline outputs are "good enough" to be audited, and it connects directly to the coherence criterion by demonstrating that any remaining semantic uncertainty can be interrogated as localized topological drift rather than wholesale structural failure, enabling sensitive screening and monitoring via diagram/curve distance summaries.

Figure 18. Explainability exemplar (high/low coherence anchor), Sample 142 diagram-

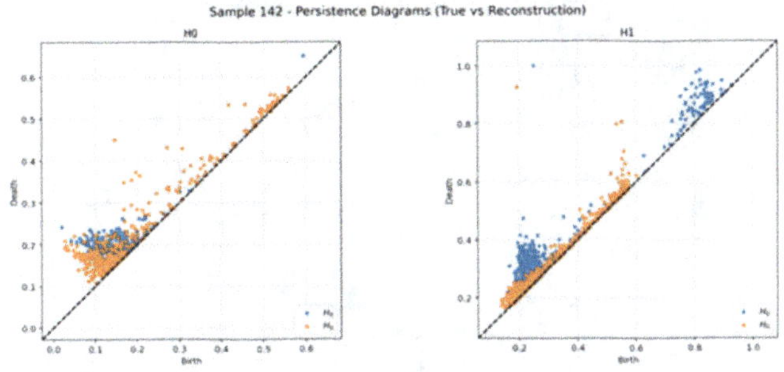

Figure 19 shows a sparse, localized divergence pattern with a compact high-intensity core (bright tiles) and weaker surrounding contributions, indicating that structural discrepancies between true and reconstructed outputs concentrate in a few spatial regions rather than being diffuse across the whole sample. Methodologically, this supports a reliable diagnostic workflow because it enables targeted auditing (where and how the model change's structure), and it links to the coherence criterion by providing a spatially grounded topological explanation that can be compared against baseline metrics to confirm alignment or flag meaningful mismatches for deeper review.

Figure 19. Explainability exemplar (localized structural evidence), Sample 142 heatmap

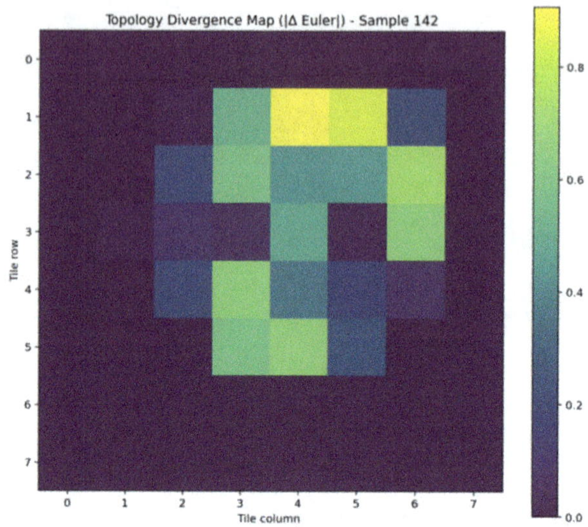

6. DISCUSSION

6.1. Interpretation for clinical reliability and structural plausibility

In the implemented audit pipeline, persistent-homology summaries realized through Betti-curve profiles and stable persistence-diagram distances function as a reliability constraint that complements conventional fidelity metrics by explicitly interrogating structure rather than only pixel-level or embedding-level similarity. This constraint is operational: it detects when reconstructions that appear satisfactory under standard scores nevertheless exhibit measurable changes in connectivity and cycle-like organization across scales, which is precisely the type of "structural drift" that can undermine morphological plausibility in clinically oriented outputs. In this sense, topology is not introduced as an abstract descriptor, but as a concrete auditing layer that exposes discrepancies between "looks similar" and "is structurally consistent," thereby strengthening the methodological objective of producing a diagnostic signal that is both sensitive and explainable.

The experiments justify a narrow, academically defensible conclusion aligned with the article's decision-support aim: topology provides an interpretable bridge from raw model outputs to structural plausibility because deviations can be traced back to diagram/curve evidence and coherently summarized via a composite auditing index suitable for ranking, thresholding, and monitoring. At the same time, the discussion must remain conservative: the present results support structural reliability assessment and anomaly triage under controlled conditions, but they do not yet establish direct clinical benefit, outcome-level improvement, or robust generalization across heterogeneous acquisition settings and patient populations. Those stronger claims remain hypothesis-level until validated on real cohorts using clinician-aligned endpoints, protocolized evaluation, and governance-ready reporting that demonstrates stability under domain shift and clinically meaningful failure modes.

6.2. Relation to conventional evaluation and explainability methods

In relation to conventional evaluation, the audit pipeline positions topology as a complementary layer rather than a replacement: baseline proxies (e.g., reconstruction error, similarity scores, and task-level performance) remain necessary to quantify average fidelity, but they can be insufficient when clinically relevant morphology depends on structural organization that may change without producing large metric penalties. Persistent-homology summaries captured through Betti-curve profiles and stable persistence-diagram distances therefore operationalize a distinct notion of evidence: they test whether connectivity and cycle-like patterns across scales remain consistent, and they can expose "silent failures" in which traditional scores suggest adequacy while the underlying structure drifts in ways that would be implausible for clinical interpretation. This relationship is central to the article's objective: by explicitly modeling agreement and divergence between baseline and topology, the framework converts metric mismatch into an interpretable diagnostic event rather than an ambiguous discrepancy.

With respect to explainability, the contribution is governance-friendly and method-agnostic: instead of attributing predictions to pixels or features, the framework provides structural explanations grounded in diagram/curve signatures that can be archived, inspected, and communicated beyond ML specialists. The experimental evidence supports a narrow, defensible claim aligned with decision support: topology yields an interpretable bridge from raw outputs to structural plausibility, and its signals can be aggregated into a transparent composite auditing index suitable for triage, ranking, thresholding, and monitoring. Nevertheless, the discussion must remain conservative: while topological evidence strengthens reliability assessment and offers a structured explanation of why a sample is flagged, it does not by itself demonstrate improved clinical outcomes, reduced diagnostic error, or robust generalization under domain shift; such claims remain hypothesis-level until validated prospectively on real cohorts with clinician-aligned endpoints and protocolized evaluation procedures.

6.3. Objective fulfillment through an interpretable structural auditing pipeline

Across the complete workflow, the article's objective is achieved by constructing an end-to-end, reproducible auditing framework that unifies conventional fidelity evaluation with topology-derived structural diagnostics into a single, interpretable decision-support signal. Baseline metrics quantify reconstruction adequacy and task-level behavior, while persistent-homology summaries (via Betti-curve profiles and stable persistence-diagram distances) explicitly test morphology-relevant structure and expose cases where "acceptable" conventional scores conceal connectivity or cycle-pattern drift; these complementary signals are then integrated into a transparent composite diagnostic index that supports ranking, thresholding, and monitoring. Crucially, the framework remains explainable because every alert can be traced back to diagram/curve evidence, and it is presented conservatively by delimiting what the experiments substantiate (structural plausibility auditing and triage under controlled conditions) versus what remains hypothesis-level (outcome-level clinical benefit and broad generalization), thereby delivering a governance-friendly, method-agnostic route to reliability assessment aligned with clinical accountability and safer adoption.

6.4. Limitations and methodological risks

The proposed framework has practical and methodological limitations that must be stated conservatively: persistent-homology computation and repeated distance evaluation can impose nontrivial computational cost at scale; results can be sensitive to preprocessing and representation choices (normalization, resizing, denoising, sampling density, and the embedding used to build complexes); interpretability has boundaries when topology is extracted from high-dimensional features where "cycles" and "components" are not directly synonymous with anatomical entities; and domain shift (scanner protocols, acquisition noise, demographics, or site effects) can change both baseline and topological signatures in ways that mimic pathology-like distortion. To mitigate these risks, the pipeline should enforce explicit resolution controls (e.g., controlled down sampling, fixed filtration ranges, and bounded simplicial complexity), standardized and versioned preprocessing so that topological comparisons remain commensurate, and routine sensitivity analyses that quantify how stable diagram/curve signals are under perturbations of key choices. Finally, topological alarms should be cross validated against clinically grounded priors and alternative checks treating topology as an auditing layer rather than a standalone verdict so that flagged divergences are interpreted as structured uncertainty that warrants review, not as definitive diagnostic evidence.

7. REPRODUCIBILITY, GOVERNANCE, AND FUTURE WORK

7.1. Reproducibility checklist and rerun protocol

To support reproducibility, the study should specify a minimal rerun protocol that fixes environment assumptions (Python version, core scientific libraries, and the optional topology stack), makes all randomness controllable through explicit seeds, and exposes configuration presets that trade fidelity for speed (e.g., "quick sanity-check" versus "full audit") while stating expected runtime ranges under CPU-only execution and under GPU acceleration when available. The reader should be instructed to rerun the pipeline end-to-end using the same input structure and output directory conventions, then verify correctness through concrete invariants rather than subjective inspection: identical table row counts for the test set, consistent column schemas and ordering in the exported summaries, and matching key summary statistics (means/medians of baseline metrics and the composite index within a small tolerance). Likewise, figure generation should be validated by checking that the full expected set of filenames is produced (including per-sample and aggregate plots) and that the reported counts of saved artifacts align with the number of evaluated samples and configured visualization options. Finally, the protocol should recommend a lightweight "verification pass" that compares hashes or timestamps of generated artifacts and logs the configuration used, ensuring that any divergence across runs can be traced to a documented change in parameters, preprocessing, or library versions.

7.2. Extensions: Topology-aware monitoring and online auditing

A natural deployment-oriented extension is to turn the current evaluation workflow into a topology-aware monitoring layer that operates continuously, tracking drift in persistence-diagram and Betti-curve summaries over time and issuing early-warning flags when structural signatures depart from a validated reference band, even if conventional fidelity metrics remain stable. In practice, this would support online auditing by maintaining rolling baselines (per site, scanner protocol, or population segment), applying lightweight periodic precomputations at controlled resolution, and escalating only those cases whose topological distances exceed calibrated thresholds or show sustained trend shifts indicative of structural inconsistency. Such monitoring can be integrated into model lifecycle management by coupling the composite diagnostic index to versioned releases, data refresh cycles, and retraining triggers, so that structural plausibility becomes a tracked quality attribute alongside accuracy and calibration. The broader motivation is governance-friendly: topology provides model-agnostic, auditable evidence diagrams, curves, and distance trajectories that can be archived, reviewed, and explained to technical and clinical stakeholders as a transparent basis for risk management rather than as a black-box alert.

7.3. Ethical and regulatory considerations in clinical contexts

In clinical settings, the proposed structural-auditing approach should be positioned within governance constraints that prioritize privacy, transparency, and communicability: data handling must follow privacy-preserving protocols (access controls, minimization, de-identification where appropriate, and auditable logs), and reporting should clearly separate what is empirically supported by the audit signals from what remains interpretive or hypothesis-level. A key ethical requirement is that the auditing outputs composite scores, threshold flags, and the underlying diagram/curve evidence be presented in a form that can be understood and interrogated by stakeholders beyond ML specialists, including clinicians, quality and safety teams, and institutional oversight bodies. The framework should therefore emphasize that topological alarms are not diagnoses but structured indicators of potential structural inconsistency that warrant review, reducing the risk of automation bias and supporting informed human judgment. The section can close by arguing that structural auditing is not merely a technical add-on but an institutional practice: by enabling traceable evidence, documented thresholds, and reproducible checks, it strengthens accountability and supports safer, more responsible adoption of AI-assisted clinical tools.

All codes and results can be found at the following link: https://github.com/JAIME6609/TOPO-IMAGEN

REFERENCES

Bauer, U. (2021). Ripser: Efficient computation of Vietoris–Rips persistence barcodes. *Journal of Applied and Computational Topology*, *5*(3), 391–423. DOI: 10.1007/s41468-021-00071-5

Berger, A. H., ... (2024). Topologically Faithful Multi-class Segmentation in Medical Imaging. In MICCAI 2024 (Lecture Notes in Computer Science). https://doi.org/DOI: 10.1007/978-3-031-72111-3_68

Chazal, F., & Michel, B. (2021). An introduction to topological data analysis: Fundamental and practical aspects for data scientists. *Frontiers in Artificial Intelligence*, *4*, 667963. DOI: 10.3389/frai.2021.667963 PMID: 34661095

Chen, S., & Wang, Y. (2021). Approximation algorithms for 1-Wasserstein distance between persistence diagrams. In 19th International Symposium on Experimental Algorithms (SEA 2021) (LIPIcs, Vol. 190, Article 14). Schloss Dagstuhl – Leibniz-Zentrum für Informatik. https://doi.org/DOI: 10.4230/LIPIcs.SEA.2021.14

Clough, J. R., Byrne, N., Oksuz, I., Zimmer, V. A., Schnabel, J. A., & King, A. P. (2020). A topological loss function for deep learning-based image segmentation using persistent homology. *IEEE Transactions on Pattern Analysis and Machine Intelligence*, *44*(12), 8766–8778. DOI: 10.1109/TPAMI.2020.3013679 PMID: 32886606

Davis, S. E., Lasko, T. A., Chen, G., Siew, E. D., & Matheny, M. E. (2022). Open questions and research gaps for monitoring and updating AI-enabled tools in clinical settings. *Frontiers in Digital Health*, *4*, 958284. DOI: 10.3389/fdgth.2022.958284 PMID: 36120717

Dey, N., Schlemper, J., Salehi, S. S. M., Zhou, B., Gerig, G., & Sofka, M. (2022). ContraReg: Contrastive learning of multi-modality unsupervised deformable image registration. In Medical Image Computing and Computer Assisted Intervention (MICCAI). https://doi.org/DOI: 10.1007/978-3-031-16446-0_7

Fu, G., El Jurdi, R., Chougar, L., Dormont, D., Valabregue, R., Lehéricy, S., & Colliot, O.The ICEBERG Study Group. (2024). Projected pooling loss for red nucleus segmentation with soft topology constraints. *Journal of Medical Imaging (Bellingham, Wash.)*, *11*(4), 044002. DOI: 10.1117/1.JMI.11.4.044002 PMID: 38988992

Gu, P., et al. (2025). TopoImages: Incorporating Local Topology Encoding into Deep Learning Models. https://doi.org/.DOI: 10.1145/3746027.3755546

Kaabachi, B., Despraz, J., Meurers, T., Otte, K., Halilovic, M., Kulynych, B., Prasser, F., & Raisaro, J. L. (2025). A scoping review of privacy and utility metrics in medical synthetic data. npj. *Digital Medicine*, *8*(1), 60. DOI: 10.1038/s41746-024-01359-3 PMID: 39870798

Kore, A., Bavil, E. A., Subasri, V., Abdalla, M., Fine, B., Dolatabadi, E., & Abdalla, M. (2024). Empirical data drift detection experiments on real-world medical imaging data. Nature Communications, 15, (Article number associated with DOI). https://doi.org/.DOI: 10.1038/s41467-024-46142-w

Levenson, R. M., Singh, Y., Rieck, B., Hathaway, Q. A., Farrelly, C., Rozenblit, J., Prasanna, P., Erickson, B., Choudhary, A., Carlsson, G., & Sarkar, D. (2024). Advancing precision medicine: Algebraic topology and differential geometry in radiology and computational pathology. *Laboratory Investigation*, *104*(6), 102060. DOI: 10.1016/j.labinv.2024.102060 PMID: 38626875

Liu, A., Guo, Y., Yong, J.-H., & Xu, F. (2024). Multi-grained radiology report generation with sentence-level image-language contrastive learning. *IEEE Transactions on Medical Imaging*, *43*(7), 2657–2669. Advance online publication. DOI: 10.1109/TMI.2024.3372638 PMID: 38437149

Liu, B., Lu, D., Wei, D., Wu, X., Wang, Y., Zhang, Y., & Zheng, Y. (2023). Improving medical vision-language contrastive pretraining with semantics-aware triage. *IEEE Transactions on Medical Imaging*, *42*(12), 3579–3589. DOI: 10.1109/TMI.2023.3294980 PMID: 37440389

Liu, B., Lu, Z., & Wang, Y. (2024). Towards medical vision-language contrastive pre-training via study-oriented semantic exploration. In *Proceedings of the 32nd ACM International Conference on Multimedia (MM '24)*. https://doi.org/DOI: 10.1145/3664647.3681531

Liu, X., Rivera, S. C., Moher, D., Calvert, M. J., & Denniston, A. K.Spirit-AI and CONSORT-AI Working Group. (2020). Reporting guidelines for clinical trials evaluating artificial intelligence interventions are needed. *Nature Medicine*, *26*, 1364–1366. DOI: 10.1038/s41591-020-1034-x PMID: 32908283

Lu, Y., & Wang, A. (2025). Integrating language into medical visual recognition and reasoning: A survey. *Medical Image Analysis*, *103*, 103514. DOI: 10.1016/j.media.2025.103514 PMID: 40023891

Mongan, J., Moy, L., & Kahn, C. E.Jr. (2020). Checklist for Artificial Intelligence in Medical Imaging (CLAIM): A guide for authors and reviewers. *Radiology. Artificial Intelligence*, *2*(2), e200029. DOI: 10.1148/ryai.2020200029 PMID: 33937821

Peng, Y., Wang, H., Sonka, M., & Chen, D. Z. (2024). PHG-Net: Persistent homology guided medical image classification. In *2024 IEEE/CVF Winter Conference on Applications of Computer Vision (WACV)*. https://doi.org/DOI: 10.1109/WACV57701.2024.00741

Pun, C. S., Lee, S. X., & Xia, K. (2022). Persistent-homology-based machine learning: A survey and a comparative study. *Artificial Intelligence Review*, *55*(7), 5169–5213. DOI: 10.1007/s10462-022-10146-z

Raminedi, S., Shridevi, S., & Won, D. (2024). Multi-modal transformer architecture for medical image analysis and automated report generation. *Scientific Reports*, *14*(1), 19281. DOI: 10.1038/s41598-024-69981-5 PMID: 39164302

Sahiner, B., Chen, W., Samala, R. K., & Petrick, N. (2023). Data drift in medical machine learning: Implications and potential remedies. *The British Journal of Radiology*, *96*(1150), 20220878. DOI: 10.1259/bjr.20220878 PMID: 36971405

Singh, Y., Farrelly, C. M., Hathaway, Q. A., Leiner, T., Jagtap, J., Carlsson, G. E., & Erickson, B. J. (2023). Topological data analysis in medical imaging: Current state of the art. *Insights Into Imaging*, *14*(1), 58. DOI: 10.1186/s13244-023-01413-w PMID: 37005938

Skaf, Y., & Laubenbacher, R. (2022). Topological data analysis in biomedicine: A review. *Journal of Biomedical Informatics*, *130*, 104082. DOI: 10.1016/j.jbi.2022.104082 PMID: 35508272

Su, Z., Liu, X., Bou Hamdan, L., & Maroulas, V. (2025). Topological data analysis and topological deep learning beyond persistent homology: A review. *Artificial Intelligence Review*, *59*(2), 58. Advance online publication. DOI: 10.1007/s10462-025-11462-w PMID: 41743488

Tralie, C., Saul, N., & Bar-On, R. (2018). Ripser.py: A lean persistent homology library for Python. *Journal of Open Source Software*, *3*(29), 925. DOI: 10.21105/joss.00925

Wadhwa, R. R., Williamson, D. F. K., Dhawan, A., & Scott, J. G. (2018). TDAstats: R pipeline for computing persistent homology in topological data analysis. *Journal of Open Source Software*, *3*(28), 860. DOI: 10.21105/joss.00860 PMID: 33381678

Wang, Z., Wu, Z., Agarwal, D., & Sun, J. (2022). MedCLIP: Contrastive learning from unpaired medical images and text. *Proceedings of the 2022 Conference on Empirical Methods in Natural Language Processing (EMNLP)*. https://doi.org/DOI: 10.18653/v1/2022.emnlp-main.256

Yang, S., Wu, X., Ge, S., Zhou, S. K., & Xiao, L. (2023). Radiology report generation with a learned knowledge base and multi-modal alignment. *Medical Image Analysis*, *86*, 102798. DOI: 10.1016/j.media.2023.102798 PMID: 36989850

Zhang, Z., & Jiang, A. (2024). Interactive dual-stream contrastive learning for radiology report generation. *Journal of Biomedical Informatics*, *157*, 104718. DOI: 10.1016/j.jbi.2024.104718 PMID: 39209086

Chapter 6
The Architecture, Capabilities, and Challenges of Vision–Language Models for Healthcare AI

M. Murali
http://orcid.org/0000-0002-4478-2820
SRM Institute of Science and Technology, India

ABSTRACT

Vision–Language Models (VLMs) are transforming healthcare by integrating visual and textual understanding for medical image analysis and clinical decision-making. Incorporating computer vision and natural language processing, vision-language models (VLMs) can manage multimodal inputs ranging from radiographic images to pathological slides and medical reports. The essence of VLMs lies in multimodal fusion, vision grounding, and medical know-how alignment, which enable reliable medical report creation, disease prediction, and anomaly discovery. The application of pre-trained models, such as CLIP, BLIP, and MedCLIP, has provided strong support for zero-shot learning and cross-modal retrieval, whereas domain-aware fine-tuning has further improved their medical adaptability and functionality. However, there are challenges related to data privacy, interpretability, and bias that need to be addressed. This paper reviews VLM architectures, training methods, and tasks, as well as challenges and directions for developing secure and clear AI for medical applications.

DOI: 10.4018/979-8-3373-7315-7.ch006

ht © 2026, IGI Global Scientific Publishing. Copying or distributing in print or electronic forms without written permission of IGI Global Scientific Publishing is prohibited. Use of this chapter to generative artificial intelligence (AI) technologies is expressly prohibited. The publisher reserves all rights to license its use for generative AI training and machine learning model development.

1. INTRODUCTION

1.1 AI in Healthcare

Artificial Intelligence (AI) has emerged as a pillar of contemporary healthcare, transforming diagnosis, treatment planning, and medical data management. AI algorithms, specifically machine learning and deep learning-based algorithms (Awadalla et al., 2023), have demonstrated tremendous success in medical imaging, predictive analytics, and personalized medicine(Thakur et al., 2022). The technologies help to analyse intricate data, such as radiology images, genomic data, and clinical records, which helps the healthcare professionals to take clinical decisions more quickly and accurately. In radiology, e.g., convolutional neural networks (CNNs) have highest accuracy in detecting abnormalities, and natural language processing (NLP) models used to summarize electronic health records (EHRs) and to identify unstructured text patterns (Al Rahhal et al., 2023). Additionally, AI-powered tools enable remote patient monitoring, telemedicine, and drug discovery by integrating large-scale data. Nonetheless, medical data is multimodal by nature, comprised of images, texts, and sensor signals, that traditional unimodal AI systems cannot process simultaneously. This has given rise to vision-language models (VLMs) merging computer vision and language comprehension (Bordes et al., 2024).

Since the relationship exists in medical images and text descriptions, AI can detect the semantic gap between visual and linguistic modalities, which allows contextual reasoning and holistic patient examination. Thus, AI can do not only the specialized task systems but comprehensive, multimodal intelligence backing strong, interpretable, and data-driven health solutions.

1.2 Vision-Language Models (VLMs)

Vision-Language Models (VLMs) define a groundbreaking step in artificial intelligence research, where vision perception and language comprehension are merged into a single learning framework. Early VLMs were motivated by dual-stream architectures one for visual processing with CNNs and another for text processing with recurrent or transformer language models (Çallı et al.. 2021). The two modalities were paired together with joint embeddings, which enabled models to relate textual notions to visual representations. Early attempts like Image Captioning and Visual Question Answering (VQA) initiated this merging, where machines could describe images and respond to questions in context (Cao et al., 2024).

The introduction of large-scale pretraining and contrastive learning, as seen in OpenAI's CLIP and Google's ALIGN models, completely changed the way of working. Based on these models, image-text pairs learned cross-modal relationships through objectives, achieved zero-shot and transfer capabilities. Constructing upon these, healthcare-specific models like MedCLIP, BioViL, and GatorTron-ViL have been developed to align medical images with clinical text, offering robust multimodal representations for diagnosis, captioning, and retrieval (Hamidieh et al., 2024).

Contemporary VLMs also draw on transformer models with attention to accomplish multimodal fusion, where visual tokens and linguistic embeddings are engaged in a joint latent space. Fine-tuning these pre-trained VLMs on clinical datasets also increases their domain interpretability and relevance. The addition of knowledge graphs, prompt tuning, and multimodal large language models (MLLMs) extended VLM capability beyond static perception to reasoning and conversation (Huang et al., 2024). In medicine, this shift enables models not just to report about a radiograph but also to interpret findings, suggest tests, or report back coherently. Therefore, VLMs are the coming together of vision, language, and medical reasoning—opening the way for a new world of intelligent and interpretable AI for clinical assistance (Liu et al., 2023).

1.3 Multimodal Understanding in Medical Domains

Naturally, healthcare data is multimodal, such as radiology images, pathology slides, clinical reports, lab tests, and patient history. AI solutions will work in one modality either analysing images or text left with disjointed insights and poor contextual awareness. Multimodal learning, as obtained through Vision-Language Models (VLMs), bridges this divide through the incorporation of visual and textual information to offer comprehensive interpretations (Parashar et al., 2024).

For example, radiology report generation involves mapping image features to diagnostic terms, and pathology analysis is improved by mapping cellular patterns to text labels. Jointly modelling such data sources improves VLMs' capacity for reasoning about medical conditions, natural language explanation of visual findings, and mapping observations across modalities. This work enhances clinical decision-making significantly, improving diagnostic accuracy and consistency. In addition to this, multimodal understanding helps automated data retrieval, and models can match text queries to medical images or vice versa (Ruggeri & Nozza, 2023).

In clinical training, VLMs are also interactive tools that can produce descriptions, draw attention to abnormalities, and offer rationales for diagnosis, hence facilitating knowledge sharing. Moreover, accuracy and multimodal models help explainability which is essential to build clinician trust. Visualization of attention maps or textual explanations enables healthcare professionals to see how and why an AI system arrived at a specific decision. Multimodal VLMs are hence a big leap towards holistic, interpretable, and context-sensitive medical AI systems (Van et al., 2024).

1.4 Fundamentals of Vision-Language Models (VLMs)

Vision-Language Models (VLMs) are at the nexus of modern multimodal AI. These models are intended to interpret, reason, and produce content involving images and text. The need for complex-data modality, incorporating images, videos, and text descriptions, has brought about the emergence of VLMs (Wang et al., 2024). In the medical field, medical images and text descriptions co-exist, and there is an unprecedented opportunity presented by VLMs to integrate medical images and text descriptions. This section explains the inner functioning of VLMs, concerning their architecture, training, pre-training, and fusion of images and text, with an emphasis on applying these models in medicine (Zhou et al., 2022).

1.5 Objectives

The aim is to discuss essential aspects of Vision-Language Models as they apply within the healthcare industry – their arrangement, functionality, and implementation. It briefly discusses how VLMs integrate various inputs such as images and texts within the medical field for improving diagnostic thinking, automated reporting, and medical knowledge retrieval. The research focuses on multimodal fusion, visual grounding, and mechanisms for aligning languages that allow VLMs tofunction in different medical domains.

Moreover, the paper explores domain-specific modifications, including fine-grained tuning strategies and use of medical datasets, that enhance VLM performance in practical healthcare environments. The paper also discusses the challenges related to data privacy, interpretability, and ethics-based deployment of such models for clinical practice. Finally, this paper aims to offer a complete picture about how VLMs are going to form the next generation of smart healthcare systems. By outlining paths for future research and summarizing the current limitations, it is expected to improve the research on vision-language modeling for safe, transparent, and clinical-strength AI, as envisioned under the value of precision medicine and human-centric AI.

2. RELATED WORKS

Paola et al. (2026) describes a methodology for systematically analyzing and understanding the behavior of vision-language models for driver gaze estimation. The methodology involves task decomposition, domain knowledge identification, and evaluation through targeted prompting. Experiments conducted on Idefics2, Qwen2-VL, Moondream, and GPT-4o identify important limitations such as sensitivity to prompts, vocabulary mismatch, image-relative spatial reasoning, and inability to reason about non-visible parts. These observations are used to develop better prompting and fine-tuning techniques, leading to performance comparable to CNN-based approaches. The methodology also enables early model filtering, informed model choice, and better understanding of model limitations, thus improving reliability. In this research (Xinming et al., 2025), Authors talked about the fusion of large language models (LLMs) and virtual reality (VR) has led to significant breakthroughs in the field of healthcare and medicine. The immersive environment provided by VR is used for surgical simulation, rehabilitation, therapy, mental health treatment, and personalized medicine. The fusion of VR and LLMs facilitates interactive medical education, better decision-making, and improved patient engagement. This study examines the current state of applications, research developments, and challenges in the convergence of LLMs and VR, emphasizing their increasing importance in the field of intelligent, accurate, and innovative healthcare.

Alexander et al. (2025) propose a privacy-preserving fitness-tracking system using only the RGB smartphone camera to facilitate remote exercise tracking. Breaking the mold of traditional models, which were limited to several exercises or were too complex to implement, their multitask neural network is capable of exercising and rep-counting on thousands of exercises. To address the data representation issue, the research also introduces the large-scale Olympia dataset, which accounts for over 1,900 exercises. Their vision-language transformer is the first to address more than one task on skeletal exercise data, achieving an exercise recognition rate of 76.5% and an off-by-one rep recognition rate of 85.3% on RGB video.

In this case, the focus is on the assessment on the various sizes and specialties of the state-of-the-art vision-language models (VLMs) for the purpose of the generation of radiology reports based on the multisequence brain MRI for patients suffering from cancer. They compared the performance of various open-source and medical VLMs in terms of expert-annotated data, objective metrics, reason-based assessors, and radiologist feedback. In this assessment, Meta-Vision 3.2 90B outperformed the large models, Meta-Vision 11B and DeepSeek-VL-2-27B outperformed the mediums, and Qwen2-VL-2B outperformed the small models. This is a groundbreaking benchmark because it highlights the power of size and specialization in a medical vision-language model.

Elshan et al. (2025) discuss the potential of combining large language models (LLMs) with vision-language models (VLMs) for the accelerated phenotyping of plant stresses. Instead of using the usual laborious and application-specific methods for analysis, VLMs combine visual understanding and commonsense reasoning for the analysis of multimodal inputs. Additionally, LLMs enhance knowledge extraction and semantic tagging as well as model interpretability using techniques such as generation augmented with retrievals. The article presents an overview of various uses and developments in the integration of LLMs and VLMs and also presents a conceptual framework for accountable and sustainable AI for agriculture.

This systematic review based on PRISMA guidelines, examined 16 studies on zero-shot VLMs for radiographic image classification, covering topics such as datasets, model architecture, language incorporation, limitations, and hyperparameter optimization. The majority of the studies were from China and the US, with no studies led by an EU country. Model architectures were very diverse, with dual-encoder and joint embedding models being the most common. Dependence on few and specialized datasets, suboptimal utilization of clinical text, and inadequate reporting of hyperparameter optimization are the limitations of the current models. This systematic review emphasizes the importance of multimodal datasets, transparent assessment, and interdisciplinary model design for robust clinical implementation. Vision and vision-language foundation models have demonstrated great potential in ophthalmology by enhancing diagnostic precision, treatment planning, and clinical processes.

This systematic review (Kai Jin et al., 2026), integrates the literature on the application of foundation models in the field of ophthalmology. The literature search covered publications between January 2020 and July 2025, and the search engines used included PubMed, Web of Science, Scopus, and Google Scholar. Among the ten studies that qualified for review, vision-based or vision-language models were applied to ophthalmology-related tasks such as retinal diseases, glaucoma, and ocular surface tumors. The studies' results were measured in terms of the performance, utility, and integration of the models, while the most important limitations were the models' large data and computational needs and lack of interpretability. Qinglong et al. (2025) introduces a generalized domain prompt learning framework that transfers recognition abilities to specific domains using limited data and resources. The framework enhances language representations by incorporating domain knowledge using quaternion networks, aligns cross-modal relationships, and adapts visual features using hierarchical vision prompts. Additionally, a low-rank adaptation approach improves domain transfer. The approach achieves state-of-the-art recognition performance in various domains, making research more sustainable and inclusive.

This technical note (Kao & Kao, 2025), gives an introduction to LLMs in radiology, describing the main applications like image interpretation, report generation, and workflow optimization. It describes the main transformer models and examples of models like GPT-4, PaLM, and Med-PaLM, focusing on the algorithms and metrics used. The technical note also deals with bias, ethics, and regulations, and gives practical advice on how to implement LLMs in radiological research and practice, aimed at both medical professionals and AI researchers. In this study (Khoriba et al., 2025), the authors explained that large language models (LLMs) and large vision models (LVMs) are revolutionizing medical image analysis by facilitating human-like report writing, better diagnostic performance, and better decision support. This paper explores the use of LLMs in image interpretation, report writing, visual question answering, and decision support systems.

3. ARCHITECTURAL FRAMEWORK OF VISION-LANGUAGE MODELS

The Vision-Language Model architecture always has three major components: the vision encoder, the language encoder, and the multimodal fusion module. These three components are used in the Vision-Language Model architecture to process the raw image and text inputs into a joint representation.

Vision Encoder: The vision encoder is responsible for processing visual data like images, videos, or medical images to derive meaningful features. Conventional vision encoders used Convolutional Neural Networks (CNNs) such as ResNet or EfficientNet, which are highly effective at modeling spatial hierarchies in images (Radford et al., 2021). But with the advent of transformer models, Vision Transformers (ViT) have become the most popular choice for the backbone. ViT splits the image into patches and learns the relationships among the patches using self-attention mechanisms, which enables the model to capture global context, an essential requirement for medical image analysis, such as MRI or histopathology images, where minute spatial relationships help detect diseases (Jia et al., 2021). Certain models, specifically designed for the healthcare sector, use hybrid models that leverage CNNs for feature extraction along with transformers for global reasoning.

Language Encoder: This processes texts, such as radiology or pathology texts, and/or patient descriptions. Transformer architectures, including BERT and its descendants, are common language encoders. They generate embeddings with context to capture word meanings and their relations. Variants of these, tailored to the healthcare domain, include BioBERT, ClinicalBERT, and PubMedBERT, and have been useful in texts containing domain jargon. This language follows the Visual Embeddings and establishes a foundation to map language along with image embeddings (Zhang et al., 2021).

Multimodal Fusion Module: The key to all vision-language models is the fusion module, which brings together visual and text inputs to a common space. This allows the model to reason about both inputs simultaneously, linking phrases from the text input (like "lung opacity") directly to regions on the image (Zhang et al., 2023). Original fusion approaches relied on simple concatenations, while more modern techniques involve cross-attention and co-attention. Cross-attention allows the text to guide the attention mechanism towards regions in the image, and vice-versa, improving semantic matching. In all medical images, the term "nodule" allows for attention to focus on the appropriate regions for the task. More modern models such as BLIP-2, ALBEF, and Flamingo use a multimodal transformer that processes both embeddings within a shared latent space (Lu et al., 2024).

Figure 1. Vision–language model architecture

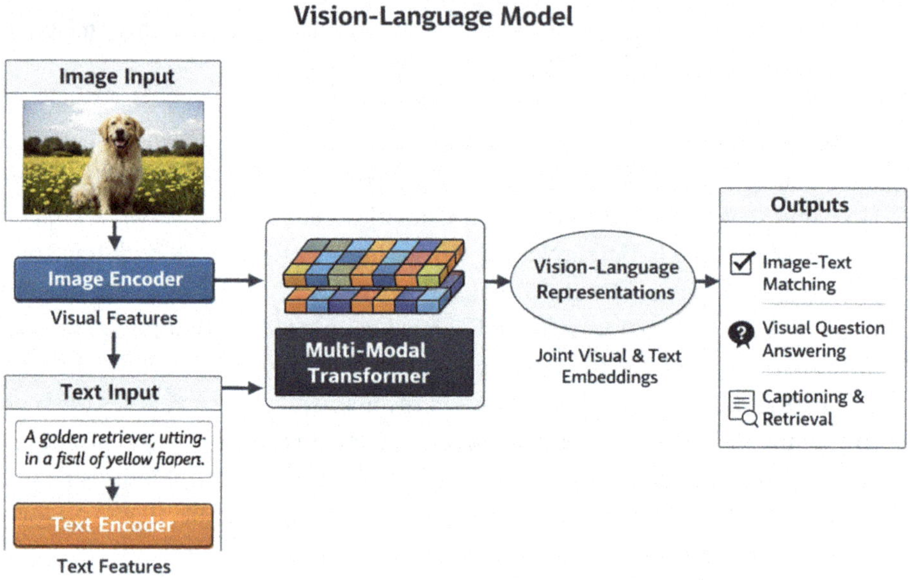

The above Figure 1 shows a canonical Vision Language Model (VLM) architecture that is designed to jointly process visual and text inputs. The processing pipeline starts with two inputs: an image input (which could be a medical image or a natural scene image) and a text input (which could be a report, a caption, or a query). The image input is fed into an image encoder, which could be a CNN (such as ResNet or EfficientNet) or a Vision Transformer (ViT), that extracts high-level visual features. At the same time, the text input is fed into a transformer-based language encoder (such as BERT).

These modality-specific embeddings are then passed to a multi-modal transformer, which is the fusion core of the model. By using self-attention and cross-attention mechanisms, this module is able to align regions of the visual modality with the appropriate linguistic tokens, thus allowing for fine-grained cross-modal reasoning. The combined vision-language representations are in a shared latent space.

Finally, these representations facilitate various downstream tasks such as image-text matching, visual question answering, and image captioning/retrieval. This architecture is very useful for the healthcare domain and other complex domains because it allows for perception, reasoning, and explanation of visual and text data.

3.1 Pretraining Paradigms and Object

The effectiveness of Vision-Language Models is highly dependent on pretraining, which enables the model to learn universal cross-modal representations before fine-tuning. The most popular paradigms for pretraining are:

Contrastive Learning: This method, made possible by the advent of models such as CLIP (Contrastive Language–Image Pretraining), involves aligning the embeddings of images and text by moving similar pairs closer together in the embedding space and pushing dissimilar pairs apart. The contrastive loss aids in pairing the descriptions with their corresponding images. In a medical context, this entails pairing descriptions such as "chest x-ray showing cardiomegaly" with images of an enlarged heart.

Image-Text Matching (ITM): ITM is essentially a binary classification task where it is determined whether the image and the text together form a pair or not. This enhances the capability to classify it as correct and incorrect pair classifications. In medical models, ITM is extensively employed to check whether the captions and the radiology images correspond correctly.

Masked Modeling: Following the framework of Masked Language Modeling from the architect of BERT, Masked Image Modeling and Masked Language Modeling are adopted in the multimodal scenario to fill the masked parts in the image and text information. In the MLM component, some words are masked, and the task is to predict them based on both the text and image information. In MIM, parts of the image are masked, and the task is to predict them based on the text information.

Generative Pretraining: Certain VLMs are trained in a generative manner, predicting either the missing captions or descriptions for the input image. Certain models such as BLIP and Flamingo incorporate this task objective, enabling the model to produce well-articulated medical reports or summaries for a given input image.

3.2 Cross-Modal Alignment and Attention Mechanisms

The key issue in VLM design is cross-modal alignment, which involves associating linguistic tokens with corresponding visual regions or features. Attention mechanisms are essential in this alignment process.

Self-Attention: This is applied to each modality to model the dependencies within each modality. In a medical image, self-attention enables the model to comprehend the relationships between different regions of the anatomy.
Cross-Attention: Connects vision and language by enabling textual features to query the visual embeddings. This attention mechanism lets the models link the textual entities to certain image regions. For instance, the expression "mass in the left upper lobe" is tied to the matching image patch through cross-attention weights.
Co-Attention Networks: These models allow for attention in both directions, i.e., from images to text and vice-versa, thereby allowing the symmetric learning of relationships between vision and language modalities. More complex models may use attention maps, which can be used as an explanation tool for medical professionals to show areas of an image that correspond to certain text outputs.

Figure 2. Cross-modal alignment and attention mechanism

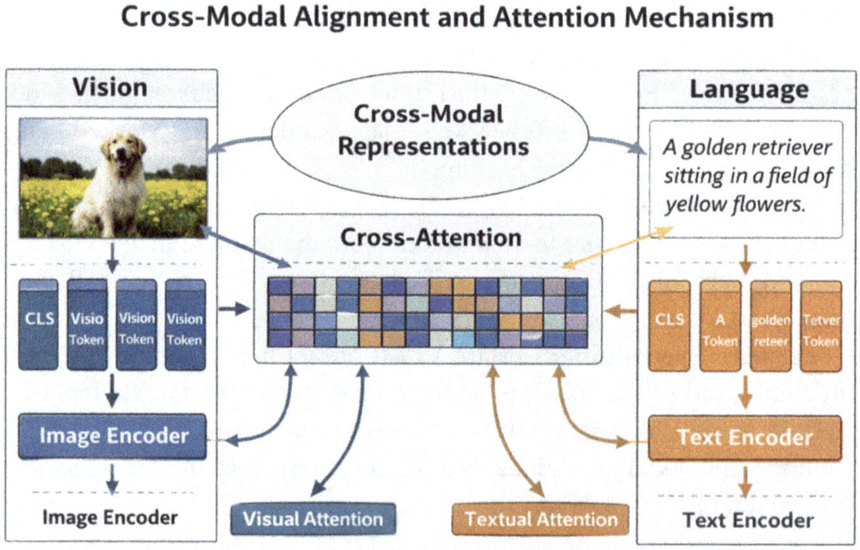

The above passage highlights the way current Vision-Language Models (VLMs) are combined via cross-modal alignment and attention. There are two concurrent paths being performed here and are referred to as the vision path and the language path. In the vision path, the input image is passed through the image encoder. This is a Vision Transformer (ViT) or a CNN-Transformer hybrid. This encodes the input image into a series of vision tokens. There is a Common Language Token (CLT) and a number of patch tokens. Every one of these is a representation of basic and detailed aspects of the image.

The text is then preprocessed in the language path by a transformer encoder such as BERT. The sentence is tokenized based on subwords and begins with a CLS token. The textual representation has embedded meanings while preserving the relationships between words and phrases.

The cross-attention module in the middle of the architecture enables interaction between the two domains. The text queries pay attention to the keys and values of the images. This enables the text elements to pay attention to the appropriate areas within the image (for example, the word "retriever" relates to the corresponding image patches of the dog). On the other hand, the image queries pay attention to the text features.

The results for both visual and text attention will point to areas in the image as well as words that guide the joint reasoning process. This finally enables cross-modal representations for fine-grained semantic alignment, which allows for reasoning, image-text matching, and question-answering, among others. This will play an essential role in domains requiring sensitivity, for instance, medical support.

3.3 Multimodal Fusion Strategies

There are various approaches to combine vision and language representations, which can be broadly classified into early, late, and hybrid fusion approaches.

Early Fusion: Combines raw image and text embeddings early in the network. Such an architecture is capable of complex and multi-faceted interaction between modalities, but its computation is quite expensive. Such an architecture is best used in cases of strongly interdependent modalities, such as pathology slide captioning.

Late Fusion: This is where separately each mode is handled, and then the resultant representations are fused. This is efficient in terms of computation but might disregard very fine, intricate relationships. This is commonly applied in the area of image and report associating, for instance, in the medical arena.

Hybrid Fusion: A combination of both methods, where partial alignment happens at various levels of the network. Models such as LXMERT and ViLT follow this strategy to achieve computational efficiency and semantic depth.

In medical applications, hybrid fusion is very useful because clinical reasoning involves both low-level image-text correlation tasks (such as locating a tumor) and high-level semantic tasks (such as identifying the progression of a disease).

Figure 3. Multimodal fusion strategies

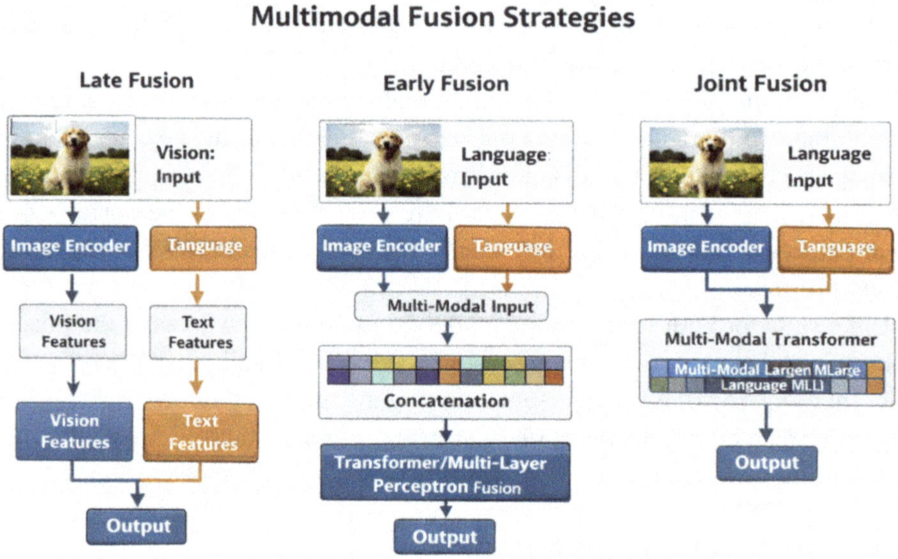

This is Figure 3, which illustrates three different methods of multimodal fusion in vision-language modeling. These approaches are Late Fusion, Early Fusion, and Joint Fusion. These approaches explain how data from different modalities, in this case visual data (images) and language data, can be combined to give a single output.

In Late Fusion, each modality is processed separately initially. The image goes through an Image Encoder to obtain its features, and the text input goes through a language encoder to obtain its features. These features are maintained separately until a point when they are combined, usually through concatenation or averaging, before the final output is produced. This method enables the independent modeling of each modality, thus avoiding any interaction between the modalities, but may not capture the subtle interactions between the modalities.

Early Fusion involves the fusion of the modalities at an earlier stage. Both the visual and text inputs are encoded and then combined using the concatenation method to form a multi-modal representation. This representation is then put through a Transformer or Multi-Layer Perceptron (MLP) layer. Early Fusion allows the network to learn the joint representations of vision and language from the beginning, which could potentially learn better cross-modal associations, but it is computationally intensive since it has to process the high-dimensional inputs.

Joint Fusion employs a multi-modal transformer to align and fuse information from both modalities in a fully end-to-end fashion. The input image and text are both encoded, and then the transformer attends jointly across the modalities to generate the output. This approach is the most advanced and captures the highest-level cross-modal interactions using attention mechanisms and is commonly employed in the latest vision-language models, such as CLIP, BLIP, and Flamingo.

In summary, the figure above illustrates the importance of fusion strategy decisions in multimodal AI systems with respect to feature interaction, model complexity, and the ability to learn cross-modal relationships.

3.4 Domain Adaptation for Healthcare

Generic VLMs are trained on big web datasets, but they don't always work with medical data because there are gaps in the domains. So, domain adaptation is necessary to make models work better for healthcare purposes. This includes:

Medical Data Pretraining: Utilizing datasets such as MIMIC-CXR, CheXpert, or MedPix that contain both images and radiology reports.
Terminology Alignment: Modifying language encoders on biomedical datasets to understand clinical terminology such as "pleural effusion" or "atelectasis."
Knowledge Infusion: Employing medical ontologies such as UMLS or SNOMED-CT to infuse domain-specific relationships into the model's knowledge.
Cross-Institutional Generalization: Applying Federated Learning or Privacy-Preserving Techniques to enhance VLMs in multiple hospitals without compromising private information.

These approaches ensure that the model is more stable, understandable, and trustworthy in a clinical setting, all of which are essential for adhering to the rules and using it for ethical purposes.

3.5 Evaluation Metrics for VLMs

To judge VLMs in healthcare, you need metrics that look at both how accurate the visuals are and how well the language flows. Some common metrics are:

Image-Text Retrieval: Recall@K and mean average precision (mAP) measure the ability of the model to link images with appropriate reports.
Caption Quality: BLEU, ROUGE, and METEOR evaluate the similarity of the language used in the generated captions and the reference captions.
Diagnostic Accuracy: Task-specific metrics such as AUC (Area Under Curve), F1-score, and sensitivity are used to determine the accuracy of a clinical test.
Explainability Metrics: Attention visualization and human evaluation by radiologists are used to measure the ease of understanding and reliability.

3.6 Interpretability and Explainability

Interpretability is vital in healthcare VLMs to ensure that predictions are clinically understandable. Techniques such as Grad-CAM, attention heatmaps, and saliency maps are used to visualize which image regions contribute to textual outputs. Moreover, models can generate textual rationales, explaining why a certain diagnosis or caption was produced. This not only improves clinician confidence but also supports regulatory transparency, aligning with medical AI governance standards.

4. EXISTING VISION–LANGUAGE MODEL METHODS

4.1 CLIP (Contrastive Language–Image Pretraining)

CLIP is one of the first vision-language models that used large-scale contrastive learning between text and images. It has two encoders: an image encoder (CNN or Vision Transformer) and a text encoder (Transformer-based). Both encoders put their inputs into a shared embedding space. A contrastive loss pulls matching image-text pairs closer together and pushes non-matching pairs apart.

CLIP has shown that it can learn without any specific training in healthcare, which means that models can recognize medical concepts without being trained on specific tasks. CLIP can link visual patterns with diagnostic labels by giving text prompts like “chest X-ray showing pneumonia.” This feature is very helpful when there isn't much labeled medical data available.

However, CLIP was initially trained on large datasets of general image-text pairs, making it less applicable in a clinical environment. Medical terminology, subtle visual cues, and specialized semantics often have poor representation, leading to poor performance on critical diagnosis tasks. Even with this flaw, CLIP is a good starting point and backbone for many medical VLMs. It makes cross-modal retrieval, image classification, and weakly supervised learning possible.

Overall, CLIP is an important part of healthcare VLM research because it is simple, scalable, and can reason without any training. However, domain adaptation and fine-tuning are necessary for clinical reliability.

4.2 BLIP (Bootstrapping Language–Image Pretraining)

BLIP builds on traditional contrastive vision-language models by adding both discriminative and generative learning goals. BLIP's architecture is different from CLIP's in that it combines image-text contrastive learning, image-text matching, and conditional language generation into one system. BLIP usually consists of a vision encoder, a language encoder, and a multimodal transformer. In the context of the healthcare industry, BLIP is useful in auto summarizing medical reports and responding to queries regarding visuals. Its capability to AutoSummarise medical visuals into coherent and clinically informed descriptions is useful in maintaining the text and visuals in sync. The goal of matching the visuals and text further maintains the semantic connection between the medical findings and the text.

BLIP's multimodal transformer is beneficial in the way it allows interaction between image patches and text in particular ways, improving model performance on visually grounded tasks. This is particularly important in the healthcare domain, where one must be able to explain why results are correct according to an AI system.

However, the complex architecture of BLIP incurs higher costs of training and utilization. Just like CLIP, for BLIP, domain-specific fine-tuning is beneficial to adapt to the medical terms and modalities. Nonetheless, BLIP is a major step forward for healthcare AI models that need to be interpretable and provide new insights.

4.3 MedCLIP

MedCLIP is a healthcare-oriented counterpart of the original CLIP developed to fill the gap between generalized vision-language models and healthcare data. MedCLIP is trained on many image and clinical reports pairing data, such as chest X-rays images and radiology reports. MedCLIP learns to associate image features and terms using a contrastive learning approach that honors healthcare domain knowledge.

One aspect that shines is the capacity for capturing specialized vocabulary in a particular field, such as terms for diseases, anatomy, and medical observations, which helps in classification, retrieval, and weakly supervised medical image diagnosis. The demonstration sets have excellent generalization capabilities without requiring much annotation.

MedCLIP relies on radiology reports to make the task of labeling scalable. The architecture of MedCLIP is also much more lightweight than other generative models of vision and language. However, the main aspect of MedCLIP is its discriminative property. In other words, MedCLIP cannot generate text by default. Because of this, it is used more for retrieval and classification than for making reports. MedCLIP is still an important step toward clinically based and reliable vision-language modelling in healthcare.

4.4 BioViL

BioViL is a biomedical vision-language model that uses region-level grounding to improve the alignment of images and text. BioViL is different from global embedding-based methods because it directly links image regions to text phrases, making it easier to understand the details. It is usually trained on biomedical images and structured clinical descriptions first.

The region-level supervision in BioViL makes it easier to identify irregularities, which is particularly helpful in pathology and radiology. The ability to connect ideas in text to specific regions in an image makes BioViL easier to understand and helps to establish trust in physicians. This is one of the largest issues with previous VLMs, which were not able to understand space.

BioViL also has the advantage of being very strong in downstream tasks such as locating medical images and locating abnormalities. However, since region-level annotations are required, data preparation becomes more complex. Additionally, the training process of BioViL is computationally intensive since it has very specific alignment goals.BioViL shows how important explainability and visual grounding are in healthcare AI, even though there are some problems with it. This makes it a useful tool for safety-critical clinical applications.

Table 1. Comparison of existing vision–language models

Model	Architecture Type	Training Objective	Generative Capability	Domain Adaptation	Explainability	Key Applications
CLIP	Dual Encoder	Contrastive Learning	No	Limited	Low	Zero-shot classification, retrieval
BLIP	Multimodal Transformer	Contrastive + Generative	Yes	⚠ Requires tuning	Moderate	Report generation, VQA
MedCLIP	Dual Encoder	Medical Contrastive Learning	No	Strong	Moderate	Medical retrieval, diagnosis
BioViL	Region-aware VLM	Grounded Alignment	No	Strong	High	Abnormality localization, explainable diagnosis

CLIP is scalable and has the capability of performing zero-shot reasoning, but it lacks any medical details. BLIP incorporates generative reasoning capabilities, which make it suitable for report generation. MedCLIP applies efficient contrastive learning to bind the medical field, and BioViL applies region-level grounding to make it easier to understand. These approaches demonstrate how VLMs are evolving into healthcare AI systems that are reliable, understandable, and task aware.

4.5 Discussion of Clinical Validation

Clinical validation is a critical discussion point in the deployment of Vision-Language Models (VLMs) for healthcare applications. Based on the document, validation must extend beyond laboratory accuracy and include real-world clinical settings such as hospitals, diagnostic centers, and multi-institutional environments. The model should be evaluated using clinically relevant metrics such as sensitivity, specificity, AUC, F1-score, and diagnostic consistency across diverse patient populations. Expert validation by radiologists, pathologists, and clinicians is essential to compare AI-generated outputs with established medical decisions and reports. In addition, the document emphasizes explainability through attention maps, grounded visual regions, and textual justifications, which are necessary to build clinician trust. Cross-institutional validation is equally important to ensure robustness across different scanners, imaging protocols, and demographic groups. Prospective validation within hospital workflows helps assess inference speed, usability, and reliability in decision support. Therefore, strong clinical validation is fundamental to ensuring patient safety, regulatory acceptance, and practical adoption of VLMs in real-world healthcare systems.

5. APPLICATIONS IN HEALTHCARE

5.1 Medical Image Interpretation (Radiology, Pathology, Ophthalmology)

Vision-Language Models (VLMs) are shaking the ground in the area of medical imaging and allowing radiology, pathology, and ophthalmology to integrate "what we see" with "what we know" in medicine. In radiology, these models interpret chest X-rays, CT scans, and MRIs together with their description to locate problems – whether it is an nodule, fracture, bleed, or enlargement. They rely upon the text descriptions in order to interpret images better through grounded images and attention maps. This is not like the traditional image-only models.

In pathology, VLMs assist in the analysis of high-resolution histopathology slides, in which diagnostic descriptions are required to assist in understanding small patterns at the cellular and tissue levels. VLMs help in tumor grading, cancer type determination, and identification of biomarkers by establishing correspondences between regions in microscopic slides to pathology notes and textual labels. Alignment among various types of data reduces the variability introduced by multiple observers-a well-known problem in pathology.

In ophthalmology, VLMs also interpret retinal fundus photos and OCT scans. They can correlate visual signals-lesions, hemorrhages, or thinning of the retina-with written diagnostic cues. That makes it easier to identify conditions such as diabetic retinopathy, glaucoma, or age-related macular degeneration. Clinicians often find it reassuring that VLMs can explain their predictions with language descriptions and attention maps.

Overall, VLMs push medical image understanding beyond the mere act of visual categorization to one that is fuller and more informative. By fusing images with medical terminology, they make diagnoses more accurate and transparent, adding practical value in heavy imaging medical fields.

5.2. Automated Report Generation

One of the most practical applications of Vision-Language Models in the healthcare sector is the automatic generation of medical reports. Medical reporting, particularly in the fields of radiology and pathology, is a time-consuming process and is also prone to inconsistencies since the level of experience and writing styles of different doctors vary. VLMs address this issue by converting the visual features extracted from medical images into text reports.

In radiology, VLMs can generate initial diagnostic reports based on X-ray images, CT scans, or MRI images by correlating visual problems with standardized medical terms. VLMs can store critical information such as the location, severity, and nature of the abnormality and generate draft reports for doctors to review and modify. This not only increases efficiency in the process, but it also reduces the time taken to generate diagnostic reports in a busy medical environment.

In pathology, the automated report writing system assists in understanding complex histological findings by correlating small visual patterns with descriptive text in diagnoses. VLMs can generate standardized pathology reports that assist in cancer diagnosis, classification, and margin analysis. The automated system assists pathologists by making their work easier while maintaining high standards in documentation.

VLMs are significant as they enhance the quality of the reports by applying multimodal reasoning. The cross-attention mechanisms in VLMs ensure that the text being produced is grounded on some aspects of the image. This ensures that the text is more accurate and does not include any false information. Additionally, the language encoders that are domain-specific ensure that the appropriate medical terms and reporting formats are applied.

Automated reports are not intended to replace doctors, but they can be very helpful tools in decision-making. VLM-based report generation systems can assist in making clinical reporting safer, faster, and more reliable by improving the ease of understanding text generation, reducing the workload, and increasing consistency.

5.3 Disease Diagnosis and Classification

Vision Language Models are very useful in the healthcare industry for the purpose of disease diagnosis and classification. Regular disease diagnosis through AI is generally done using images as input data, which may not be a correct representation of the entire scenario. This is resolved by the Vision Language Models since they combine visual evidence as well as textual knowledge.

In the process of diagnosis by medical images, the VLMs combine information presented in the images with clinical observations and prior knowledge of medicine. Take, for example, chest imaging, where the VLMs associate imaging patterns of chest images with symptoms of conditions such as pneumonia, tuberculosis, cardiomegaly, and lung cancer.

VLMs used for pathology-based diagnosis integrate image characteristics at a cellular level with text related to diagnoses. VLMs help with cancer identification, gradings, and sub-type classification of cancer. These models work by using attention and text-based explanation capabilities for justifying predicted outcomes, which is an important aspect of their functionality and approval for medical applications.

VLMs in ophthalmology help to classify retinal disorders by associating images from the fundus or OCT with labels, thus improving screening accuracy and earlier diagnosis. Also, VLMs eliminate biases in their applications by considering various distributions, rather than using information from a single distribution.

Overall, VLMs optimize the process of disease diagnosis by performing context-aware classification, improved generalization abilities, as well as efficient decision-making processes. VLMs are quite unique tools for the field of precision medicine and AI-supported clinical practices because they combine perception understanding with reasoning based on language.

5.4 Patient Record Summarization and Retrieval

Vision-Language Models can also be applied to the summarization and retrieval of patient data, particularly when dealing with large electronic health records. Healthcare data is multimodal in nature, including images, text, lab results, and past reports. VLMs enable the linking of visual data to text stories, which allows for the analysis of all these different types of data in one place.

VLMs can be used to provide a compact clinical abstract of the patient history that can be constructed from images of diagnoses, opinions of doctors, and past results. This can enable doctors to have a quick idea of the patient's status, progress of the disease, and past treatments, particularly in the ICU and ER.

These search engines also facilitate multi-modal searches in patient data, whether it's done through text inputting or images. A physician, for example, may search previous instances relevant to "chest X-ray with bilateral opacities" by either searching the text or displaying an actual picture to search for similar instances and findings.

Apart from the images, the VLMs allow longitudinal analysis since they associate imaging sessions done at different times with the corresponding changes in the medical history. Thus, it becomes simple to determine the success of the treatment and the progress of the disease. Furthermore, with the use of explicable retrieval techniques, all becomes clear since the physician knows the visual or text indicators that contributed to the retrieval.

Overall, VLMs increase clinical efficiencies, help reduce information overflow, and facilitate informed care by enabling easier access, summarization, and extraction of patient information.

6. CHALLENGES AND LIMITATIONS

6.1 Data Privacy and Ethical Issues

Privacy and ethics management remains quite an important consideration for Vision-Language Models (VLMs), especially when applied to the healthcare domain. Medical Vision-Language Models, for instance, depend on massive amounts of highly sensitive and multimodal data. This could range from images, radiology results, and pathology comments to electronic health records. Such data often involves direct identifiers and protected health information. For this reason, privacy regulations such as HIPAA, GDPR, and others need to be satisfied. Storing and processing such data files could result in leakage, unauthorized access, and even patient re-identification.

The pre-training of the VLMs using centralized data sources is ethically dubious, since obtaining data from various institutions can violate patient confidentiality. This is because even when using anonymized data sources, they might be susceptible to reverse reconstruction and membership inference attacks, in which malicious parties use pre-trained VLMs to harvest highly personal information. Additionally, having VLMs capable of generating text is potentially dangerous due to the concern of transmitting highly personal patient information through report generation.

Informed consent and data rights extend the list of ethical considerations. Patients are not informed that their health data can be utilized to develop large-scale multimodal models of artificial intelligence. The development of volume-based models in health care support systems imposes a variety of duties concerning accuracy, accountability, and trust. Ineffective validation of the models can lead to misrepresenting data as actual results.

Handling such problems requires very effective privacy-preserving strategies, including federated learning, differential privacy, sound data management, and very tight security controls. To promote the proper, secure application compatible with patient rights as well as medical ethics, there is a need for ethical guidelines for the application of AI.

6.2 Bias and Fairness in Medical Datasets

Bias and fairness holdbacks keep Vision–Language Models from being reliably generalizable in healthcare. When we train VLMs, medical data are surrounded by gaps: differences in who's included, which institutions are represented, and socioeconomic backgrounds. This overrepresentation of certain populations or the types of diseases, imaging devices, and regions makes models perform worse for the underrepresented groups, which leads to unequal or inaccurate clinical outcomes.

In addition, the bias in imaging data originates from different acquisition protocols, types of scanners, and annotation preferences of various hospitals. Clinical text also contains subjective language, clinician preferences, and perhaps historical biases that could already be present in records. If VLMs learn such biases, then they will propagate them and increase the gap in diagnosis, risk prediction, and treatment recommendations.

The language side of the VLMs is particularly vulnerable: these models may associate certain medical conditions with demographic descriptors or fail to generalize across underserved populations. That can cause systematic misclassification or lower diagnostic accuracy for minority populations, worsening health disparities instead of reducing them.

In multimodal fusion, the bias compounds because image and text biases interact in complex ways. It is challenging to identify and correct a multimodal bias since one can hardly say which modality contributed to the error. All these issues may only appear in a deployment context without fairness-focused evaluation.

To reduce bias, we need diverse, representative datasets; transparent reporting of who's in the data and how it's collected; and training methods that explicitly address fairness. Guaranteeing wide benefit involves regular audits for bias, checks on subgroup performance, and engagement with domain experts. The development of trusting VLMs supporting the creation of fair and ethical healthcare requires active thematicization of bias.

6.3 Model Interpretability and Explainability

One of the key deterrents in Vision-Language Models associated with healthcare is the difficulty of interpretability and explainability: Clinical decisions require complete clarity, sound justification, and auditable trails. However, VLMs are based on large deep networks featuring millions or even billions of parameters driven by multimodal transformers. This in itself puts a barrier to trace how conclusions are arrived at. As long as the process is not open, the clinicians find it difficult to instil their trust in the system, and the regulators face huge barriers to justify the approval of the same.

Some insight is provided by the attention mechanisms and visual grounding, but they only go that far. Attention weights do not reliably map to true causal reasoning, and the highlighted areas in the images or generated rationales may look convincing while not really providing the actual decision path. This can foster unwarranted trust in AI's results, which is dangerous in high-stakes medical areas of operation.

Things are even harder to explain in multimodal settings. The interaction of visual and textual representations is too complex; most of the aspects related to how specific image features influence text outputs or vice versa, or vice versa, remain unsettled. For example, in automatic report generation, a model is found to have generated fluent plausible descriptions lacking strong support in the provided visual evidence. That raises concerns about hallucinations and questions the reliability of diagnoses.

From a clinical perspective, explanations must be aligned with the medical reasoning rather than just technical metrics. Clinicians need clear, clinically meaningful justifications that tie predictions to anatomical regions, recognizable disease patterns, or established medical concepts. Current explainability techniques very often miss this alignment.

Causally grounded and clinically interpretable explainability methods are necessary for studies moving forward. This might be in the form of human-centered evaluations, explanation benchmarks, or medical knowledge graphs. For clinicians to be able safely and ethically to adopt VLMs in healthcare, and for patient safety, they must be understandable.

6.4 Computational Complexity and Deployment Issues

Vision-Language Models face immense difficulties when adapted to real-world applications in the healthcare industry, because of their intensive processing and deployment issues. Vision-Language Models comprise large vision encoder models plus transformer-based models and multimodal model layers, requiring large amounts of memory and processing capacity. It takes immense processing power and memory and is not feasible to train in smaller healthcare setups.

Another very important consideration is the inference speed, which is particularly important in a clinical setting, where time is of the essence. The inference speed may become a bottleneck in a clinical application, limiting the utility of VLMs for these types of problems. Higher resolution images also make the computation even more expensive.

Infrastructure needs, data security needs, and interoperability issues further make the deployment complex. Compatibility of the VLMs with the present IT infrastructure of hospitals, PACS, and EHR needs sound engineering practices. Deployment on the cloud involves newer issues of privacy as well as those of healthcare regulations. Deployment on the device has hardware limitations.

Model updates and maintenance further increase complexity. Though learning from additional data would prove excellent, privacy issues hinder this process of continuous learning because of potential performance issues. Achieving robustness, reliability, and consistency amid various environments is still a challenge.

These problems require techniques of model compression, efficient architectures, edge cloud collaboration, and optics. But there is a need for scaled down VLM models.

7. FUTURE RESEARCH DIRECTIONS

7.1 Integration with Foundation and Multimodal Large Language Models

Integration of Vision-Language Models with foundation models and multimodal big language models is a promising area to take the future of health care AI forward. The foundation models developed on a large multimodal dataset have been observed to generalize and understand the context. Thus, incorporating medical vision language models into it would provide the benefit of not only understanding images, but the ability to converse and provide explanations.

Future research should emphasize the further integration of visual encoders with very large language models for biomedicine. This combination allows the model to analyze medical images, review the patient's medical record, and provide medical findings based on the context. Learning and instruction tuning with the prompt method could ease the transition into different medical tasks. It would make retraining less necessary. Health knowledge graphs could add precision to medical predictions and prevent hallucinations.

Nevertheless, there are certain challenges that have been existing in the context of the benefits that need to be stabilized for clinical reliability, controllability of generative tasks, and the function being aligned with clinical practices. Efficient multimodal alignment techniques will be critical. Integrating VLMs and multimodal foundation and LLMs may revolutionize healthcare AI into interactive clinical companions for diagnosis, teaching, and decision-making assistance.

7.2. Federated Learning for Privacy-Preserving Healthcare

Federated Learning FL is a reliable way to overcome privacy and governance issues associated with healthcare Vision-Language Models. FL enables joint VLM training by all relevant institutions across their networks while allowing them to retain their patient data, which is a critical aspect of FL because a healthcare VLM network draws a wide variety of data from various hospitals, devices, and patients.

Future directions should involve federated learning methods geared towards multimodal data. These methods should handle problems associated with multimodal data. Methods of personalizing federated learning strategies would help in adjusting models derived from around the globe for more precise clinical environments. This would enable improvements in generalization and privacy. The introduction of differential privacy into secure aggregation would help in preventing a leakage of information.

However, federated learning brings about its own set of difficulties in FL, making system management even more complicated, the time to reach convergence even more considerable, and, more significantly, making debugging even more complicated in the case of multimodal models. There is considerable scope for work in developing efficient FL architectures and methodologies for parameter sharing in federated VLMs. Federated learning hence serves to promote large-scale, ethical, and inclusive development of healthcare VLMs.

7.3 Human–AI Collaboration for Clinical Decision Support

Collaborations between human and AI are one of the key ways forward to make the Vision-Language Models useful for clinical decision support. Whatever this may be, VLMs are not meant to replace the doctor but rather augment them as smart assistants by making it easier for clinicians to derive insights, explanations, and suggestions in a multitude of ways. Safe and effective integration of AI into real workflows of clinics and how they think and reason remains important.

In the future, research should stress the need for interactive and intuitive interfaces that allow clinicians to query VLMs regarding their opinion, check what visual grounding is employed for a particular opinion, and trace the line of reasoning. Human-in-the-loop allows doctors to assess, modify, or upgrade AI outputs to increase reliability and accountability. As these systems learn from constant active feedback by clinicians, their performance and trust should increase accordingly.

Another critical frontier is uncertainty estimation: VLMs need to convey their degree of confidence while flagging ambiguous cases that merit expert review. Embedding ethical guidelines and clinical protocols into decision-support pipelines will help ensure responsible AI use. Ultimately, the refinement of human–AI collaboration will turn VLMs into dependable clinical partners that will underpin health decisions having accuracy, clarity, and a focus on patients.

8. CONCLUSION

Vision-Lang Models (VLMs) represent an important milestone in AI applications in the healthcare industry because they enable doctors to learn from visual biological data and text simultaneously. Unlike previous solutions where the system relies on multiple sources independently, VLMs integrate what images express and what is said in clinical reports. This facilitates reasoning similar to what happens in real environments where doctors have to make decisions based on different sources.

Vision-Lang Models integrate vision encoders, language encoders, and multimodal fusion techniques.

This article explores the architectural essences of VLMs and highlights crucial components like cross-modal attention, multimodal transformers, and spectrum pre-training: contrastive and generative. It traces how models like CLIP, BLIP, MedCLIP, and BioViL convey an indication of a shift from general multimodal learning towards clinically informed and explainable models focused on a particular biological domain. Models of this type have immense potential in radiology, pathology, ophthalmology, or clinical note analysis.

Nevertheless, amidst these accomplishments, there still exist major hurdles to actualize in applications. These include concerns over data privacy, ethics, biases within datasets, interpretability, and computational complexity. Remedying these requires the use of privacy-preserving frameworks in machine learning, fair datasets, interpretable machine learning designs, and applications adapted to healthcare settings.

The future of VLMs will depend on directions such as the integration of the foundation and multimodal large language models, the role of Federated Learning for secure cooperation, and human-AI-centered clinical decision-making tools in improving the safety and accuracy of VLMs in the context of health outcomes. Vision-Language Models will be the underpinning of the next breakthrough in smart, ethical, and patient-focused systems in the context of health outcomes.

REFERENCES

Al Rahhal, M. M., Bazi, Y., Elgibreen, H., & Zuair, M. (2023). Vision-language models for zero-shot classification of remote sensing images. *Applied Sciences (Basel, Switzerland)*, *13*(22), 12462. DOI: 10.3390/app132212462

Alexander, A. M., Fitzgibbons, L. M., Kunz, H. E., Ortiz Correa, Z. K., Nair, K. S., Port, J., & Lanza, I. R. (2025). Intermuscular adipose tissue in healthy human aging—Effects of exercise training and implications to metabolic health. *Journal of Applied Physiology (Bethesda, Md.)*, *139*(5), 1300–1308. DOI: 10.1152/japplphysiol.00719.2025 PMID: 41115067

Awadalla, A., Gao, I., Gardner, J., Hessel, J., Hanafy, Y., Zhu, W., Marathe, K., Bitton, Y., Gadre, S., Sagawa, S., Jitsev, J., Kornblith, S., Koh, P. W., Ilharco, G., Wortsman, M., & Schmidt, L. OpenFlamingo. (2023). An open-source framework for training large autore-gressive vision-language models, URL https://arxiv.org/abs/2308.01390. arXiv:2308.01390.

Bordes, F., Pang, R. Y., Ajay, A., Li, A. C., Bardes, A., Petryk, S., et al. (2024). An introduction to vision-language modeling. arXiv preprint

Çallı, E., Sogancioglu, E., Van Ginneken, B., Van Leeuwen, K. G., & Murphy, K. (2021). Deep learning for chest X-ray analysis: A survey. *Medical Image Analysis*, *72*, 102125.

Cao, W., Zhang, J., Xia, Y., Mok, T. C., Li, Z., Ye, X., & Zhang, L. (2024). Bootstrapping chest ct image understanding by distilling knowledge from x-ray expert models. In *Proceedings of the IEEE/CVF Conference on Computer Vision and Pattern Recognition* (pp. 11238-11247). DOI: 10.1109/CVPR52733.2024.01068

Elshan, E., Binzer, B., & Winkler, T. J. (2025). From Software Users to Software Creators: An Exploration of the Core Characteristics of the Citizen Developer Role and the Related Re-and Upskilling Programs: From Software Users to Software Creators.... *Business & Information Systems Engineering*, *67*(1), 31–53. DOI: 10.1007/s12599-024-00915-1

Guerrero-Tamayo, A., Oleagordia-Ruiz, I., & Garcia-Zapirain, B. (2025). Vision-language zero-shot models for radiographic image classification: A systematic review. *Machine Learning with Applications*, •••, 100826.

Hamidieh, K., Zhang, H., Gerych, W., Hartvigsen, T., & Ghassemi, M. (2024). Identifying implicit social biases in vision-language models. vol. 7, In *Proceedings of the AAAI/ACM conference on AI, ethics, and society* (pp. 547–561). Conference paper. DOI: 10.1609/aies.v7i1.31657

Huang, C., Jiang, A., Feng, J., Zhang, Y., Wang, X., & Wang, Y. (2024). Adapting visual-language models for generalizable anomaly detection in medical images. In *Proceedings of the IEEE/CVF conference on computer vision and pattern recognition* (pp. 11375–11385). Conference paper. DOI: 10.1109/CVPR52733.2024.01081

Jia, C., Yang, Y., & Xia, Y.. (2021). Scaling up visual and vision-language representation learning with noisy text supervision. In *International Conference on Machine Learning (PMLR)*, pp. 4904-4916.

Jin, K., Yu, T., Ying, G., Ge, Z., Li, K. Z., Zhou, Y., Shi, D., Wang, M., Goktas, P., & Grzybowski, A. (2026). A systematic review of vision and vision-language foundation models in ophthalmology. *Advances in Ophthalmology Practice and Research*, *6*(1), 8–19. DOI: 10.1016/j.aopr.2025.10.004 PMID: 41532028

Kao, J. P., & Kao, H. T. (2025). Large Language Models in radiology: A technical and clinical perspective. *European Journal of Radiology Artificial Intelligence*, *2*, 100021. DOI: 10.1016/j.ejrai.2025.100021

Khoriba, G., Nouman, M., & Rashed, E. A. (2025). Large language models in medical image understanding. In: Cutting-edge artificial intelligence advances and implications in real-world applications. CRC Press, p. 32 Pages. DOI: 10.1201/9781032632483-7

Liu, B., Lu, D., Wei, D., Wu, X., Wang, Y., Zhang, Y., & Zheng, Y. (2023). Improving medical vision-language contrastive pretraining with semantics-aware triage. *IEEE Transactions on Medical Imaging*, *42*(12), 3579–3589. DOI: 10.1109/TMI.2023.3294980 PMID: 37440389

Lu, M. Y., Chen, B., Williamson, D. F., Chen, R. J., Liang, I., Ding, T., Jaume, G., Odintsov, I., Le, L. P., Gerber, G., Parwani, A. V., Zhang, A., & Mahmood, F. (2024). A visual-language foundation model for computational pathology. *Nature Medicine*, *30*(3), 863–874. DOI: 10.1038/s41591-024-02856-4 PMID: 38504017

Paola, J. D., Martikainen, J., Farahani, H., Lötjönen, K., & Rovamo, H. (2026). Drawn Futures: How Finland's Diverse Youth Visualise Tomorrow. *Journal of Community & Applied Social Psychology*, *36*(2), e70253. DOI: 10.1002/casp.70253

Parashar, S., Lin, Z., Liu, T., Dong, X., Li, Y., Ramanan, D., & Kong, S. (2024). The neglected tails in vision-language models. In *Proceedings of the IEEE/CVF Conference on Computer Vision and Pattern Recognition* (pp. 12988-12997).

Qinglong, L., Xiaodong, W., Song, X., Xiang, X., & Bo, P. (2025). Analysis of distribution network reliability based on distribution automation technology. *Energy Informatics*, *8*(1), 27. DOI: 10.1186/s42162-025-00478-9

Radford, A., Kim, J. W., Hallacy, C., Ramesh, A., Goh, G., Agarwal, S., & Sutskever, I. (2021, July). Learning transferable visual models from natural language supervision. In *International conference on machine learning* (pp. 8748-8763). PmLR.

Ruggeri, G., & Nozza, D. (2023). A multi-dimensional study on bias in vision-language models. In J. Rogers, & N. Okazaki (Eds.), *Findings of the association for computational linguistics: ACL, 2023* (pp. 6445–6455). Association for Computational Linguistics. DOI: 10.18653/v1/2023.findings-acl.403

Thakur, P. S., Khanna, P., Sheorey, T., & Ojha, A. (2022). Trends in vision-based machine learning techniques for plant disease identification: A systematic review. *Expert Systems with Applications*, *208*, 118117. DOI: 10.1016/j.eswa.2022.118117

Van, M.-H., Verma, P., & Wu, X. (2024). *On large visual language models for medical imaging analysis: An empirical study. In 2024 IEEE/ACM conference on connected health: applications, systems and engineering technologies. 172–176.*

Wang, Y., Yu, Z., Wang, J., Heng, Q., Chen, H., Ye, W., Xie, R., Xie, X., & Zhang, S. (2024). Exploring vision-language models for imbalanced learning. *International Journal of Computer Vision*, *132*(1), 224–237. DOI: 10.1007/s11263-023-01868-w

Xinming, X. U., Haoxuan, L. I., Zhouyu, G. U. A. N., Dian, Z. E. N. G., Yiming, Q. I. N., Yang, W. E. N., & Weiping, J. I. A. (2025). Urgent needs, opportunities and challenges of virtual reality in healthcare and medicine in the era of large language models. *Virtual Reality & Intelligent Hardware*, *7*(5), 453–467. DOI: 10.1016/j.vrih.2025.08.001

Zhang, P., Li, X., Hu, X., Yang, J., Zhang, L., Wang, L., & Gao, J. (2021). Vinvl: Revisiting visual representations in vision-language models. In *Proceedings of the IEEE/CVF conference on computer vision and pattern recognition* (pp. 5579-5588). DOI: 10.1109/CVPR46437.2021.00553

Zhang, X., Wu, C., Zhang, Y., Xie, W., & Wang, Y. (2023). Knowledge-enhanced visual-language pre-training on chest radiology images. *Nature Communications*, *14*(1), 4542. DOI: 10.1038/s41467-023-40260-7 PMID: 37507376

Zhou, K., Yang, J., Loy, C. C., & Liu, Z. (2022). Learning to prompt for vision-language models. *International Journal of Computer Vision*, *130*(9), 2337–2348. DOI: 10.1007/s11263-022-01653-1

Chapter 7
The Challenges of Vision Language Models (VLMs)

Apoorav Sharma
http://orcid.org/0009-0002-9966-7691
Lovely Professional University, India

Lovleen Marwaha
Lovley Professional University, India

ABSTRACT

Vision Language Models (VLMs) can be viewed as one of the most important developments in artificial intelligence where visual and linguistic modalities are combined to improve the analysis of medical imaging and the clinical decision-making process. This chapter is an in-depth discussion of the importance of VLMs in future healthcare, and the fact that such systems are capable of handling complex multimodal information like medical images and related clinical texts. The discussion outlines the disruptive value of VLMs in enhancing the accuracy of diagnoses, automatic generation of reports, and individualising treatment planning. Nevertheless, the application of VLMs to healthcare is followed by significant challenges. Limitations to technical issues are low and nonhomogeneous medical data, large computational costs, and interpretable domain-specific model adaptation.

I. INTRODUCTION

a. Overview of Vision Language Models (VLMs)

Vision Language Models (VLM) are also advanced artificial intelligence systems that combine and process both visual and textual information in parallel, allowing

DOI: 10.4018/979-8-3373-7315-7.ch007

ht © 2026, IGI Global Scientific Publishing. Copying or distributing in print or electronic forms without written permission of IGI Global Scientific Publishing is prohibited. Use of this chapter to generative artificial intelligence (AI) technologies is expressly prohibited. The publisher reserves all rights to license its use for generative AI training and machine learning model development.

interpretation, analysis and creation of multimodal content, which is a combination of images and text (Ryu et al., 2025). With their help, VLMs overcome the divide between computer vision and natural language processing, enabling sophisticated multimodal thinking and perception with the help of high-level deep learning, employing methods of transformer-based architectures in particular. These models can learn both visual and linguistic contextual representations with relationships that are jointly learned, which are also used to carry out image captioning, visual question answering, and cross-modal retrieval with greater accuracy and flexibility. Development of VLMs has been changing considerably in the past years. The initial works were concentrated on single tasks such as image caption generation and visual question answering with the help of comparatively simple architectures and small datasets. Advances were made with the advent of large-scale pre-trained models based on large multimodal datasets and transformer-based models, which made it possible to perform zero-shot and few-shot learning. This has been enabled by advances in model architecture, methods of training vision and language tasks together, and the existence of a variety of datasets and various large-scale datasets that more accurately reflect the complexity of real-world multimodal data. The significance of VLMs in healthcare can also be explained by the fact that these systems can integrate high-quality visual data provided by medical imaging with textual clinical data, including radiology report and patient records. Such integration helps to promote more accurate diagnosis, automatic report creation, and more individualised treatment plan. VLMs provide the insights of complex medical data by allowing multimodal analysis to overcome the limitations of unimodal systems and can be considered critical to the next-generation health care technologies. Recent advances in Vision Language Models include architectures such as CLIP (Contrastive Language–Image Pretraining), BLIP (Bootstrapping Language-Image Pretraining), and domain-specific systems like Med-PaLM and LLaVA-Med, which extend multimodal reasoning capabilities to clinical contexts.

b. Significance of VLMs in Next-Generation Healthcare

The potential medical imaging and diagnosis VLM VLM has the potential to transform the field because it allows visual and textual data to be processed and interpreted simultaneously. In medical imaging, VLMs would have the ability to identify and characterise abnormalities of different modalities of X-rays, computed tomography (CT), and magnetic resonance imaging (MRI). VLMs can be used to support end-to-end diagnostic processes, including unimodal analysis, through the integration of image data with related clinical text, including radiology reports, patient history, and clinical notes (Fang et al., 2025; Ryu et al., 2025). This multimodal feature provides a better way of detecting subtle pathological features, aids in the differentiating diagnosis and supports the elaboration of detailed, clinically relevant diagnostic reports. Also, VLMs may support cross-modal retrieval operations, allowing clinicians to query images with a natural language or produce interpretive descriptions so that access to information and decision-making are simplified. The importance of VLMs in enhancing patient care and treatment planning is also important. These models can be used to personalise insights by synthesising visual and textual data to support the adoption of precision medicine by correlating imaging detection with clinical parameters and recorded response of previous treatments based on patient records (Carroll et al., 2024; Quidwai and Lagana, 2024). As an example, VLMs can be used to suggest specific treatments based on patient-specific contexts by comparing the results of imaging with clinical parameters and prior treatment responses as reported in patient records. More so, the clinical workflows may be enhanced with VLMs that minimize diagnostic turnaround times by automatically generating reports and detecting anomalies and can thereby provide swift clinical decision-making. Such an increase in efficiency is crucial in healthcare settings with high demands where timely interventions can have a significant difference in patient outcome. VLMs can also be promising in assisting longitudinal patient tracking through sequential imaging along with the changing clinical data that take into account the early disease progression or the response of treatment. Although these are promising applications, the implementation of VLMs in the healthcare setting has a number of challenges. Heterogeneity and complexity of medical information is one of the greatest challenges, as medical data differ significantly in format, quality, and annotation standards across institutions and imaging activities. Such variability makes it cumbersome to train models and generalize them, which requires domain-specific adaptation and resilient preprocessing pipelines. Also, the implementation of VLMs in current clinical settings cannot be considered non-trivial; its ability to be compatible with various medical imaging devices, electronic health records (EHRs), and healthcare IT standards is required so that the workflow is not disrupted. The other severe issue is the interpretability and explainability of VLM results because clinicians need to have a clear-cut rationale to have trust and utilise AI-driven knowledge properly. Finally, strict regulatory standards and ethical issues, including patient privacy, data confidentiality and reduction of bias, should be strictly pursued to enable safe, fair and within the rules of practise deployment of VLMs in clinical practise. Figure 1 illustrates an overview of how Vision Language Models (VLMs) integrate multimodal data streams medical imaging and clinical text to perform diagnostic interpretation, report generation, and treatment recommendation tasks. For example, Med-PaLM has demonstrated the ability to answer medical visual questions and generate clinically relevant explanations from radiological images.

Figure 1. The diagram illustrates how Vision Language Models integrate visual inputs (such as X-rays, MRIs, CT scans, and pathology images) with textual inputs (including clinical notes, radiology reports, and patient history) through a multi-modal encoder and transformer fusion mechanism

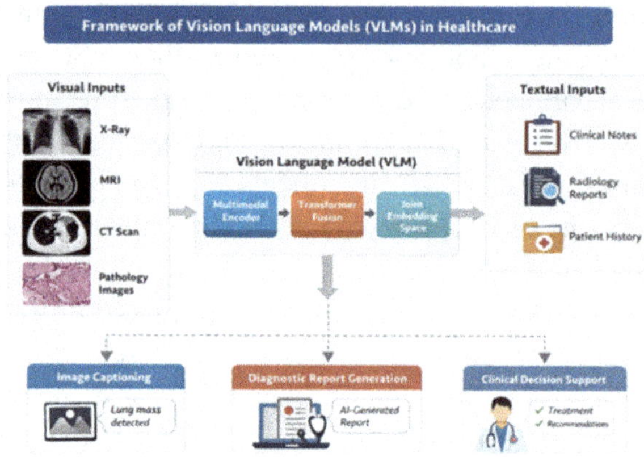

II. TECHNICAL CHALLENGES

a. Data Quality and Availability

Access to high-quality, diverse, and fully annotated medical imaging datasets is the key to the success of effective Vision Language Models (VLMs) in the health-care environment. Nevertheless, there are a few intrinsic problems in this field that impede the process of data acquisition, maintenance, and usage, thus affecting the performance and applicability of VLMs. (Shad et al., 2021) The small size and the lack of diversity in medical image datasets are among the most significant ones. In contrast to general-purpose image datasets, medical imaging data is usually not abundant since medical procedures are highly specialised and data collection is not only costly but also complex. Most of the datasets are specific to the institution and include specific patient demographics, imaging devices and clinical protocols, limiting the representativeness of the data. Such a dearth of diversity may result in models that are effective when using data of particular sources but not when generalising to other populations or other clinical settings. Moreover, medical images belong to many modalities X-rays, computed tomography (CT), magnetic resonance imaging

(MRI), ultrasound, and pathology slides have different characteristics and diagnostic value. This heterogeneity leads to more complexity in the compilation of the datasets and training of the models as it necessitates specialised preprocessing and normalisation methods to coordinate data to be able to learn effectively in multimodals. Another important issue is the level of annotation and consistency. The process of medical image annotation is labour intensive and cannot be done without expert knowledge usually given by radiologists or pathologists among others. The end result is that subjective nature of certain diagnostic interpretations may lead to inter and intra- observer variability, which causes discrepancies in labels and ground truth data. Also, the granularity of annotation can be either coarse (image-level labels) or fine-grained (pixel-level segmentations) and this suggests which kinds of learning tasks can be facilitated by annotation. Supervised learning methods are hampered by the lack of high-quality richly annotated datasets, which are fundamental in the process of model training and validation. This difficulty is further complicated by the fact that the cost and time needed to obtain expert annotation is very high, causing a bottleneck in the process of expanding the dataset and developing models (Duan et al., 2025; Xue et al., 2020).

Data availability is further complicated because of privacy issues and regulatory limitations. In the United States, the Health Insurance Portability and Accountability Act (HIPAA) and in the European Union, the General Data Protection Regulation (GDPR), establish strict rules, including a high level of consent of patients, anonymization of data, and safe operations. Such regulations tend to restrict the transportation of medical imaging information across the institutions and borders which lead to fragmented and siloed datasets. This cannot pool large scale and heterogeneous data which impedes the creation of strong VLMs that need a lot of training data to obtain complex multimodal associations. Additionally, the issue of patient privacy and data security requires the adoption of the state of the art de-anonymization methods, which will reduce the amount of personally identifiable information and ensure the retention of clinically significant data characteristics. There are also logistical and ethical issues associated with getting quality labelled medical data. The process of annotation will require cooperation between AI researchers and clinical experts and may need feedback loops to make labeling processes more accurate and relevant to clinical settings. There are issues of ethical concerns in making sure that data collection and annotation do not burden the patients and that care is not compromised. Moreover, medical knowledge is dynamic and thus annotations and diagnostic criteria change over time and require constant updates and validation of datasets to guarantee clinical validity. This time dimension creates even more complexity in dataset handling and retraining of the models(Arunachalam et al., 2024; Elendu et al., 2023). These data related issues cannot be solved in a single-faceted manner. More sophisticated data augmentation methods can increase both size and variety of datasets by synthesizing realistic perturbations of the current images and thus overfitting can be reduced and better generalization of models achieved. The semi-supervised and self-supervised learning approaches make use of unlabeled or partially labels data to minimize the use of expensive annotations. Transfer learning allows pre-trained models using large general-domain datasets to be fine-tuned using smaller medical datasets and converge faster and achieve higher performance. The tools of federated learning and privacy preserving machine learning potentially provides a viable way to train models across institutions without revealing confidential data, which will eliminate the obstacle of data sharing and still remain compliant with the data protection rules. To conclude, the quality and presence of medical imaging data is one of the key bottlenecks in the creation and implementation of VLMs in health care. The challenges of dataset size, diversity, annotation quality, privacy and ethical concerns will have to be overcome to create robust, accurate, and generalizable models and provide valuable clinical insights. Cooperation between clinicians, data scientists and policymakers is essential to introduce the standard data curation guidelines, ethical principles and technical solutions enabling high-quality and secure data sharing and data annotation practises. Public datasets such as MIMIC-CXR, CheXpert, and ROCO have been widely used for training medical VLMs; however, they suffer from annotation inconsistencies and demographic bias. These limitations directly affect model generalization and fairness across diverse patient populations.

b. Model Architecture and Complexity

Vision Language Models (VLMs) used in healthcare are supposed to be both practical and efficient in clinical settings in terms of the complexity and computational requirements and the domain-specific adaptability. These paradigms are mostly based on big-scale transformer-based models which have proven to be extremely successful in the process of modelling the multimodal associations of visual and text data. The introduction of such architectures to healthcare however presents a number of critical issues associated with the size of the model, the need of computational resources, domain adaptation, and interpretability. The tradeoff between the size of the models and computation is a soluble issue in the development of VLMs in healthcare applications. Millions and billions of parameters Transformer architectures are large in terms of memory and processing power to train and run. Although large models have the advantage of improved ability to learn multimodal representation that is complex, in practise they cannot be practically used in clinical settings, which are often limited in hardware infrastructure. Hospitals and clinics might not have the high-performance GPUs or cloud computing resources to support such models especially in resource-constrained settings or rural healthcare facilities(Cascella et al., 2024; Lamaakal et al., 2025) and near or real-time inference may be a critical component of clinical processes, and slow outputs may prevent timely decision-making. Thus, it is urgent to maximize VLM architectures to minimize the size of models and the computational overhead without affecting the precision. Such methods as model pruning, quantization, knowledge distillation, and efficient transformer variants (e.g., Linformer, Performer) are actively studied in order to develop lightweight but performant models useful in the healthcare domain. There is also an additional layer of complexity in filling the requirements of domain-specific adaptations. General-purpose VLMs that are trained on a large dataset such as COCO or Visual Genome are more generalised to visual and linguistic knowledge, but do not tend to be specific to medical conditions. Medical images also have their own unique features, medial texture, anatomical structure, and pathological patterns, which differ greatly with natural ones. Similarly, clinical languages are specialised, which means that they include terminology and abbreviations domain specific and containing contextual subtleties, non-existent in general corpora. Therefore, to customise VLMs to healthcare, it is necessary to adjust elements or redesign them to be effective in encoding visual and textual medical elements. This adaptation can take the form of using domain knowledge of the form of specialised embeddings, attention mechanisms that attend to clinically relevant regions, or multi-task learning models that simultaneously learn diagnostic and linguistic tasks. Moreover, the lack of annotated medical datasets makes it necessary to use transfer learning methods based on using pretrained weights, however, adjusted to the healthcare-specific distributions. Model architectures can be more interpretable and perform better by adding expert knowledge (e.g. medical ontologies or hierarchical anatomical representations), although architectural choices should be made carefully when constructing such hybrid models. Explainable and interpretable VLM architectures are a strict clinical adoption issue. Deep learning models and especially multimodal transformers are inherently complex, which makes their decision-making process opaque, which may be challenging to trust by clinicians, affecting the process of clinical validation, regulatory conditionality, and ethical accountability (Srinivasulu et al., 2025). The creation of VLMs that are inherently interpretable means including mechanisms that indicate salient image regions or textual phrases that led to predictions. Concentrating on visualisation and saliency maps, as well as gradient-based attribution, allow obtaining partial information about model areas of focus but might not be clinical-specific or consistent. More sophisticated methods attempt to produce natural language explanations that agree with clinical reasoning to give interpretable explanations that can be assessed by clinicians. This can also architecturally demand the use of modular designs that decouple feature extraction and decision logic or include interpretable intermediate representations. Complexity versus transparency Often, trade-offs are present between making models complex and easy to explain and making them simple and black-box. The creation of architectures with a high quality of diagnostic accuracy and with high explanatory capabilities is a research frontier.

In addition, they are compounded by the multimodality of VLMs. The necessity to closely intertwine vision and language modalities requires architectural innovations to provide consistent interactions of cross-modes. Cross-attention, co-attentional transformers or joint embedding spaces are the strategies that are used to align visual and textual features. Nevertheless, these mechanisms make architecture more complicated and more expensive to calculate. Further design constraints are the need to ensure that such fusion processes are interpretable and are clinically meaningful. Considering an example, models should not contain the spurious correlations of the image regions and textual tokens that may be deceiving in terms of clinical interpretation. To conclude, the complexity and architecture of VLMs in healthcare require an amicable tradeoff between scalability, domain specificity, and interpretability. It is essential to reduce computational requirements with the help of efficient model design to deploy it in practice and domain adaptation to make it relevant to medical data properties. At the same time, there is an increase in explainability that allows building clinician trust and regulatory compliance. To effectively solve all these interconnected issues, AI researchers, clinicians, and healthcare engineers have to cooperate on developing VLM architectures that are powerful and yet, accessible, reliable, and transparent in a clinical setting. Figure 2 summarizes the hierarchical taxonomy of challenges faced in deploying Vision Language Models (VLMs) across healthcare. It visually distinguishes technical, ethical, regulatory, and clinical domains, each encompassing unique but interdependent constraints influencing AI readiness. Most VLMs follow a dual-encoder architecture consisting of a vision encoder (e.g., Vision Transformer) and a language encoder (e.g., Transformer-based LLM), aligned through contrastive learning or cross-attention mechanisms.

Figure 2. This diagram categorizes the multidimensional challenges associated with Vision Language Models into four key domains—technical, ethical, regulatory, and clinical

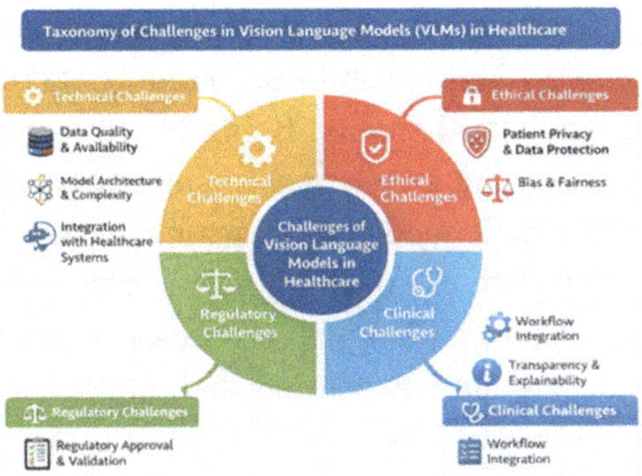

c. Integration with Existing Healthcare Systems

The deployment of Vision Language Models (VLMs) into the current healthcare system is a complex of issues that encompass not only the development of the model but also the implementation of the research in the clinics. These issues mainly include compatibility with existing medical imaging systems, perfect integration with electronic health records (EHRs) and interoperation across different healthcare systems. The necessity to deal with these issues is important to achieve clinical utility of VLMs and integrate them successfully in healthcare practise without affecting a conventional practise (Hartsock and Rasool, 2024; Ryu et al., 2025). One of the major technical challenges is compatibility with the existing medical imaging technologies. The imaging modalities of healthcare institutions are diverse in nature including X-rays, computed tomography (CT), magnetic resonance imaging (MRI), ultrasound and pathology imaging and they yield data in a variety of formats and resolutions. These images get frequently stored and transmitted by standards such as DICOM (Digital Imaging and Communications in Medicine) which contains both image data and metadata that are critical in clinical interpretation. VLMs should be in a position to accept and process these heterogeneous data formats correctly. Nevertheless, the inconsistencies between imaging protocols, types of scanners and imaging acquisition parameters among various vendors and institutions make the standardisation of model inputs challenging. Moreover, medical imaging can be full of patient identifiers or institution identifiers which need to be handled with caution to ensure compliance with privacy. To be able to preprocess and normalise and interpret such varied imaging data without sacrificing important diagnostic information, advanced data processing pipelines, which must be reliable enough in clinical terms, are required. The other fundamental issue is seamless integration with electronic health records (EHRs). Architecture, data models, and interoperability EHR systems are highly heterogeneous in both architecture and data model and often mirror healthcare IT infrastructure heterogeneity. Being based on visual and textual data, VLM should be able to search and match imaging information with relevant clinical descriptions, laboratory findings, medication history, and other patient data, located in EHRs. To retrieve useful textual information in unstructured or semi-structured clinical notes, sophisticated natural language processing (NLP) features specific to medical language are needed such as dealing with abbreviations, medical jargon, and terminology based on context. Additionally, EHRs are highly regulated and secured, which requires VLM integration to be in line with data protection requirements and ensure low latency and high availability. Integrating it may necessitate application programming interfaces (APIs) or specialized interfaces to connect VLM frameworks to EHR databases, either of which may be complex to both write and maintain technically. Moreover, the timely and accurate delivery of information is required in clinical workflows; therefore, the outputs of VLM should be displayed in EHR user interfaces in a way that will not disrupt clinician decision-making but contribute to alert fatigue (Hossain et al., 2024). Interoperability between various healthcare systems is critical to expand the use of VLM in environments other than individual ones. Healthcare ecosystems are generally made up of a number of software systems, devices, and databases sold by different vendors that have proprietary standards and communication protocols. Interoperability will be achieved based on the widely accepted standards of healthcare IT including HL7 (Health Level Seven), FHIR (Fast Healthcare Interoperability Resources), and IHE (Integrating the Healthcare Enterprise) profile. These standards will support orderly data transfer, semantic integrity, and collaborative processes, and the insights created by VLM could have access to and be used in different clinical units and hospitals. Nevertheless, there is a technical challenge with mapping VLM outputs which are usually multimodal and high-dimensional into standardised clinical terminologies and formats. As an illustration, the semantic alignment and validation of model-generated diagnostic impressions or image annotations into codified data (e.g., SNOMED CT, LOINC) coded data that is compatible with the patient records involves complex processes. Furthermore, interoperability requires constant change to ensure that standards, software version, and clinical uses are up to date. In addition to the technical compatibility, integration should take into account the system scalability, reliability and maintainability. The healthcare systems work with strict uptime specifications and any AI solution should be capable of working with these boundaries. The implementation of VLMs in clinical settings implies setting up of efficient infrastructure to serve models, monitor and control their versioning, making sure that the clinical services are not disrupted by updating or retraining. Also, to meet regulatory requirements, integration workflows should be capable of supporting audit trails and logging in order to examine AI-assisted decision-making post-hoc. The nature of the clinical settings also requires the use of user-centred design methods to make sure that VLM tools are compatible with clinical workflows and provide an easy interface and useful insights instead of overloading the user with raw data or other complicated results of the analysis. Overall, to integrate Vision Language Models with the current healthcare systems, one will have to face significant issues with data compatibility, EHR interoperability, and compliance with healthcare IT standards. It requires full technical solutions that include data preprocessing pipelines that can support heterogeneous imaging modalities, robust and secure interfaces with heterogeneous EHR systems, as well as standard communication protocols that can support smooth data exchange among platforms. It is necessary to overcome these difficulties to incorporate VLMs into the clinical practise and to make sure that all their high-tech multimodal features can be converted into real gains in the quality of diagnostics, productivity of work, and patient care. As outlined by recent studies, the technical challenges surrounding VLMs extend across data integrity, architectural efficiency, and system interoperability, all of which directly influence clinical reliability and scalability (Table 1). For instance, recent implementations integrate AI models with PACS and EHR systems to enable automated radiology report drafting and decision support within clinical workflows. The deployment of large-scale VLMs involves significant computational costs, including GPU infrastructure, storage, and maintenance, which may limit adoption in resource-constrained healthcare settings. However, these costs may be offset by improvements in diagnostic efficiency, reduced clinician workload, and faster turnaround times, leading to potential long-term cost savings for healthcare institutions. Federated learning offers a cost-efficient alternative by enabling decentralized model training across institutions without requiring centralized data storage, thereby reducing data transfer costs and enhancing privacy compliance.

Table 1. Comparative overview of technical challenges in Vision Language Models (VLMs)

No.	Technical Challenge	Description	Impact on Healthcare VLMs	Potential Solutions
1	Data Quality and Availability	Limited, heterogeneous, and poorly annotated medical datasets hinder model training and generalization.	Reduces diagnostic accuracy and causes poor model robustness across populations.	Federated learning, semi/self-supervised learning, synthetic data generation, and standardized data curation.
2	Model Architecture and Complexity	Transformer-based VLMs require massive computational power and domain adaptation for medical use.	Limits clinical deployment, increases latency, and reduces interpretability.	Model compression, knowledge distillation, domain-specific embeddings, and explainable architectures.
3	Integration with Healthcare Systems	Difficulties aligning with imaging formats (DICOM), EHR standards, and interoperability protocols.	Workflow disruption, data silos, and lack of real-time utility.	Adoption of HL7/FHIR standards, secure APIs, and modular AI-EHR interfaces.

III. ETHICAL AND REGULATORY CHALLENGES

a. Patient Privacy and Data Protection

Regulatory requirements in healthcare data, including the Health Insurance Portability and Accountability Act (HIPAA) in the United States, as well as the General Data Protection Regulation (GDPR) in the European Union, are required when implementing Vision Language Models (VLMs) in healthcare. These rules require stringent conditions regarding the gathering, storage, processing and distribution of patient information in an attempt to safeguard personal privacy as well as the security of the data. HIPAA requires the security of protected health information (PHI) in which administrative, physical, and technical methods are to be implemented to avert unauthorised access and breach. In a similar manner, GDPR focuses on minimization of data, restrictions of purpose and direct patient consent, and patient rights, data access, and data removal. These regulatory frameworks should be integrated into the design and operation protocols of VLM to ensure that they comply with the law and act ethically (Conduah et al., 2025). Effective anonymization and de-identification of patient information is an important technical and procedural issue to consider in the deployment of VLM. Medical imaging data typically includes embedded identifiers in metadata as well as in the images (e.g. patient names on scans). Powerful de-identification strategies should eliminate or obscure all personally identifiable data without negatively affecting the clinical value of the data. It is a fine line because overmasking data may lead to poor quality and context in order to train and infer an accurate model. Additionally, anonymization processes should be up-to-date continuously to overcome the progress of re-identification threats, particularly with progress in data linkage and inference attacks. Privacy-sensitive approaches like differential privacy, secure multiparty computation and federated learning models can also be used to further improve the protection of data as well as allow institutions to collaboratively develop models. Overcoming the concerns regarding unauthorised access and data breaches is the priority due to the sensitivity of healthcare data and the effects that such exposure has. VLM systems need to instal elaborate cybersecurity provisions such as data at rest and data in transit encryption, role-based access control, audit log, and intrusion detection solutions. Deployments in the cloud would also need other specifications like secure authentication measures and adherence to cloud security measures. Regular security cheques and incident response plans are necessary to detect the vulnerabilities and reduce them in time. Moreover, technical controls are strengthened by organisational policy that regulates data governance, trainings and controls over accountability to reduce human error and insider threats. The open dialogue with patients and other stakeholders regarding the use and protection of data practises helps build trust and implement AI in healthcare ethically (Hasan and Ahmed, 2025). Combined, these elements of patient privacy and data protection represent a challenging yet inseparable basis of responsible development and clinical implementation of VLMs. Regular compliance with regulatory provisions, application of stringent anonymization methods, and high levels of security are all the measures that assure that the rights of patients are honoured and that confidential health data is preserved throughout the AI lifecycle. Bias in VLMs can be quantitatively evaluated using fairness metrics such as demographic parity, equalized odds, and subgroup performance variance.

b. Bias and Fairness in VLMs

Prejudice and equity are essential ethical issues pertaining to implementing Vision Language Models (VLMs) in healthcare because these machines directly affect the diagnostic process and patient outcomes. Prejudices with VLMs are mainly caused by the training data and model development process, which are likely to inherently contain or even increase existing healthcare disparities. It is important to identify and reduce such biases to make sure that the model will operate fairly in various patient groups and avoid the promotion of health disparities. One of the key bases of bias is associated with the construction of training datasets. Clinical text and medical imaging datasets tend to be underrepresented with respect to demographic groups that may be based on age, gender, ethnicity, socioeconomic status, and geographic location. This underrepresentation has the potential to make VLMs be suboptimal when it comes to minority or marginalised populations, resulting in an imbalance in the accuracy of the diagnosis and recommendations of treatment. Besides, biases can be caused by uneven distribution or severity of diseases in datasets, which will cause the model sensitivity to be biassed towards more prevalent diseases or patient groups. The heterogeneity of the healthcare delivery systems and regional differences in the clinical practice also introduce bias in the datasets, which impact the generalizability of the models (Hilling et al., 2025; Restrepo et al., 2024). Reducing bias is a complex process that demands complex measures that can be supported by starting with curating the entire dataset in a way that focuses on diversity and representativeness. This entails intentional incorporation of diverse patient groups and clinical conditions in data gathering and annotation and standardisation of labelling procedures to minimise subjectivity. Class imbalances can be dealt with with data augmentation and/or synthetic data generation methods and attention has to be paid to maintain clinical realism. Besides data-level interventions, algorithmic methods, like fairness-conscious learning, adversarial debiasing, and training sample reweighting are used to decrease training model bias. These techniques seek to be able to balance performance measures amongst the subgroups without a reduction in total accuracy. The provision of fair performance among the varied populations of patients implies also strict evaluation procedures that evaluate model behaviour on stratified test sets to mirror demographic and clinical heterogeneity. The post-deployment should be continuously monitored to identify any emerging bias due to the changes in patients or clinical practise. Clinician-patient feedback loops may also give qualitative information regarding model fairness and update the iterative process. The solutions to the possible inequality in healthcare outcomes of the VLM biases are not limited to technical mitigation but also ethically and with regard to regulations. Comprehensiveness in model development, such as publication of dataset structure and recognized constraints, are associated with informed clinical practice and patient confidence. The regulatory systems are also placing more importance on the assessment of fairness during the approval of AI-based medical devices, and developers must prove equitable efficacy. Ethical standards favor the inclusion of design and responsible systems to avoid the harm caused by AI and assist in health equity. Overall, patient groups cannot be served equally in VLMs because of unfair data criteria and biases that require intentional approaches to data curation, model training, evaluation, and governance. The interdisciplinary effort of the AI researchers, clinicians, ethicists, and policymakers is essential in coming up with solid frameworks that are able to detect, reduce, and track the bias, thus preventing disparities and promoting trust in AI-based healthcare solutions. Figure 3 illustrates the convergence of ethical, regulatory, and clinical dimensions required for responsible Vision Language Model (VLM) deployment in healthcare. This integrated framework emphasizes that only through cross-domain alignment can VLMs achieve true clinical trustworthiness and equitable adoption.

Figure 3. The figure illustrates the intersection between three foundational pillars: Ethical Readiness, Regulatory Validation, and Clinical Integration that collectively underpin the development of trustworthy and deployable Vision Language Models (VLMs) in healthcare

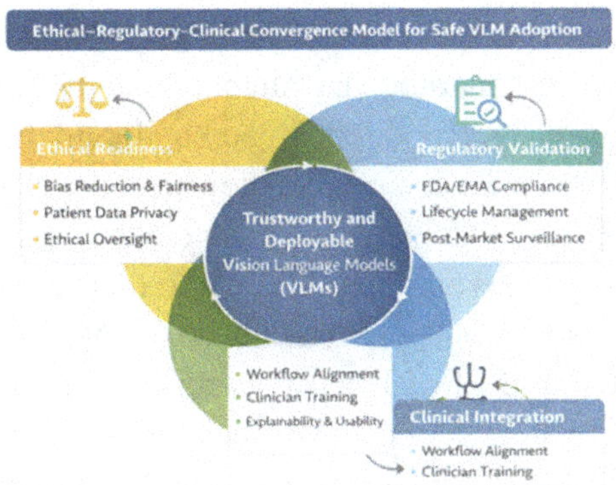

c. Regulatory Approval and Validation

The regulatory environment to Vision Language Models (VLMs) in the healthcare sector entails resolving the challenges of categorising, certifying, and licencing AI-based diagnostic systems to be operated within the current medical device systems. Relevant to the software discussed as a medical device (SaMD), VLM should be able to meet the strict regulatory requirements of the authorities, including the U.S. Food and Drug Administration (FDA), the European Medicines Agency (EMA), and other local governments. Such agencies demand detailed records that prove safety, efficacy, and reliability and ensure clinical implementation. Nonetheless, the adaptive and dynamic form of the AI/ML models such as VLMs which might be continually learning or updating creates a challenge to the traditional regulatory paradigms which were created in response to inanimate devices. The developers are thus required to work with the changing regulatory advice that is progressively taking into account risk-based, lifecycle-driven methods to AI/ML-based medical technologies. Clinical validation of VLM-based diagnostic tools has been a major challenge since it involves strict demonstration of how the model will be applied in various patient groups and or clinical situations with consistency. Validation studies are commonly completed in multi-center clinical trials or in retrospective studies where the product of VLM is compared to gold standards of established gold, e.g., expert radiologist interpretations or biopsy findings (Mccoy et al., 2025). The heterogeneity of clinical documentation, variability in imaging modalities, complexity of multimodal data integration require well-crafted protocols in order to evaluate diagnostic accuracy, sensitivity, specificity, and clinical utility. Also, VLMs should be analysed using the criteria of strength against confounding variables like imaging artefacts, demographic heterogeneity and comorbidities. Validation also considers the interpretability of model output since clear reasoning can be accepted by clinical and regulatory reviews. Post-market surveillance systems are also fundamental to observe the actual performance, model drift, and maintain the safety margins in the future (Chukwu et al., 2019). To ensure that they meet the changing AI/ML regulations, developers must ensure that they have a system that is comprehensive in terms of quality management systems and, in this context, must include such sub-systems as model development, validation, deployment and maintenance. Regulatory frameworks are being adjusted to deal with AI-related issues, focusing on transparency, explainability and risk reduction in the AI lifecycle. As an example, the proposed regulatory scheme of AI/ML-based SaMD by the FDA includes a premarket review of the algorithm alterations, an in-time monitoring, and a post-market performance reports. Equally, the AI Act proposed by the European Union presents the conditions of high-risk AI systems, such as healthcare apps, which require the conformity assessment and documentation of the risk management process. The compliance deals with the adherence to data governance policies, cybersecurity standards, and patient safety regulations as well. Cooperation with regulatory specialists, clinicians, and ethicists is essential to be able to work effectively through these changing demands and to achieve timely access to the market and provide protection to the patient (Muralidharan et al., 2024). Overall, the regulation of VLMs in the spheres of healthcare requires a complex strategy that can tackle the exceptional features of AI-based diagnostic devices. To make VLMs safe, effective, and trustworthy so that they can be used clinically, it is important to overcome challenges in clinical validation, adjust to dynamic regulatory frameworks, and put in place robust quality management and post-market surveillance systems. Ethical and regulatory dimensions form the backbone of trustworthy AI in healthcare. Table 2 consolidates the principal governance areas privacy, fairness, and validation and the corresponding mitigation pathways that ensure responsible VLM deployment (Table 2)

Table 2. Ethical and regulatory dimensions of vision language models in healthcare

No.	Ethical/Regulatory Dimension	Core Issue	Risk in Clinical Use	Mitigation and Best Practices
1	Patient Privacy & Data Protection	Ensuring compliance with HIPAA, GDPR, and protection against re-identification.	Breach of confidential patient data; legal and ethical violations.	De-identification, differential privacy, federated learning, robust cybersecurity, and governance policies.
2	Bias and Fairness	Underrepresentation of demographic groups in training datasets.	Health disparities, inaccurate predictions for minorities.	Diverse datasets, fairness-aware learning, and continuous post-deployment monitoring.
3	Regulatory Approval & Validation	Lack of clear frameworks for adaptive AI medical devices.	Delays in clinical deployment; unclear accountability.	Lifecycle-based FDA/EMA compliance, robust clinical validation, and post-market surveillance.

IV. CLINICAL IMPLEMENTATION CHALLENGES

a. Clinical Workflow Integration

The implementation of the Vision Language Models (VLM) into an established clinical practise should be thoroughly adaptive to guarantee that the emerging AI solutions will not interfere with the current healthcare provider activities but instead serve as an addition to them. Clinical practises tend to be complicated with several procedures, procedures, and stakeholders being part of them; such as radiologists, clinicians, technicians and administrative personnel. The effective implementation of VLMs requires these workflows in order to be aligned to ensure that the operation of VLM is efficient and contributes to the smooth adoption. The process of adjustment of VLMs to fit the current clinical workflows requires the comprehension of the particular operating conditions under which medical workers are operating. This involves determining where VLM outputs can be employed to add value to VLM, e.g., to automated anomaly detection in imaging, initial draught of reports, or decision support in diagnosis. VLM interfaces are to be designed in a manner that takes usability into consideration and even present results in a way that is both understandable and practical to clinicians. Integration needs to reduce the extra cognitive load, or workflow disruption, without causing too much in the way of additional alerts or redundancy in the information displayed to clinicians, potentially leading to fatigue. By integrating outputs of VLM into the current clinical information systems, including Picture Archiving and Communication Systems (PACS), and Electronic Health Records (EHRs), it will be easier to access and use regularly. Besides, it needs to be flexible to fit various clinical environments raanging between large-volume hospitals to smaller outpatient clinics with a variety of workflow constraints (Kim et al., 2025; Vankayala, 2025). The key to the benefits of VLM-based tools is to train healthcare professionals to be able to use them efficiently. Clinicians need to learn how to use the VLM interfaces not only technically but also understand the scope of the interfaces and their limitations and the way to interpret the outputs of AI-generated outputs. The training programmes must focus on the utilisation of VLMs as assistive technology and not as substitutes of clinical judgement to create a human-AI partnership. Sustained competency is enabled by continuous learning, such as the revision of models, and their developments. Also, the integration of clinicians during the development and implementation stages may enhance the design of the tools, making them user friendly and easily adaptable to the requirements of users. One of the most important issues in clinical implementation is the balancing of automation and the human expertise and decision-making. Whereas VLMs have the capability to automate some routine or time-intensive tasks, e.g., image triaging or report generation, the responsibility of diagnosis and treatment choice should remain with the healthcare professionals. To be successful in the integration process, it is necessary to create clear limits to AI autonomy and clarify cases of when human intervention is a requirement. Those workflows that are based on a combination of automated preliminary analyses and clinician review are the most efficient but maintain safety and accountability. VLM outputs, like confidence scores and explainability characteristics, will help clinicians consider AI recommendations with a critical view. Moreover, the plans of managing the discrepancies between the AI results and the assessment of the clinician have to be created to guarantee patient safety and prevent mistrust. Overall, integrating VLMs into the clinical workflow requires a human-driven strategy that would help align AI opportunities with the current health procedures, extensive training to empower medical workers, and a strong approach to the balance between automation and human control. These factors will have to be addressed to implement VLMs successfully into the clinical practise and make it more efficient with regard to patient care and diagnostic results in the absence of clinical judgement and workflow integrity. Potential failure modes include incorrect report generation, hallucinated findings, and misalignment between image features and textual descriptions, which can adversely impact clinical decisions.

b. Interpretability and Explainability

It is essential to develop interpretability and explainability techniques when working with Vision Language Models (VLMs) in healthcare to address the intrinsic black box-like nature of complex multimodal AI systems and guarantee the transparency of the clinical decision-making process by them. Architectures of VLM are based on complex transformer-based architectures that take the high-dimensional visual and textual data in as inputs and generate visual and textual outputs, which are not always intuitive to clinicians to comprehend or make judgments about. Such a lack of transparency is a major clinical adoption hindrance, since healthcare practitioners need to have understandable, reliable explanations to legitimise AI-generated knowledge and have the ability to employ it without apprehension into patient care (Weiner et al., 2025).. As a solution to this, several techniques have been suggested and are currently being developed to clarify VLM outputs to healthcare providers. Attention maps and saliency visualisation are two visual explanation methods that can be used to show the parts of an image that the model relies on the most to make its prediction, allowing a clinician to determine whether the model is highlighting clinically or pathologically significant anatomical or pathological characteristics. On the same note, text-based explanations may detect the important phrases or parts of clinical notes or reports that impacted the thought process of the model. Using a multimodal explanation model, a combination of these visual and textual attributions will facilitate a more comprehensive insight into the process of decision-making of the model, which corresponds to the clinical situation (Ghadekar et al., 2025). Higher-order methods seek to produce natural language accounts which are similar to that of a human clinical reasoning process, and which give interpretable explanations as to why a certain diagnosis or recommendation was made. These descriptions can be put into clinically useful terms including pertinent imaging results and matching textual data. Architecturally, this can be by constructing modular VLMs equipped with purposeful explanation generation modules or by setting explainability goals during training to motivate explainable model behaviour. These approaches do not only increase the trust of clinicians but also simplify the analysis of errors and refinement of models by helping to become more visible the modes of failure. Although these progresses have been achieved, there are still problems in making sure that there is consistency, fidelity, and clinical relevance in explanations. The visual saliency techniques are also prone to identifying non-specific or spurious areas that give false meaning. Explanation in written form can be simplistic to complex model reasoning, or not reflect finer medical understanding. Thus, interpretability methods should be strictly tested against clinical judgement and against user centred design principles, so that explanations can support, and not be counter-productive to clinical working processes. The concept of transparency in VLM-aided clinical decision-making will not be limited to the technical methodology of explaining the models, but also to the explicit provision of model constraints, confidence, and uncertainty values. The provision of clinicians with quantitative values of the reliability of the predictions is useful in adjusting the trust and making decisions regarding the perception when to trust AI outputs or consult additional human evaluation. Also, to implement models ethically and in compliance with laws, transparent records of the model creation, the nature of training data, and discovered biases are necessary

(Salimparsa et al., 2025). To conclude, a complex approach to interpretability, which involves the integration of visual and textual explanation techniques, natural language justification, quantification of uncertainties, and effective communication can be used to address the black box issue of VLMs in healthcare. They are necessary to promote clinician trust, make informed decisions, and make VLMs effective and accountable instruments in clinical practise. Common explainability techniques include Grad-CAM for visual attribution and SHAP values for feature importance analysis in multimodal settings.

c. Performance Evaluation and Quality Assurance

Proper benchmarks and standards of Vision Language Models (VLMs) in healthcare need to be established to provide objective data on the diagnostic accuracy of VLM, its reliability, and its clinical utility. In contrast to traditional AI models, VLMs use multimodal data, and assessment systems are necessary to determine both visual and textual interpretation and the combination of the two. Benchmarking requires standardized data set representing the richness of clinical scenarios, imaging modalities and patient demographics. These datasets must include well-labelled ground truths that have been certified by expert clinicians so as to be clinically relevant. Measures should not just be based on traditional accuracy measures but have sensitivity, specificity, area under the receiver operating characteristic curve (AUC-ROC) and task-specific measures such as the quality of report generation or cross-modal retrieval precision. Other benchmarking protocols must also pay attention to noise robustness, imaging artifacts, and domain shifts to approximate the real-world variability (Parida et al., 2024; Ryu et al., 2025). Provision of continuous monitoring and updating systems to deployed VLMs is essential to ensure performance after some time of operation in the dynamically evolving clinical setting. Model drift may arise as a result of patient population change, upgrade in imaging technology or changing clinical practise, which may worsen VLM accuracy and safety. Continuous quality assurance systems entail real-time monitoring of performance based on the incoming clinical information, feedback mechanisms of the medical practitioners and automated detection of abnormal outputs. Training or fine-tuning only after every period using new data will guarantee that models change their distribution as new knowledge is gained. To record update in the model and aid in regulatory compliance, version control and audit trail needs to be maintained. Also, the alerting mechanisms should be provided to the monitoring systems that will indicate when the performance deviates significantly so that the intervention could be implemented in time. To resolve the difficulties related to comparing VLM performance to human experts the validation studies should be well designed and representation of the clinical decision-making complexities should be considered.

Comparison of participants on a head-to-head basis should take into consideration the variability in expert interpretation and the inter-observer differences. Having ground truths of consensus or having annotations by a number of experts maximizes the rigor of evaluation. The comparative studies need to assess not just the accuracy of diagnostic but also such factors as the speed of the diagnostic, its consistency, and its effect on clinical workflow. Mixed evaluation procedures that involve quantitative and qualitative measurements of clinicians will offer a holistic explanation of the VLM potential and constraints. Moreover, the explicit description of uncertainty estimates and confidence intervals related to VLM predictions can help clinicians to put AI results in perspective in comparison to human judgement. It is important to note that VLMs are not substitutes but aid in the workflow, and its performance should be evaluated in the framework of human-AI products (Lettner et al., 2024). Overall, stringent performance measurement and quality assurance systems that are designed to meet the multimodal and clinical characteristics of VLMs are essential to protect the safety, efficacy, as well as reliability of healthcare implementation. These structures should include standardized benchmarks, constant monitoring plans and subtle human expert comparisons to make certain that VLMs provide consistent, clinically meaningful value throughout their life cycle. Standardized benchmarking of Vision Language Models in healthcare should include evaluation on datasets such as MIMIC-CXR and CheXpert. Performance metrics must extend beyond accuracy to include F1-score, Area under the Curve (AUC-ROC), precision-recall, and clinically relevant sensitivity-specificity trade-offs. These metrics provide a more comprehensive assessment of diagnostic reliability and robustness across patient populations.

Evaluation of VLMs should include:

- Diagnostic accuracy (AUC, sensitivity, specificity)
- Multimodal alignment (CLIPScore)
- Bias assessment
- Clinical usability metrics

V. FUTURE DIRECTIONS AND POTENTIAL SOLUTIONS

a. Advancements in VLM Architectures

The future of Vision Language Models (VLMs) in the healthcare context is the development of models specific to healthcare needs, which can help eliminate the existing limitations and realise all their potential in practise. The intricacy and particularity of medical information require new architectural advances that are capable of capturing the delicacies of visual medical images and rich clinical text without sacrificing computational power and interpretability and flexibility. A potential direction is to develop new architectures that incorporate domain-specific inductive biases and medical expertise into the architecture. In contrast to general-purpose VLMs that are trained on natural images and on common every-day language, healthcare-oriented VLMs have an advantage of using anatomical priors, disease ontologies and clinical terminologies in order to direct the learning process. As an illustration, hierarchical representations of anatomical structures or pathology-specific features may be incorporated into the model to make the model pay attention to clinically relevant regions and patterns to improve the accuracy of a diagnosis. These architectures can incorporate convolutional modules that are trained to handle the characteristics of medical images together with transformer layers that can handle clinical narratives to more accurately conduct multimodal fusion. Separable feature extraction, cross-modal interaction, and decision-making parts can be useful in achieving interpretability and simpler adaptation to new medical fields or tasks (Acharya et al., 2024; Gu et al., 2024). Another important direction is the development of more efficient and less heavyweight VLM models, which can be deployed in resource-limited clinical settings. Transformer based models are powerful large-scale models that are not always practical because they are computationally and memory intensive. Studies of compressible models like pruning, quantization and knowledge distillation can lead to smaller model sizes and lower inference latency, with only minor performance loss. Besides, other types of transformers, like sparse attention mechanisms, linear transformers, or hybrid models of convolutional and transformer layers may be studied to provide architectures that are more adapted to the high-resolution and high-dimensional imaging in medicine. Smaller models allow real-time inference and can be integrated into point of care devices, allowing greater access to high-quality AI diagnostics than tertiary care centres. The exploration of multi-modal strategies, which go beyond the vision and language to include other types of healthcare data, is a new frontier. Imaging and textual data used with structured electronic health record (EHR) meta-data, lab results, genomics, or physiological measurements can be used to offer a more comprehensive picture of clinical decision-making. Disease characterization, prognosis prediction, and individual treatment plans can be enhanced with the help of multi-modal fusion strategies that are successful in merging heterogeneous data sources. The architectural aspect of this involves adaptable frameworks which can absorb a wide range of data modalities, synchronise temporal and semantics and different data quality. As an example, the relationships among clinical entities can be modelled with the help of graph neural networks, whereas the relative significance of the various modalities can be dynamically weighted with the help of attention-based mechanisms. The multimodal VLMs of this type are likely to provide a holistic representation of patients to capture the complexity of clinical situations. Besides, the future architectures can be designed with continual learning and domain adaptation mechanisms in response to new clinical knowledge and data distributions. This has online updating features where the models learn on new data whilst maintaining previous knowledge hence they do not require complete retraining. Architectures that enable explainability through design, e.g. disentangled latent space architectures or explainable intermediate layers, will contribute to clinical trust and regulatory compliance. To conclude, the future of VLM architectures in healthcare is a complex process: the domain-specific knowledge is to be integrated in order to enhance clinical functionality, lightweight and efficient models are to be implemented to facilitate practical use, and the multimodal integration is to be extended to a wider range of patient-related data. All these innovations will help VLMs provide correct, interpretative, and context insight that can be easily implemented in various healthcare environments.

Future research should prioritize:

1. Lightweight VLMs for edge deployment
2. Explainable multimodal reasoning
3. Standardized medical datasets

b. Collaborative Data Sharing and Standardization

The creation of strong systems of safe and ethical sharing of medical data is inherent to the further development of Vision Language Models (VLMs) in healthcare because these models strongly require extensive and high-quality data sets. Data sharing with other parties demands consideration of strict privacy laws and regulations like HIPAA and GDPR that address privacy of patient data and mandate strict requirements in access and transfer over data. Safe systems should have modern privacy-maintaining technologies such as federated learning, differential privacy, and secure multiparty computation implemented in their design to allow institutions to train models across their premises without having to access raw patient data. Such methods assist in breaking data silos and at the same time, adhere to legal and ethical provisions. Moreover, the governance systems that include effective data use arrangements, audit systems, and responsibility of stakeholders are necessary to build trust between the involved parties and patients. Standardization of medical image annotation and labeling is also essential to achieve consistency, quality and interoperability across datasets to be used in training VLM. Medical imaging annotation is a complicated task because it requires specialist clinical judgement, diagnostic variability, and annotation granularity (e.g. image level versus pixel segmentation). Conventionally, standard guidelines should specify annotation schemas, labelling conventions and quality control instructions to minimise inter and intra observer variability. Semantic interoperability can be achieved by harmonizing terminologies with the help of structured ontologies, including SNOMED CT or RadLex. Also, the annotation tool must provide collaborative workflow that allows making repeated expert review and consensus. It is also feasible to have benchmark datasets that have standardised annotations to give a basis of fair comparison and validation of models (Chen et al., 2025). Developing massive, heterogeneous, and high-quality healthcare data to be used in training VLM requires the concerted actions between institutions and regions to reflect a wide range of patients, imaging modalities, and clinical settings. The heterogenous datasets reduce the biases and improve the generalizability of the models, which will ensure the fair performance of the models on populations. The curation of data should focus on the extensive metadata, the imaging parameters, clinical histories, and outcome measures to augment multimodal learning. Synthetic data generation and augmentation are some of the strategies that can be used to supplement real-world data, especially where the disease is rare or underrepresented. Cross-institutional consortia and public-private partnerships are critical in sharing resources, standardizing and harmonization of data. After all, it is these big datasets that support the creation of efficient and clinically viable VLMs that can handle the intricacy of healthcare situations.

CONCLUSION

The introduction of Vision Language Models in healthcare represents an enormous potential and a considerable degree of complexity at the same time. The chapter has clarified the complex issues that cut across technical, ethical, regulatory and clinical issues that need to be confronted in order to maximise the use of VLMs. The limited, heterogeneous data, computer resource constraints, and the necessity of domain-specific and interpretable architectures are among the technical difficulties that support the relevance of specialised model development. The smooth connexion with the existing medical imaging systems and EHRs require compliance with the interoperability standards and effective data exchange protocols. The ethical requirements are focused on protecting patient privacy, reducing biases, and equitable performance in the context of a wide range of populations, and to overcome the changing regulatory environment, stringent validation is required and life cycles managed. The clinical implementation issues imply the need to integrate VLMs into the current workflows, encourage the development of the trust between clinicians and explainability, and find the balance between automation and human attention. The chapter supports the future directions such as architectural innovation to embrace medical understanding, effective model designs that fit various clinical environments, and interoperable structures to enable safe and standard data sharing. Laws and ethical standards are also required to adapt to allow responsible AI usage. Interdisciplinary collaboration will be essential in the achievement of the transformative potential of VLMs in healthcare, involving the bridging of AI research, clinical expertise, ethics, and policy. By focusing on these interrelated issues as a whole picture, VLMs have the potential to transform the way medical imaging is analysed and clinical decisions are made, which will ultimately bring precision medicine and enhance patient outcomes in all parts of the world.

REFERENCES

Acharya, A., Shrestha, S., Chen, A., Conte, J., Avramovic, S., Sikdar, S., Anastasopoulos, A., & Das, S. (2024). Clinical risk prediction using language models: Benefits and considerations. *Journal of the American Medical Informatics Association : JAMIA*, *31*(9), 1856–1864. DOI: 10.1093/jamia/ocae030 PMID: 38412328

Arunachalam, P., Usharani, R., Thirumal, S., Swarnalatha, A. P., & Maheswari, B. U. (2024). *Study on AI-Powered Advanced Drug Discovery for Enhancing Privacy and Innovation in Healthcare*. Igi Global., DOI: 10.4018/979-8-3693-3212-2.ch003

Carroll, A. N., Storms, L. A., Malempati, C., Shanavas, R. V., & Badarudeen, S. (2024). Generative Artificial Intelligence and Prompt Engineering: A Primer for Orthopaedic Surgeons. *JBJS Reviews*, *12*(10). Advance online publication. DOI: 10.2106/JBJS.RVW.24.00122 PMID: 39361780

Cascella, M., Semeraro, F., Montomoli, J., Bellini, V., Piazza, O., & Bignami, E. (2024). The Breakthrough of Large Language Models Release for Medical Applications: 1-Year Timeline and Perspectives. *Journal of Medical Systems*, *48*(1), 22. Advance online publication. DOI: 10.1007/s10916-024-02045-3 PMID: 38366043

Chen, J., Duan, H., Zhang, X., Gao, B., Grau, V., & Han, J. (2025). From Gaze to Insight: Bridging Human Visual Attention and Vision Language Model Explanation for Weakly-Supervised Medical Image Segmentation. *IEEE Transactions on Medical Imaging, PP, 1*. Advance online publication. DOI: 10.1109/TMI.2025.3616598 PMID: 41052168

Chukwu, S. C., Rafii, M. Y., Ramlee, S. I., Ismail, S. I., Oladosu, Y., Okporie, E., Onyishi, G., Utobo, E., Ekwu, L., Swaray, S., & Jalloh, M. (2019). Marker-assisted selection and gene pyramiding for resistance to bacterial leaf blight disease of rice (Oryza sativa L.). *Biotechnology, Biotechnological Equipment*, *33*(1), 440–455. DOI: 10.1080/13102818.2019.1584054

Conduah, A. K., Ofoe, S., & Siaw-Marfo, D. (2025). Data privacy in healthcare: Global challenges and solutions. *Digital Health*, *11*, 20552076251343959. Advance online publication. DOI: 10.1177/20552076251343959 PMID: 40475296

Duan, J., Zhang, M., Song, M., Xu, X., & Lu, H. (2025). Eye Tracking-Enhanced Deep Learning for Medical Image Analysis: A Systematic Review on Data Efficiency, Interpretability, and Multimodal Integration. *Bioengineering (Basel, Switzerland)*, *12*(9), 954. DOI: 10.3390/bioengineering12090954 PMID: 41007199

Elendu, C., Amaechi, D. C., Elendu, T. C., Jingwa, K. A., Okoye, O. K., John Okah, M., Ladele, J. A., Farah, A. H., & Alimi, H. A. (2023). Ethical implications of AI and robotics in healthcare. *Revista de Medicina (São Paulo), 102*(50), e36671. DOI: 10.1097/MD.0000000000036671 PMID: 38115340

Fang, M., Wang, Z., Pan, S., Feng, X., Zhao, Y., Hou, D., Wu, L., Xie, X., Zhang, X.-Y., Tian, J., & Dong, D. (2025). Large models in medical imaging: Advances and prospects. *Chinese Medical Journal, 138*(14), 1647–1664. DOI: 10.1097/CM9.0000000000003699 PMID: 40539307

Ghadekar, P., Gupta, N., Samgir, S., Umbare, S., Rathod, K., Deshpande, N., & Chaudhari, L. (2025). *Transparent Clinical Support Through Cross-Modal Fusion and Aligned Explanations*. Springer Science Business Media Llc. DOI: 10.21203/rs.3.rs-6636328/v1

Gu, X., Chen, Y., & Tong, W. (2024). KARAN: Mitigating Feature Heterogeneity and Noise for Efficient and Accurate Multimodal Medical Image Segmentation. *Electronics (Basel), 13*(23), 4594. DOI: 10.3390/electronics13234594

Hartsock, I., & Rasool, G. (2024). Vision-language models for medical report generation and visual question answering: A review. *Frontiers in Artificial Intelligence, 7*, 1430984. Advance online publication. DOI: 10.3389/frai.2024.1430984 PMID: 39628839

Hasan, M. T., & Ahmed, I. (2025). AI-DRIVEN ANOMALY DETECTION FOR DATA LOSS PREVENTION AND SECURITY ASSURANCE IN ELECTRONIC HEALTH RECORDS. *Review of Applied Science and Technology, 04*(03), 35–67. DOI: 10.63125/dzyr0648

Hilling, D. E., Ihaddouchen, I., Buijsman, S., Townsend, R., Gommers, D., & Van Genderen, M. E. (2025). The imperative of diversity and equity for the adoption of responsible AI in healthcare. *Frontiers in Artificial Intelligence, 8*, 1577529. Advance online publication. DOI: 10.3389/frai.2025.1577529 PMID: 40309720

Hossain, M., Mahabub, S., Masum, A., & Jahan, I. (2024). Natural Language Processing (NLP) in Analyzing Electronic Health Records for Better Decision Making. *Journal of Computer Science and Technology Studies, 6*(5), 216–228. DOI: 10.32996/jcsts.2024.6.5.18

Kim, H., Lee, S.-Y., You, S. C., Huh, S., Kim, J.-E., Kim, S.-T., Ko, D.-R., Kim, J. H., Lee, J. H., Lim, J. S., Park, M. S., & Lee, K. Y. (2025). A Bilingual On-Premises AI Agent for Clinical Drafting: Implementation Report of Seamless Electronic Health Records Integration in the Y-KNOT Project. *JMIR Medical Informatics, 13*(8), v13i8e76848. Advance online publication. DOI: 10.2196/76848 PMID: 41284981

Lamaakal, I., Maleh, Y., El Makkaoui, K., Ouahbi, I., Pławiak, P., Alfarraj, O., Almousa, M., & Abd El-Latif, A. A. (2025). Tiny Language Models for Automation and Control: Overview, Potential Applications, and Future Research Directions. *Sensors (Basel)*, *25*(5), 1318. DOI: 10.3390/s25051318 PMID: 40096098

Lettner, J., Królikowska, A., Ramadanov, N., Oleksy, Ł., Hakam, H. T., Becker, R., & Prill, R. (2024). Evaluating the Reliability of MyotonPro in Assessing Muscle Properties: A Systematic Review of Diagnostic Test Accuracy. *Medicina (Kaunas, Lithuania)*, *60*(6), 851. DOI: 10.3390/medicina60060851 PMID: 38929468

Mccoy, L. G., Bihorac, A., Celi, L. A., Elmore, M., Kewalramani, D., Kwaga, T., Martinez-Martin, N., Prôa, R., Schamroth, J., Shaffer, J. D., Youssef, A., & Fiske, A. (2025). Building health systems capable of leveraging AI: Applying Paul Farmer's 5S framework for equitable global health. *BMC Global and Public Health*, *3*(1), 39. Advance online publication. DOI: 10.1186/s44263-025-00158-6 PMID: 40312417

Muralidharan, V., Adewale, B. A., Huang, C. J., Nta, M. T., Ademiju, P. O., Pathmarajah, P., Hang, M. K., Adesanya, O., Abdullateef, R. O., Babatunde, A. O., Ajibade, A., Onyeka, S., Cai, Z. R., Daneshjou, R., & Olatunji, T. (2024). A scoping review of reporting gaps in FDA-approved AI medical devices. *NPJ Digital Medicine*, *7*(1), 273. Advance online publication. DOI: 10.1038/s41746-024-01270-x PMID: 39362934

Parida, A., Jiang, Z., Packer, R. J., Avery, R. A., Anwar, S. M., & Linguraru, M. G. (2024). QUANTITATIVE METRICS FOR BENCHMARKING MEDICAL IMAGE HARMONIZATION. *Proceedings. IEEE International Symposium on Biomedical Imaging*, 2024, 1–5. DOI: 10.1109/ISBI56570.2024.10635289

Quidwai, M. A., & Lagana, A. (2024). *A RAG Chatbot for Precision Medicine of Multiple Myeloma*. Cold Spring Harbor Laboratory. DOI: 10.1101/2024.03.14.24304293

Restrepo, D., Wu, C., Vásquez-Venegas, C., Matos, J., Gallifant, J., Celi, L. A., Bitterman, D. S., & Nakayama, L. F. (2024). *Analyzing Diversity in Healthcare LLM Research: A Scientometric Perspective*. Cold Spring Harbor Laboratory. DOI: 10.1101/2024.06.18.24309113

Ryu, J. S., Kang, H., Chu, Y., & Yang, S. (2025). Vision-language foundation models for medical imaging: A review of current practices and innovations. *Biomedical Engineering Letters*, *15*(5), 809–830. DOI: 10.1007/s13534-025-00484-6 PMID: 40917147

Salimparsa, M., Sedig, K., Lizotte, D. J., Abdullah, S. S., Chalabianloo, N., & Muanda, F. T. (2025). Explainable AI for Clinical Decision Support Systems: Literature Review, Key Gaps, and Research Synthesis. *Informatics (MDPI)*, *12*(4), 119. DOI: 10.3390/informatics12040119

Shad, R., Cunningham, J. P., Ashley, E. A., Langlotz, C. P., & Hiesinger, W. (2021). Designing clinically translatable artificial intelligence systems for high-dimensional medical imaging. *Nature Machine Intelligence*, *3*(11), 929–935. DOI: 10.1038/s42256-021-00399-8

Srinivasulu, A., Agrawal, A., & Vedaiyan, R. (2025). Overcoming diagnostic and data privacy challenges in viral disease detection: An integrated approach using generative AI, vision transformers, explainable AI, and federated learning. *Frontiers in Virology*, *5*, 1625855. Advance online publication. DOI: 10.3389/fviro.2025.1625855

Vankayala, V. Venkata Naga Mahesh Kumar Vankayala. (2025). Auditing AI Access to Electronic Health Records: HIPAA Compliance, Challenges, Solutions, and Future Directions. *Journal of Computer Science and Technology Studies*, *7*(8), 458–464. DOI: 10.32996/jcsts.2025.7.8.51

Weiner, E. B., Dankwa-Mullan, I., Nelson, W. A., & Hassanpour, S. (2025). Ethical challenges and evolving strategies in the integration of artificial intelligence into clinical practice. *PLOS Digital Health*, *4*(4), e0000810. DOI: 10.1371/journal.pdig.0000810 PMID: 40198594

Xue, C., Deng, Q., Li, X., Dou, Q., & Heng, P.-A. (2020). *Cascaded Robust Learning at Imperfect Labels for Chest X-ray Segmentation*. Springer., DOI: 10.1007/978-3-030-59725-2_56

Chapter 8
Vision Language Models for Medical Imaging:
Foundation Models for Diagnostic Reasoning, Reporting, and Clinical Workflow Intelligence

Vipin Tyagi
http://orcid.org/0000-0003-4994-3686
Jaypee University of Engineering and Technology, Guna, India

ABSTRACT

Vision language models (VLMs) represent a transformative paradigm in medical artificial intelligence, enabling joint reasoning over clinical images and textual information. Their ability to integrate radiology scans, pathology slides, ultrasound frames and structured/unstructured medical text positions them at the center of the next generation of intelligent diagnostic systems. This chapter provides a comprehensive and unified exploration of VLMs for medical imaging, beginning with foundational principles, covering architectural advances, discussing clinical applications, identifying challenges such as hallucination risks and mapping future research directions. The chapter integrates conceptual explanations, empirical trends and clinically informed insights with detailed figures, diagram sketches and tables. The aim is to equip researchers, clinicians and developers with a complete understanding of how vision language models can responsibly and effectively support next-generation medical imaging pipelines.

DOI: 10.4018/979-8-3373-7315-7.ch008

ht © 2026, IGI Global Scientific Publishing. Copying or distributing in print or electronic forms without written permission of IGI Global Scientific Publishing is prohibited. Use of this chapter to generative artificial intelligence (AI) technologies is expressly prohibited. The publisher reserves all rights to license its use for generative AI training and machine learning model development.

1. INTRODUCTION

Medical imaging sits at the heart of modern clinical care. Chest radiographs, CT scans, MRIs, ultrasound, retinal imaging and digital pathology slides are used daily to detect disease, monitor treatment and guide interventions. At the same time, healthcare systems face rising imaging volumes and a shortage of specialists, particularly radiologists and pathologists. This mismatch creates a clear need for trustworthy, scalable AI support.

For the past few years, most medical imaging AI tools have been "vision-only" convolutional neural networks (CNNs) trained to classify diseases or segment organs. These systems can be powerful, but they also have limitations. They typically require carefully curated labels and their outputs often remain difficult for clinicians to interpret. In real clinical work, radiologists do not just look at images, they analyze images and language: reports, patient histories, prior examinations, lab results and guidelines. Vision-language models (VLMs) bridge that gap. Rather than treating imaging and text as separate streams, VLMs provide a shared representation space where images align with clinical descriptions. This multimodal alignment allows a single system to support a broad range of tasks: report generation, medical visual question answering (Med-VQA), cross-modal retrieval and grounded explanation. VLMs can also learn from "free supervision" in the form of paired clinical reports, reducing reliance on expensive human labeling (Zhang et al., 2023).

The rise of VLMs in medicine builds on breakthroughs in general-domain vision language learning (Radford et al., 2021) and the rapid scaling of transformers. Importantly, medical VLMs must meet higher standards than general models: reliability, fairness, robustness, transparency and patient safety.

2. IMPORTANCE OF COMBINING VISION AND LANGUAGE IN CLINICAL IMAGING

2.1 The nature of clinical interpretation

Radiology and pathology are inherently multimodal disciplines because the final clinical meaning emerges from an interaction between visual evidence and linguistic reasoning. A radiology report is not a simple caption of an image. It is a structured clinical argument that integrates image observations with patient context, prior studies and diagnostic logic. A typical medical report contains:

- **Findings**: descriptive observations available in the image (e.g., "right lower lobe consolidation")

- **Impression**: the diagnostic synthesis and prioritization of likely etiologies
- **Comparison**: temporal reasoning across prior studies (e.g., "increased since 03/12/2025")
- **Uncertainty language**: calibrated confidence statements (e.g., "cannot exclude," "may represent," "suggestive of")
- **Negation**: explicit ruling out of critical conditions (e.g., "no pneumothorax," "no intracranial hemorrhage")

These linguistic patterns are not stylistic choices. They encode clinical reasoning, risk management and communication norms that support decision-making, triage and follow-up. According to clinical NLP research, negation and uncertainty are essential for accurately interpreting medical text, particularly in radiology where many key statements describe absence of findings or limited confidence. In practice, misinterpreting "no evidence of pneumonia" as positive pneumonia can be as harmful as missing a lesion in the image.

Pathology is similarly multimodal: the diagnostic workflow often combines whole-slide imaging and microscopic patterns with textual metadata (clinical history, specimen type, immune histochemistry results) and the final diagnosis is frequently a structured narrative with qualifiers and differential diagnoses.

Because the clinical meaning is expressed jointly through what is seen and how it is described, models trained only on image labels are constrained to a narrow supervision signal. They often miss the richness of reasoning present in reports, including differential diagnosis, borderline findings, uncertainty calibration and temporal evolution.

2.2 Paired image-text data as supervision

A major advantage in medical imaging is that images are routinely paired with expert-generated text as part of standard care. Radiology images are associated with reports, pathology slides are associated with diagnostic sign-out and many institutions maintain longitudinal imaging histories. These paired data enable self-supervised and weakly supervised learning without requiring expensive pixel-level annotation or curated labels.

Contrastive learning is particularly well-suited for this application. The main idea is to learn representations by bringing paired image and text closer in embedding space while rejecting mismatched pairs. This uses the report as a naturally available supervisory signal, even when explicit labels are incomplete or inconsistent. ConVIRT showed that contrastive pretraining on radiograph-report pairs improves performance on multiple downstream tasks while reducing the amount of labeled data required (Zhang et al., 2023). Similar principles were later reinforced by general-domain work such as CLIP, which demonstrated that contrastive image-text pretraining can produce transferable representations across diverse tasks (Radford et al., 2021).

This strategy benefits the medical domain for following reasons:

- **Dense semantic coverage**: reports contain many clinically relevant facts per study, including non-target findings that typical labels ignore.
- **Natural clinical vocabulary**: supervision is grounded in real clinical language and uncertainty patterns.
- **Scalability**: hospitals generate large volumes of paired studies, supporting large-scale pretraining.
- **Label efficiency**: pretraining can reduce the dependency on scarce expert annotations for downstream tasks.

However, paired clinical text is also noisy and variable. Reports can contain hedging, templated sections and clinically irrelevant boilerplate. This requires careful preprocessing and clinical NLP techniques and it also motivates large-scale learning where models can average out idiosyncratic phrasing and learn consistent multimodal signals (Johnson et al., 2019).

2.3 Transformers and multimodal representation learning

Transformers provide a natural architecture for multimodal learning because they treat inputs as sequences of tokens and learn global interactions using attention. This is crucial in medical imaging where clinically meaningful patterns may be subtle, distributed and context-dependent.

Vision Transformers (ViTs) split an image into patches and encode them as tokens, enabling attention across the entire image rather than relying only on local receptive fields as in traditional convolutional networks (Dosovitskiy et al., 2021). ViTs have proven highly effective in large-scale environment and are increasingly used in medical imaging, including radiology and digital pathology, where global context and long-range dependencies matter.

On the language side, transformer models capture contextual meaning and are strong at representing complex clinical phrases, including negation and uncertainty. BERT introduced bidirectional contextual encoding and became the foundation for domain-adapted medical language models (Devlin et al., 2019). ClinicalBERT showed that further pretraining on clinical notes improves performance on clinical NLP tasks, reflecting the importance of domain-specific language patterns (Alsentzer et al., 2019).

By aligning the latent representations of visual and textual tokens, Vision-Language Models (VLMs) can learn joint embeddings that capture clinically meaningful semantics. This enables:

- **Cross-modal retrieval:** retrieving relevant images given text queries, or retrieving reports given images
- **Zero-shot and few-shot transfer**: adapting to new tasks with minimal labeled data
- **Grounded reasoning**: linking report statements to image evidence
- **Better uncertainty modeling**: using hedging and negation as part of the learning signal

Transformers also support more explicit fusion strategies, such as cross-attention between image tokens and text tokens, which can help models learn to attend to image regions relevant to particular clinical phrases. This is especially valuable in settings like chest radiography where statements such as "no pleural effusion" depend on attending to specific anatomical regions and subtle cues and where clinical text contains many negated findings that must be grounded appropriately (Johnson et al., 2019).

Many clinically relevant tasks lack large, clean annotation sets. Even when labels exist, they often represent simplified endpoints such as "pneumonia present" rather than the full reasoning process. By learning from paired image–report data at scale, VLMs can acquire richer representations that transfer better to new tasks and new clinical environments, improving performance when labeled examples are limited (Zhang et al., 2023; Radford et al., 2021). This is particularly valuable in healthcare settings where distribution shifts are common due to differences in scanners, protocols, patient populations and reporting styles.

Radiology reports routinely compare current images against prior studies and this temporal reasoning is central to assessing progression or treatment response. VLMs trained on report language that encodes comparison and change may learn features that better represent disease trajectory, rather than static classification alone. Publicly available datasets such as MIMIC-CXR explicitly include report text and metadata that enable research into longitudinal modeling and multimodal clinical reasoning (Johnson et al., 2019).

In practice, clinicians often search for similar prior cases, relevant information files, or evidence-based references. Joint embeddings learned by VLMs enable cross-modal retrieval, for example retrieving radiographs similar to "right apical pneumothorax," or retrieving reports that match a given image. This can support education, audit and rapid second-opinion workflows, especially when integrated with curated uncertainty handling and quality control.

Report generation is a basic VLM application, but its clinical value depends on accuracy, grounding and calibrated uncertainty. Large radiology datasets such as CheXpert introduced the idea of explicit uncertainty labels, highlighting that uncertainty must be modeled rather than ignored. VLMs that learn from real report language may better capture the distribution of hedging, negation and impression-style summarization. This can eventually support structured reporting assistance, draft impressions and consistent phrasing, provided that outputs are rigorously validated and constrained to avoid hallucinations.

The same principles extend to digital pathology, where text supervision includes diagnosis, grading, specimen type and immunohistochemistry context. Transformers have been increasingly adopted for pathology due to the need to model large context and long-range spatial dependencies and multimodal training can connect microscopic patterns with diagnostic narratives. This suggests a unified VLM perspective across imaging specialties, where models learn shared clinical semantics while adapting to modality-specific evidence.

3. ARCHITECTURE FAMILIES OF VISION-LANGUAGE MODELS

Medical VLMs can be categorized into four major architectural families, differing in how they combine visual and textual information, what training objectives they use, and what clinical tasks they support best. In medicine, performance trade-offs depend less on raw model size and more on alignment quality, grounding fidelity and robustness to clinical language conventions like negation and uncertainty.

3.1 Dual-Encoder Contrastive Models

Dual-encoder models use two separate encoders: one for images, one for text, and align their outputs using a contrastive objective that pulls matched image-text pairs together and pushes mismatched pairs apart. CLIP popularized this at scale using internet image-text pairs, demonstrating strong transfer and zero-shot behavior (Radford et al., 2021). ConVIRT adapted the same principle to radiology, using image-report pairs to achieve strong downstream performance with fewer labels (Zhang et al., 2023).

- **Best suited for:** cross-modal retrieval, zero-shot classification, large-scale pretraining from routine report pairs.
- **Strengths:** scalable and efficient; embeddings can be computed offline and indexed; strong general-purpose representations with good zero-shot behavior.

- **Limitations:** limited fine-grained grounding (the model may match "right lower lobe opacity" without localizing it); weaker compositional reasoning across multiple findings; false negatives in contrastive training, since mismatched pairs may still be clinically similar.

MedCLIP addressed the false negative problem by leveraging unpaired data, improving performance in low-label settings particularly relevant in healthcare where large paired datasets are often privacy-restricted.

3.2 Fusion Models

Fusion models allow direct token-level interaction between image patches and text tokens through cross-attention layers, making them better suited for tasks requiring precise grounding and reasoning. A typical pipeline includes a vision backbone producing patch tokens, a language encoder producing word tokens, and a fusion module where cross-attention learns their relationships; an approach demonstrated effectively in ViLBERT and LXMERT (Lu et al., 2019; Tan and Bansal, 2019).

This matters in medicine because clinical language often refers to localized findings: "right lower lobe opacity," "no pleural effusion," "enlarged cardiac silhouette." BioViL showed that improving medical language modeling and aligning it with imaging substantially strengthens biomedical VLP (Boecking et al., 2022).

- **Best suited for:** phrase grounding, clinical VQA, evidence-aligned explanation, multi-finding reasoning.
- **Strengths:** better grounding; supports contextual multi-finding reasoning; more suitable for explainability tools like attention maps.
- **Limitations:** heavier computation; harder to scale; region-level or phrase-level supervision is often unavailable in clinical data.

3.3 Encoder-Decoder Generative Models

Encoder-decoder VLMs generate text conditioned on visual representations — an image encoder produces a latent representation, and a decoder generates text autoregressively. Inspired by frameworks like T5 (Raffel et al., 2020), this architecture is the natural fit for radiology report generation, impression writing, and structured summarization.

- **Best suited for:** automatic report drafting, impression generation, structured finding lists, follow-up recommendations, longitudinal summarization.

- **Strengths:** outputs naturally resemble clinical language; can model uncertainty and hedging style; supports multi-sentence reasoning across findings.
- **Limitations and risks:** hallucination is a serious failure mode; a falsely generated "no pneumothorax" is as dangerous as a missed one. Generated reports can appear authoritative even when the model is uncertain. Report similarity metrics don't always reflect clinical correctness, making clinically informed evaluation essential. Safe deployment typically requires grounding checks, uncertainty calibration, and verification modules.

3.4 LLM-Backed Multimodal Assistants

These models connect a vision encoder to a large language model via projection layers, adapters, or cross-attention, using the LLM as a general reasoning and instruction-following engine. Flamingo demonstrated how visual conditioning via cross-attention enables strong few-shot multimodal learning (Alayrac et al., 2022).

LLaVA-Med adapted a general visual instruction-tuned model to the biomedical domain through biomedical concept alignment and self-supervised instruction tuning, enabling complex clinical instruction-following and multi-turn visual conversations (Li et al., 2023). Med-PaLM M extended this further, training a single model across 14 biomedical tasks; from radiology report generation to mammography, dermatology, and genomic variant calling. A clinician evaluation found physicians preferred Med-PaLM M-generated chest X-ray reports over radiologist-authored ones in up to 40.5% of cases across 246 chest X-rays (Tu et al., 2024).

- **Best suited for:** conversational clinical Q&A, interactive reporting assistance, multi-step workflows, multimodal decision support prototypes.
- **Strengths:** flexible natural language interaction; unified interface for retrieval, summarization, QA, and drafting; supports iterative refinement and multi-turn context.
- **Limitations and safety concerns:** highest hallucination risk; the LLM can generate confident but incorrect clinical statements; the model may reason well linguistically while losing grounding in image evidence; clinical deployment requires careful validation, monitoring, and scope definition. Safe usage typically requires retrieval augmentation, uncertainty estimation, evidence citation, and robust abstention for out-of-distribution queries.

These systems are most trustworthy when used as assistive tools rather than autonomous diagnosticians.

Figure 1 shows a general VLM architecture overview for medical imaging.

Figure 1. General architecture of a vision-language model for medical imaging

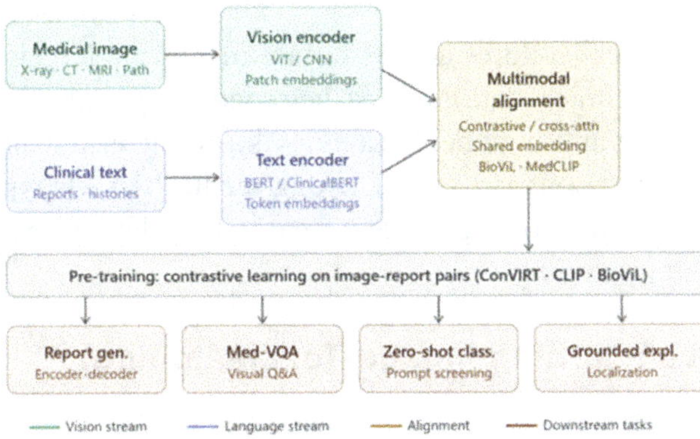

3.5 Selecting an Architecture

No single architecture dominates across all clinical settings. Selection of architecture depends on the task, available supervision, interpretability requirements, and safety constraints.

Generative and LLM-backed models require extra safeguards in clinical deployment; grounding mechanisms, uncertainty calibration, conservative decoding, and safety checks, because plausible clinical language can easily mask incorrect statements. Table 1 provides a comparison of main medical VLMs.

Table 1. Comparative summary of representative medical VLMs

Model	Year	Architecture	Key Dataset(s)	Primary Task(s)	Key Reference
ConVIRT	2020	Dual-encoder contrastive	CheXpert, RSNA	Zero-shot classification, retrieval	Zhang et al., 2023
CLIP (general)	2021	Dual-encoder contrastive	400M web image-text pairs	Zero-shot transfer across tasks	Radford et al., 2021
MedCLIP	2022	Dual-encoder and semantic decoupling	MIMIC-CXR, CheXpert	Classification (unpaired data)	Wang et al., 2022
BioViL	2022	Fusion (cross-attention)	MIMIC-CXR	Phrase grounding, report generation	Boecking et al., 2022
CheXzero	2022	Dual-encoder contrastive	MIMIC-CXR	Zero-shot multi-label detection	Tiu et al., 2022
LLaVA-Med	2023	LLM-backed assistant	PMC-15M (biomedical)	Clinical VQA, instruction following	Li et al., 2023
Med-PaLM M	2024	LLM-backed generalist (PaLM-E)	MultiMedBench (14 tasks)	Report generation, VQA, genomics	Tu et al., 2024

4. PRE-TRAINING OBJECTIVES AND ALIGNMENT STRATEGIES

A medical VLM's capabilities and its failure modes are largely shaped during pre-training. Because clinical data is scarce, heterogeneous, and institution-specific, the choice of objectives and alignment strategies is a key determinant of downstream performance, generalization, and safety. Strong medical VLMs typically combine multiple objectives: contrastive alignment, masked modeling, instruction tuning, and retrieval-based grounding.

4.1 Contrastive Learning (Image-Text Matching)

Contrastive learning trains a model to pull matched image-text pairs together (e.g., a chest X-ray with its report) and push mismatched pairs apart, learning a shared embedding space where aligned modalities cluster; typically via an InfoNCE-style loss. This is important in medical VLMs because:

- Learns generalizable representations that transfer across classification, report generation, QA, and retrieval tasks
- Encourages features that survive variation in scanners, protocols, and patient demographics supporting cross-site generalization
- Scales naturally from routine (image, report) pairs without manual labeling

  Key challenges in this are:
- Report noise: hedged language ("likely," "cannot exclude") and omitted negatives create imperfect supervision
- Shortcut learning: models may latch onto portable X-ray markers or hospital-specific formatting rather than pathology
- Weak negatives: two pneumonia cases are still semantically similar; hard-negative mining helps but adds complexity

Contrastive pretraining remains the dominant strategy in medical VLM research and has been extended to include richer negative sampling, semantic-aware loss functions, and federated contrastive objectives (Zhang et al., 2023).

4.2 Masked Language and Masked Image Modeling

Masked modeling forces the model to reconstruct missing input rather than memorize surface patterns; building deeper understanding of structure and meaning.

Masked Language Modeling (MLM) masks random tokens in clinical text for the model to predict. This builds mastery of medical vocabulary, abbreviations, and structured phrases, and improves handling of negation, uncertainty, and temporal language; ultimately benefiting downstream QA and report summarization.

Masked Image Modeling (MIM) masks image patches for the model to reconstruct. This teaches anatomical priors, captures texture and geometry (especially valuable in CT/MRI), and reduces label dependence through self-supervision.

Together, masked modeling strengthens both encoders: language encoders gain clinical fluency; vision encoders gain structural sensitivity (Dosovitskiy et al., 2021).

4.3 Instruction Tuning

Instruction tuning adapts a pre-trained model to follow natural language commands like *"Describe the findings in this X-ray"* or *"Is there a pleural effusion?"* moving from alignment to clinically useful, structured outputs. Its importance is due to:

- Fixes "prompt brittleness" models can be strongly pre-trained but still respond poorly to real-world queries
- Enables one model to handle QA, report drafting, localization descriptions, and triage explanations
- Can incorporate refusal behaviors, uncertainty reporting, and "I don't know" responses when done carefully

Key design choices for instruction tuning are:

- Instruction datasets need diverse clinical prompts with expert-verified target answers
- Output format can be enforced: Findings -> Impression -> Differential
- Must be paired with grounding strategies, since fluent but incorrect outputs remain a risk

Instruction tuning transforms a strong representation learner into a reliable clinical assistant.

4.4 Knowledge Grounding and Retrieval Augmentation

Clinical decision-making depends on guidelines, textbooks, and protocols; not just pattern recognition. Even a well-trained model can hallucinate or give outdated recommendations. Retrieval-Augmented Generation (RAG) addresses this by retrieving relevant evidence (guideline excerpts, references, structured knowledge bases) and conditioning outputs on it. Importance of grounding in healthcare is due to:

- Reduces hallucination by anchoring outputs to explicit supporting text
- Keeps responses aligned with current standards as guidelines evolve
- Improves transparency through evidence snippets or citations

- Helps with rare conditions where robust model encoding may be weak

Key challenges in knowledge grounding are:

- Poor retrieval degrades generation
- Correctly retrieved text can still be misapplied
- Clinical retrieval systems must respect privacy and access controls

RAG-based grounding can substantially reduce hallucination and improve reliability (Lewis et al., 2020).

4.5 Best-Practice Pre-training Pipeline

Strong medical VLMs follow a multi-stage pipeline rather than a single objective:

Stage 1: Foundation pre-training: Large-scale contrastive alignment and masked modeling (MLM/MIM) build robust visual and language encoders with minimal dependence on curated labels.

Stage 2: Domain adaptation: Further training on in-domain clinical corpora (radiology reports, discharge summaries, biomedical literature) sharpens medical vocabulary, negation handling, and institution-specific phrasing. Hard-negative contrastive refinement reduces shortcut learning.

Stage 3: Instruction tuning: The model is adapted to real-world clinical prompts using expert-written or carefully filtered instruction-response datasets, improving output consistency and enabling multi-task behavior.

Stage 4: Retrieval augmentation: Integration with curated sources (textbooks, guidelines, protocols) conditions generation on retrieved evidence, improving factual accuracy and transparency.

Stage 5: Safety and calibration tuning: Targeted tuning improves uncertainty calibration, refusal behavior for out-of-scope queries, and adherence to clinical constraints, generally using clinician feedback, adversarial evaluation, and institution-specific validation.

This sequence: representation learning - instruction alignment - grounding - safety tuning - has become the standard blueprint for medical VLMs that balance generalization, usability, and clinical trustworthiness.

5. MEDICAL IMAGING DATASETS FOR VLMS

Datasets are the foundation of medical VLMs; they determine what clinical concepts a model learns, how well it generalizes, and how safely it can be evaluated. Three structural realities shape this space: imaging studies are routinely paired with expert text, privacy constraints are strict, and clinical practice is highly variable. Progress tends to follow datasets that combine scale, report availability, and clinically meaningful labeling.

5.1 Chest X-ray Datasets

Chest radiographs dominate early medical VLM research because they fulfill all requirements for multimodal pretraining: high volume, standardized acquisition, and paired radiology reports. They also cover high-impact conditions like pneumothorax, pleural effusion, and cardiomegaly.

MIMIC-CXR is in important resource having a large set of de-identified chest radiographs paired with free-text reports. Its strength lies in diverse inpatient populations and authentic clinical language, helping models learn the structure of clinical reasoning and uncertainty phrasing (Johnson et al., 2019).

CheXpert is widely used for benchmarking, offering report-derived labels with explicit uncertainty handling. This reflects a core clinical reality: radiologists frequently use hedged, ambiguous language that can't be reduced to binary truth values, making CheXpert valuable for robustness evaluation.

Chest X-ray datasets work well due to:

- Scale supports large model training with stable visual patterns
- Reports provide rich supervision, including negation and uncertainty
- Standard views simplify learning compared to full-body CT
- Downstream tasks are clinically relevant and well-defined

It has following key limitations:

- Single modality; no broader imaging diversity
- Label noise from automated report labelers
- Performance drops across institutions with different scanners or reporting styles
- Models may learn spurious correlations (e.g., portable imaging markers, ICU artifacts)

These limitations make cross-institutional validation essential and caution warranted when generalizing chest X-ray results to broader medical settings.

5.2 CT and MRI

CT and MRI add significant complexity; they're volumetric, often multi-sequence or multi-phase, and each study can involve hundreds of slices. This strains both vision and language components.

Key differences from chest X-ray:

- Findings may span many slices (volumetric structure)
- Higher dimensionality increases compute demands
- Protocol and sequence diversity matters, especially in MRI
- Reports describe multiple organs and findings in greater detail

Common modeling approaches:

- Slice-based modeling: simple and efficient, but loses 3D spatial coherence
- 3D tokenization / 3D transformers: preserves structure but is computationally heavy
- Hierarchical attention: balances efficiency and performance by aggregating local features into study-level representations

Public CT and MRI datasets are generally smaller than chest X-ray datasets, and privacy concerns are more severe given the identifiable anatomy they may contain. This makes self-supervised and weakly supervised learning especially important.

To address these challenges, recent research has focused on scaling VLMs to handle volumetric and high-resolution modalities.

5.2.1 Scaling to 3D and High-Resolution Modalities

A standard CT chest scan may contain 300–600 axial slices, processing all of them simultaneously exceeds most current hardware limits. Early approaches processed slices independently, but this creates a critical gap: losing 3D spatial coherence means losing the ability to detect lesions spanning multiple slices or reason about anatomy in three dimensions.

Emerging architectures are able to address this issue. 3D Vision Transformers (3D-ViT) extend patch tokenization into the axial dimension, enabling attention across all three planes simultaneously (Dosovitskiy et al., 2021). Hierarchical attention models process small 3D sub-volumes locally, then aggregate chunk-level representations into study-level embeddings; preserving local 3D structure while remaining computationally feasible. Protocol-aware conditioning (providing metadata about sequence type, acquisition phase, or slice thickness) further improves alignment between visual features and report language.

In digital pathology, the analogous challenge is gigapixel whole-slide images. Patch-based multiple instance learning pipelines extract features from thousands of tiles and aggregate them via attention-weighted pooling; connecting slide-level visual representations to pathology report text without requiring tile-level labels.

5.3 Digital Pathology

Whole-slide images present extreme scale challenges; gigapixel resolution far exceeds what standard transformers can process end-to-end. Yet pathology reports offer rich supervision: tumor subtype, grade, margins, biomarkers, and staging context.

Pathology works well for VLMs as:

- Text supervision is diagnostic and structured
- Visual patterns map strongly to language labels like grade or subtype
- Multimodal context is natural; diagnosis depends on morphology plus clinical metadata

Standard pipeline for Whole-Slide Images (WSI):

1. Split the slide into patches at one or more magnifications
2. Encode each patch using a vision backbone
3. Aggregate patch features via attention or pooling into slide-level embeddings
4. Align embeddings with pathology report text or diagnostic labels

The key challenge is that diagnostic signal is often localized to a small tissue region within a heterogeneous slide. Naive aggregation can dilute these features, making attention-based aggregation and multiple instance learning essential.

5.4 Dataset Challenges

Dataset size and label quality don't tell the whole story. Several deeper issues determine whether a model can safely generalize beyond its training distribution. These issues are:

- Privacy constraints: Strict regulations make de-identification costly and imperfect, limiting public dataset diversity and concentrating research around a few benchmarks.
- Institutional bias and domain shift: Imaging protocols, devices, patient populations, and reporting styles vary across hospitals. Models trained on one dataset may fail in another (Johnson et al., 2019).
- Label noise and ambiguity: Automated labelers introduce noise through ambiguous language, incomplete documentation, and uncertain findings. CheXpert explicitly accounts for this, reflecting that many clinical statements can't be treated as binary.
- Spurious correlations: Models may learn shortcuts like patient positioning, portable scanner artifacts, or ICU-specific markers — inflating benchmark scores while reducing real-world reliability.

- Evaluation limitations: Good evaluation requires clinically grounded correctness, appropriate uncertainty handling, cross-institutional validation, and sensitivity to rare but critical findings. Combining multiple metrics and clinician-reviewed assessments helps.

5.4.1 Dataset Selection Criteria for VLM Pretraining

Choosing datasets isn't just about size; it requires matching dataset properties to architecture, training objective, and clinical task. Below are practical selection criteria.

Paired text availability datasets like MIMIC-CXR are valuable because they provide large-scale report pairing and realistic clinical language (Johnson et al., 2019). To select dataset for pretraining, consider free-text reports paired with images, clear findings/impression separation, and coverage of negation, uncertainty, and comparison phrasing. Such datset is best suited for dual-encoder contrastive pretraining, fusion-based grounding, report generation. Associated risks are boilerplate text and templated phrases can teach non-informative shortcuts.

Scale is important for contrastive learning, but only if diversity is real. MIMIC-CXR offers wide clinical diversity (Johnson et al., 2019), but single-institution datasets risk encoding institution-specific artifacts and shortcuts. It is best suitable for dual-encoder models, broad representation learning. Associated risks are overfitting to setting-specific distributions (e.g., ICU vs. outpatient).

Collapsing uncertainty into binary labels distorts clinical truth. CheXpert's uncertainty-aware labeling framework is a key reason it remains the standard for robustness evaluation. It is best suitable for benchmarking, uncertainty-sensitive tasks, calibration studies. Associated risks are automated labelers introduce systematic errors, especially for subtle findings.

Modality complexity and dimensionality CT and MRI datasets are generally smaller and more protocol-diverse, making weak supervision and self-supervised learning especially important. Architecture choice (slice-based, 3D, hierarchical) depends heavily on data volume and compute availability. It is best suitable for hierarchical fusion models, 3D VLM research. Associated risks are protocol heterogeneity creates hidden distribution shifts; many public datasets are too small for large-scale end-to-end training.

Region-level annotations (bounding boxes, segmentation masks, phrase-level alignments) are essential for grounded models. Without them, visual explanations may appear grounded without truly linking phrases to image evidence. These are best suitable for fusion models, explainability-aligned systems, safety-critical workflows. Associated risks are: grounding labels are rare and expensive; absence can produce misleading explanations.

Report style varies across institutions and individual radiologists. MIMIC-CXR reflects real clinical variability (Johnson et al., 2019), making it useful for studying generalization under language shift. It has risk of overfitting to template phrases; performance can degrade under new reporting conventions even when imaging distribution is stable.

Pathology-specific criteria WSI datasets differ fundamentally from radiology. Diagnostic signal may occupy a small area within a heterogeneous slide, making multiple instance learning and attention aggregation critical. The most valuable datasets include rich diagnostic sign-out text or structured pathology reports. These are suitable for patch-based dual-encoder pretraining, fusion models for region-to-diagnosis grounding, multi-scale VLMs. Associated risks are slide-level labels are often coarse and noisy; stain and scanner differences can cause severe domain shift.

6. CLINICAL APPLICATIONS OF MEDICAL VLMS

Medical Vision-language Models are increasingly being used as clinical support systems that connect imaging evidence to text-based reasoning. Their value comes from two unique strengths: they can learn directly from paired image-report data at scale and they can support both discriminative tasks like screening and generative tasks like report drafting. At the same time, clinical use requires careful attention to safety, uncertainty and reliability because errors in interpretation can propagate into downstream decisions.

6.1 Radiology report generation

Radiology report generation uses an image-conditioned model to produce a draft report or a structured output such as a findings list and impression summary. In a typical workflow, the model produces a preliminary report that a radiologist reviews, edits and finalizes. This positions report generation as a documentation and efficiency tool rather than a fully autonomous diagnostic system.

It is useful in medical applications because a substantial portion of radiology work involves repetitive phrasing and standardized descriptions, especially for normal studies or routine follow-up exams. Used responsibly, report generation can:

- reduce time spent on dictation and editing
- promote standardized phrasing and structured reporting
- reduce variability in normal or straightforward cases
- help trainees by providing consistent reporting templates

Report generation systems may produce clinically plausible but incorrect statements. Hallucinations can include both false positive findings and false negatives such as incorrectly stating “no pneumothorax.” In clinical settings, the risk is amplified because generated text sounds authoritative. Therefore, responsible use typically requires:

- strict human review as the default
- uncertainty-aware output formatting
- evidence grounding and consistency checks
- conservative design that encourages abstention when confidence is low

A more proactive approach to managing hallucination involves grounded reasoning and knowledge graph integration. Rather than evaluating a generated report only at the output level, grounded systems link every clinical claim in the generated text to a specific entity or spatial coordinate in the source image. Tools such as RadGraph; a structured graph representation that extracts clinical entities (such as findings, anatomy, and attributes) and relations from radiology reports provide a framework for this kind of verification (Jain et al., 2021). A grounding-aware generation pipeline can use RadGraph-style entity extraction to check whether each assertion in the model output is supported by an identifiable image region or a retrieved clinical fact. If a generated report states 'right lower lobe consolidation,' the system can attempt to localize the corresponding region in the image and flag the assertion as unverified if no supporting evidence is found. This approach shifts the safety boundary from post-hoc review to inline verification, reducing the risk that fluent but incorrect clinical language reaches the radiologist without a warning.

In many realistic cases, report generation is most useful as:

- an auto-complete assistant that suggests sentence-level templates
- a structured output tool that proposes a consistent findings summary
- a draft generator limited to specific modalities and stable workflows

This bounded use case helps reduce risk while capturing productivity gains.

6.2 Medical visual question answering (Med-VQA)

Medical VQA enables clinicians or students to ask questions about an image and receive answers grounded in the image and associated knowledge. This interaction can take many forms, including binary questions, localization queries, comparison questions and explanation-style prompts. Relevant question examples are:

- "Is there a pneumothorax?"
- "Where is the lesion?"
- "What findings support pulmonary edema?"
- "Has this opacity improved compared to the prior scan?"

Med-VQA is useful because Med-VQA supports workflows where rapid clarification is important such as:

- triage and preliminary review
- clinician-to-radiologist communication
- education and self-testing for trainees
- audit and quality review
- patient-facing explanation support when carefully constrained

Med-VQA systems can answer confidently even when the question is underspecified or when the image quality limits interpretation. They may also fail to model uncertainty appropriately, which is central to clinical imaging. Safer Med-VQA requires:

- calibrated confidence estimates
- explicit handling of uncertain answers
- grounding visual evidence
- integration with priors and metadata when appropriate

6.3 Zero-shot classification and screening

Zero-shot screening uses a pretrained Vision-language model to detect findings without requiring explicit labeled training data for the target task. Instead of training a classifier for each pathology, the model evaluates similarity between an image embedding and text prompts such as "pleural effusion present". It is useful as it:

- reduces dependence on expensive expert labels
- supports rapid adaptation to new findings and terminology
- enables evaluation and deployment prototypes quickly
- can generalize to findings that were not explicitly labeled during training

CheXzero demonstrated that contrastive image–text pretraining on chest X-rays and radiology reports enables zero-shot multi-label pathology detection, showing performance comparable to radiologists on external evaluation datasets for common chest pathologies (Tiu et al., 2022).

Performance claims must be interpreted carefully. Even when a model achieves strong AUC scores on benchmarks, real-world screening requires:

- calibration across sites
- handling of prevalence shifts
- robust performance on rare but critical findings
- consistent performance across patient subgroups
- integration with clinical workflows and follow-up pathways

Zero-shot screening is most reliable when used as a decision support layer, for example prioritizing studies for review or flagging potential abnormalities, rather than making final clinical calls.

6.4 Retrieval and case-based reasoning

VLM embeddings enable searching by text, searching by image similarity, or retrieving similar multimodal cases. This supports case-based reasoning, which is a natural form of clinical decision support. Its clinical and educational value is in:

- retrieving similar cases for comparison
- building teaching sets linked to real report language
- supporting second-opinion workflows
- enabling multi-institution audit and cohort discovery when governed appropriately
- helping trainees learn pattern recognition and reporting conventions

    In such cases, Dual-encoder contrastive models are especially effective because:

- embeddings can be precomputed and indexed
- retrieval is fast and scalable
- image and text queries map into the same semantic space

This application is one of the safer VLM use cases because it supports clinicians by surfacing relevant examples rather than generating new clinical facts.

6.5 Grounded explanations and localization

Grounded explanation aims to connect generated language to image evidence. Fusion-based or cross-attention VLMs can:

- highlight image regions relevant to a statement
- produce explanations aligned with those regions

- support interpretability for clinicians and auditors

Trust in clinical AI depends on whether outputs are supported by evidence. If a model says "right lower lobe opacity," it should also provide a map or localization cue that demonstrates where this signal exists. Grounding supports:

- interpretability
- error analysis
- education
- more reliable workflow integration

Visual explanations can be misleading if they are not truly causal and attention maps are not always reliable explanations. For clinical deployment, grounded explanations are strongest when combined with:

- explicit localization supervision when available
- consistency checks between text claims and image evidence
- clinician review and audit trails

Clinical deployment of medical VLMs requires more than strong benchmark performance. A deployment pipeline is shown in Figure 2. Hospitals and regulators evaluate these systems across the entire lifecycle, including data governance, workflow integration, prospective validation and post-deployment monitoring. Because VLMs can generate text and may appear authoritative, monitoring is essential to reduce hallucination risk, manage uncertainty and ensure clinicians remain in control.

Figure 2. Clinical deployment pipeline for medical VLMs

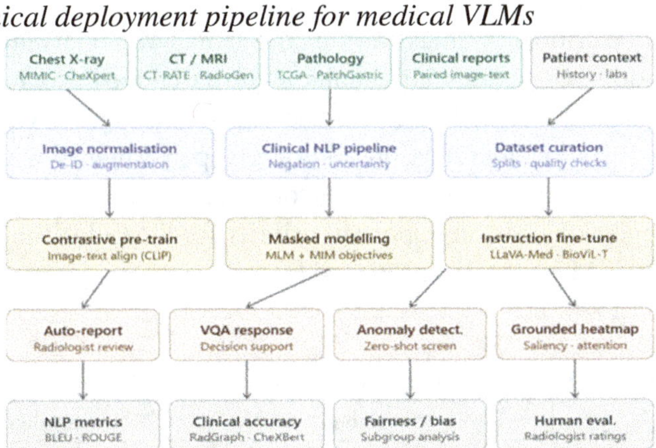

6.6 Human-in-the-Loop Clinical Workflows

The most effective deployment model for medical VLMs is not one in which the system operates as an autonomous diagnostician, but one in which it functions as an interactive collaborator within a clinician-supervised workflow. In this human-in-the-loop (HITL) paradigm, a radiologist does not simply review a model-generated report; they engage in a dynamic conversation with the system: requesting clarification, challenging a finding, asking for alternative interpretations, or narrowing the model's attention to a specific anatomical region. LLM-backed assistants are particularly well-suited to this interaction style because they support multi-turn dialogue and instruction following (Li et al., 2023). However, interactive AI systems introduce a risk that is distinct from simple factual error: automation bias. Automation bias describes the tendency of human operators to over-rely on automated decision support, accepting machine outputs with insufficient scrutiny even when those outputs are incorrect (Goddard et al., 2012). In radiology, automation bias is especially concerning because VLMs can produce reports that are fluently written, appropriately hedged, and structurally conventional, all of which may reduce a clinician's vigilance toward potential errors. A radiologist who reviews 50 AI-drafted reports per shift may become anchored to the model's language and less likely to catch a hallucinated finding or a missed lesion. Designing HITL systems that actively counter automation bias requires deliberate engineering choices. These include surfacing explicit uncertainty flags at the point of review rather than only in a confidence score buried in metadata, requiring active clinician acknowledgment of model-identified critical findings, varying the format of model outputs to prevent over-familiarization, and conducting regular audit-based feedback loops that allow the clinical team to evaluate model performance and flag disagreements. Prospective clinical validation studies that measure radiologist performance with and without AI assistance and that specifically track errors that occur when clinicians accept incorrect AI suggestions; are an important priority for the field. Table 2 shows key risks in medical VLMs and mitigation strategies.

Table 2. Key risks in medical VLMs and mitigation strategies

Risk	Description	Mitigation Strategy
Hallucination	False clinical statements	Grounding, RAG amd verification
Automation bias	Over-reliance by clinicians	HITL workflows and audits
Dataset bias	Poor subgroup performance	Diverse datasets and validation
Domain shift	Performance drop across hospital	Cross-site testing
Uncertainty miscalibration	Over/under confidence	Calibration and abstention

7. EVALUATION OF MEDICAL VLMS

Evaluation is one of the hardest problems in medical Vision-language modeling because the outputs are often long, structured and clinically nuanced. A medical report is not only a description of an image. It is a safety-critical document that contains negation, uncertainty, differential diagnosis and follow-up recommendations. This means that evaluation must measure not only linguistic quality, but also clinical correctness, grounding and harm potential.

Traditional NLP metrics such as BLEU, ROUGE and METEOR measure surface-level similarity between generated text and reference text. They are useful for evaluating fluency and overlap, but they often fail in clinical imaging for several reasons.

- A generated report can match the reference report closely while still making a clinically dangerous error. For example: a report that says "no pneumothorax" instead of "small pneumothorax" may still share many overlapping phrases. a report may correctly describe most findings but hallucinate one high-risk condition. two valid radiology reports may use different wording and structure, leading to low BLEU or ROUGE despite clinical correctness
- Radiologists can legitimately produce different reports for the same image, depending on clinical context, reporting style and the level of detail required. This one-to-many mapping breaks the assumption behind overlap metrics that there is a single correct reference.
- A single token or phrase can invert meaning such as "no pleural effusion" versus "pleural effusion", "cannot exclude pneumonia" versus "pneumonia present"

  Overlap metrics are not designed to treat these high-impact semantic flips as catastrophic errors.
- Impression sections often prioritize urgent findings. A model may mention correct entities but in a misleading or unsafe way by downplaying the most urgent issue.

Therefore, traditional metrics are acceptable for reporting baseline linguistic similarity, but they must never be used alone to claim clinical readiness. Table 3 provides a comparison of evaluation metrics for medical VLMs.

Table 3. Comparison of evaluation metrics for medical VLMs

Metric	Measures	Strengths	Limitations
BLEU/ROUGE	Text similarity	Easy benchmarking	Ignores clinical correctness
CheXpert label	Clinical labels	Clinically meaningful	Label noise
RadGraph	Entity relations	Captures structure	Misses uncertainty nuance
Human review	Clinical judgment	Gold standard	Expensive, subjective

Clinically meaningful evaluation focuses on whether the output captures medically relevant facts correctly, handles uncertainty appropriately and avoids harmful errors. Many evaluation protocols combine several layers, from automated extraction to clinician judgment.

Rather than evaluating full text, entity-level evaluation extracts clinically meaningful units such as:

- findings such as "pleural effusion," "pneumothorax," "consolidation"
- anatomy such as "right lower lobe," "left apex"
- modifiers such as severity, size, laterality and temporality

Approaches like RadGraph-style extraction aim to represent reports as structured sets of entities and relations. This allows evaluation to measure whether the model identified the correct clinical concepts and linked them properly, even if phrasing differs. It is able to observe perfectly:

- presence or absence of key findings
- laterality and anatomical grounding in text
- omission errors where key entities are missing

But it may skip capturing:

- subtle semantic cues such as uncertainty calibration
- reasoning quality in impression statements
- phrasing risks that might mislead clinicians

This approach converts reports into standardized labels and compares them for agreement. A common strategy is to use a labeler such as CheXpert-style labeling and compute agreement between generated and reference reports for selected pathologies and has following advantages:

- easier benchmarking across papers
- aligns evaluation with clinically meaningful categories
- supports comparison to image-based classifiers

At the same time following limitations also exist:

- depends on the accuracy of the labeler
- may miss clinically important context and rare findings

- can reward generic outputs that mention common labels without specificity

Clinical evaluation should not treat all errors equally. Many pipelines separate errors into severity categories such as:

- critical errors: missed pneumothorax, missed intracranial hemorrhage, incorrect laterality in urgent findings
- major errors: incorrect presence of pneumonia, missing pulmonary edema, wrong device placement
- minor errors: small wording mistakes, non-impactful omissions, stylistic differences

Severity scoring supports a safety-first approach because even a low error rate becomes unacceptable if critical errors occur.

For real clinical utility, evaluation should include clinician review and in some settings, linkage to downstream outcomes such as follow-up imaging, interventions, or discharge decisions. Although outcome-based evaluation is complex and often infeasible for early research, it is the closest proxy to clinical value.

Two reports with similar factual content can have very different clinical effects depending on wording and prioritization.

7.3 Human evaluation

Human evaluation remains essential in medical VLM assessment because clinical correctness depends on context, subtlety and pragmatic communication. Human review is also necessary for verifying that the model is not hallucinating, omitting urgent findings, or producing misleading certainty. The VLM assessment should be evaluated by:

- radiologists for radiology report generation and imaging interpretation tasks
- pathologists for pathology slide interpretation tasks
- clinicians such as emergency physicians and intensivists for triage-oriented outputs
- medical educators for learning tools and case-based tutoring applications

A strong human evaluation protocol typically includes:

- correctness of key findings
- correctness of negation and uncertainty
- appropriateness of impression summary
- clinical actionability and safety
- whether the model output would mislead or anchor a clinician

Human review should report inter-rater agreement because even experts can disagree, especially in borderline imaging cases. A robust evaluation design often includes:

- multiple reviewers per case
- blinded review, where feasible
- adjudication by a senior radiologist or consensus panel
- explicit labeling of disagreements as uncertainty rather than forcing a single ground truth

The most important principle is that evaluation must emphasize errors that matter clinically. For example, missing a pneumothorax, misclassifying intracranial hemorrhage, or hallucinating a pulmonary embolism carries far higher harm potential than minor descriptive inaccuracies.

Robust evaluation frameworks are essential to ensure that medical VLMs are not only accurate but also safe, reliable, and clinically deployable.

8. FUTURE RESEARCH

Two forces will shape the future of medical vision–language modeling: the push for larger, more capable multimodal models, and the urgent need for safety, governance, and real-world clinical trust. In healthcare, capability alone isn't enough but models must be reliable under uncertainty and fit seamlessly into clinical workflows. Recent studies emphasize multimodal clinical reasoning as a key frontier in AI-enabled healthcare systems (Tu et al., 2024).

Whole-patient reasoning is the next important aspect. Today's medical VLMs typically focus on one modality, like chest X-rays, but clinicians never work that way. They weigh imaging alongside labs, notes, medications, and history across time. Future systems will need to do the same; summarizing patient timelines, catching cross-modality inconsistencies, and supporting differential diagnoses from multiple data sources. The hard part is aligning noisy, uneven data types while keeping outputs transparent and auditable.

Federated learning will become critical as valuable clinical datasets remain siloed in hospitals due to privacy laws and institutional barriers. Training across sites without moving raw data can improve generalization, reduce institutional bias, and expand representation for underserved populations. But it comes with real challenges site variability, compute costs, privacy-utility tradeoffs, and the need for regulatory buy-in.

3D and temporal reasoning are also overdue. Most clinical imaging is volumetric or time-varying; CT, MRI, ultrasound, fluoroscopy, yet most VLMs still treat images as static 2D snapshots. Future models will need to track disease progression, assess treatment response, and flag new versus chronic findings. Real-time streaming VLMs could assist during ultrasound or interventional procedures, though they raise serious safety concerns given their influence on live decisions.

Finally, knowledge-grounded assistants address a gap that pure perception models can't: reasoning and communication failures. Retrieval-augmented systems that cite clinical guidelines, reference similar cases, and constrain outputs to trusted sources can reduce hallucinations, improve transparency, and support evidence-based care without retraining the full model every time medical knowledge evolves.

8.1 Infrastructure and Operational Feasibility:

A practical barrier that shapes the adoption of medical VLMs is the hardware and latency cost of inference. Hospital administrators and clinical informatics teams must balance diagnostic reasoning depth against the real-time constraints of radiology and pathology workflows. Lightweight dual-encoder models such as CLIP-style contrastive architectures can typically be served on a single GPU with 8-16 GB of VRAM and respond in under 100 milliseconds per query, making them suitable for high-throughput retrieval, triage flagging, and zero-shot screening pipelines. Their reasoning depth is limited to global image-text alignment and they cannot generate explanatory text or follow complex instructions. Full LLM-backed assistants such as those in the LLaVA-Med or Med-PaLM M class require substantially more compute. Depending on model size and quantization, inference may require 40-80 GB of VRAM across multiple GPUs, and response latency for a full radiology report can range from several seconds to over a minute. This class of system is appropriate for asynchronous workflows such as report drafting assistance, but is currently unsuitable for real-time triage in high-volume emergency settings without purpose-built inference infrastructure. Encoder-decoder generative models occupy a middle ground: they can produce structured report drafts at moderate latency and VRAM cost, making them a practical choice for overnight batch reporting or semi-automated impression generation. Integration with hospital information systems (HIS) and electronic health records (EHR) adds further requirements: HL7 FHIR compatibility, DICOM standards compliance for imaging data, role-based access controls, and audit logging to satisfy clinical governance requirements. Institutions planning to deploy medical VLMs should evaluate feasibility across all of these dimensions before committing to a model architecture.

Beyond regulatory compliance, the responsible deployment of medical VLMs raises broader ethical considerations that the field must address systematically. Data privacy is a foundational concern: even de-identified imaging datasets can be re-identified when combined with other data sources, and model weights trained on private clinical data can encode patient-level information that may be recoverable through model inversion attacks. Bias in multimodal datasets is equally serious: if training data overrepresents patients from particular demographic groups, institutions, or geographic regions, model performance will be systematically worse for under-represented populations; a disparity that can propagate into clinical decision support at scale. Explainability is a third dimension: clinicians are ethically and legally accountable for their diagnostic decisions, and deploying AI systems whose reasoning cannot be audited or explained places them in an untenable position. The interpretable models literature has argued that, in high-stakes decision contexts, the goal should be to make models that are intrinsically interpretable rather than to add post-hoc explanations to opaque ones (Rudin, 2019). For medical VLMs, this principle supports the development of architectures that produce evidence-linked outputs as a first-class design requirement rather than an afterthought. Regulatory approval pathways for AI clinical tools including the FDA's 510(k) and De Novo routes for software as a medical device; require prospective validation evidence that current medical VLM benchmarks rarely provide, highlighting the gap between research publication standards and clinical deployment readiness.

Finally, progress in medical VLMs will depend on standardization and benchmarking. The field currently suffers from inconsistent evaluation protocols, differences in dataset splits, and varying definitions of safety, making it difficult to compare results across papers and assess true clinical readiness. Priority needs include shared benchmark tasks spanning multiple modalities rather than only chest X-ray, standardized reporting of subgroup performance across demographics and acquisition settings, consistent evaluation of negation and uncertainty handling, standardized hallucination and critical error metrics for report generation, and external validation requirements with cross-site generalization reporting. Strong benchmarks should measure clinical correctness rather than text similarity, severity-weighted error rates, calibration and abstention behavior, robustness under distribution shift and rare critical cases, and grounding quality such as phrase-to-region faithfulness. Without such standardization, high benchmark scores can mask unsafe behavior and meaningful clinical progress becomes hard to measure, while shared benchmarks also strengthen reproducibility, an essential requirement for high-stakes deployment.

A parallel and equally urgent priority is alignment with emerging regulatory frameworks. On January 7, 2025, the U.S. Food and Drug Administration (FDA) published draft guidance titled 'Artificial Intelligence-Enabled Device Software Functions: Lifecycle Management and Marketing Submission Recommendations,' which applies a Total Product Life Cycle (TPLC) approach to AI-enabled medical device software (Food and Drug Administration, 2025). This guidance requires manufacturers to address AI-specific documentation across the entire device lifespan from initial design and validation through post-market performance monitoring; and explicitly identifies transparency, bias mitigation, and human factors engineering as core requirements for premarket submissions. For developers of medical VLMs, this framework has direct technical implications. Uncertainty quantification is not merely a desirable model property; under the TPLC approach it constitutes a regulatory compliance mechanism, because the FDA requires that device labeling accurately represent model performance limitations and known failure modes. Similarly, hallucination mitigation and grounding strategies can be positioned as tools for satisfying the FDA's requirements for risk management and output transparency. Framing technical capabilities as regulatory compliance tools substantially increases their relevance for industry practitioners, clinical informaticists, and hospital procurement teams who must evaluate AI systems against both clinical and regulatory standards.

9. CONCLUSION

Vision-language models are reshaping medical imaging AI by bringing together visual evidence and clinical language in a shared reasoning framework. They offer the promise of scalable report generation, interactive question answering, improved retrieval and broader generalization through self-supervised learning. The field has rapidly evolved from dual-encoder contrastive systems toward generalist multimodal assistants capable of open-ended clinical reasoning, as demonstrated by models such as LLaVA-Med and Med-PaLM M (Li et al., 2023; Tu et al., 2024). Yet clinical deployment requires careful handling of hallucinations, bias and reliability challenges that are now actively addressed through grounded reasoning, retrieval augmentation, and knowledge graph integration. Equally important are the ethical, regulatory, and operational dimensions of deployment: ensuring fairness across patient populations, meeting the FDA's Total Product Life Cycle requirements, managing automation bias in human-in-the-loop workflows, and integrating VLMs with existing hospital information systems. The most successful VLM systems will be those designed for collaboration: they augment clinician expertise rather than replace it, include robust grounding and verification mechanisms and are evaluated using clinically meaningful standards that go beyond surface-level text similarity. With responsible development, rigorous prospective validation, and alignment with emerging regulatory frameworks, VLMs can become core engines of next-generation healthcare; reducing workload, improving quality and supporting better outcomes.

REFERENCES

Alayrac, J. B., Donahue, J., Luc, P., Miech, A., Barr, I., Hasson, Y., Lenc, K., Mensch, A., Millican, K., Reynolds, M., Ring, R., Rutherford, E., Cabi, S., Han, T., Gong, Z., Samangooei, S., Monteiro, M., Menick, J., & Borgeaud, S.. (2022). Flamingo: a visual language model for few-shot learning. In *Proceedings of the 36th International Conference on Neural Information Processing Systems (NIPS '22)*. Curran Associates Inc., Red Hook, NY, USA, Article 1723, 23716–23736. DOI: 10.52202/068431-1723

Alsentzer, E., Murphy, J. R., Boag, W., Weng, W. H., Jin, D., Naumann, T., & McDermott, M. B. A. (2019). Publicly available clinical BERT embeddings. *Proceedings of the 2nd Clinical Natural Language Processing Workshop*, 72–78. Minneapolis, Minnesota, USA. Association for Computational Linguistics. DOI: 10.18653/v1/W19-1909

Boecking, B., (2022). Making the Most of Text Semantics to Improve Biomedical Vision-Language Processing. In Avidan, S., Brostow, G., Cissé, M., Farinella, G. M., & Hassner, T. (Eds.), Lecture Notes in Computer Science: Vol. 13696. *Computer Vision – ECCV 2022. ECCV 2022*. Springer., DOI: 10.1007/978-3-031-20059-5_1

Devlin, J., Chang, M., Lee, K., & Toutanova, K. (2019). BERT: Pre-training of Deep Bidirectional Transformers for Language Understanding. *North American Chapter of the Association for Computational Linguistics*. 4171–4186. DOI: 10.18653/v1/N19-1423

Dosovitskiy, A., Beyer, L., Kolesnikov, A., Weissenborn, D., Zhai, X., Unterthiner, T., Dehghani, M., Minderer, M., Heigold, G., Gelly, S., Uszkoreit, J., & Houlsby, N. (2021). An image is worth 16x16 words: Transformers for image recognition at scale. *International Conference on Learning Representations (ICLR)*. DOI: 10.48550/arXiv.2010.11929

Food and Drug Administration. (2025). Artificial intelligence-enabled device software functions: Lifecycle management and marketing submission recommendations (Docket No. FDA-2024-D-4488). U.S. Department of Health and Human Services. https://www.fda.gov/media/184856/download

Food and Drug Administration (FDA). (2021). *Good Machine Learning Practice for Medical Device Development: Guiding Principles.*

Goddard, K., Roudsari, A., & Wyatt, J. C. (2012). Automation bias: A systematic review of frequency, effect mediators, and mitigators. *Journal of the American Medical Informatics Association: JAMIA*, *19*(1), 121–127. DOI: 10.1136/amiajnl-2011-000089 PMID: 21685142

Jain, S., Agrawal, A., Saporta, A., Truong, S. Q., Nguyen Duong, D., Bui, T., Chambon, P., Lungren, M., Ng, A., Langlotz, C., & Rajpurkar, P. (2021). RadGraph: Extracting Clinical Entities and Relations from Radiology Reports (version 1.0.0). *PhysioNet*. RRID:SCR_007345.

Johnson, A. E. W., Pollard, T. J., Berkowitz, S. J., Greenbaum, N. R., Lungren, M. P., Deng, C.-Y., Mark, R. G., & Horng, S. (2019). MIMIC-CXR, a de-identified publicly available database of chest radiographs with free-text reports. *Scientific Data*, *6*(1), 317. Advance online publication. DOI: 10.1038/s41597-019-0322-0 PMID: 31831740

Li, C., Wong, C., Zhang, S., Usuyama, N., Liu, H., Yang, J., Naumann, T., Poon, H., & Gao, J. (2023). LLaVA-Med: Training a large language-and-vision assistant for biomedicine in one day. *In Proceedings of the 37th International Conference on Neural Information Processing Systems (NIPS '23)*. Curran Associates Inc., Red Hook, NY, USA, *Article 1240,* 28541–28564.

Lu, J., Batra, D., Parikh, D., & Lee, S. (2019). ViLBERT: Pretraining task-agnostic visiolinguistic representations for vision-and-language tasks. *Proceedings of the 33rd International Conference on Neural Information Processing Systems.* Curran Associates Inc., Red Hook, NY, USA, *Article 2,* 13–23.

Radford, A., Kim, J. W., Hallacy, C., Ramesh, A., Goh, G., Agarwal, S., Sastry, G., Askell, A., Mishkin, P., Clark, J., Krueger, G., & Sutskever, I. (2021). Learning transferable visual models from natural language supervision. Proceedings of the 38th International Conference on Machine Learning (ICML), PMLR 139, 8748–8763.

Raffel, C., Shazeer, N., Roberts, A., Lee, K., Narang, S., Matena, M., Zhou, Y., Li, W., & Liu, P. J. (2020). Exploring the limits of transfer learning with a unified text-to-text transformer. [JMLR]. *Journal of Machine Learning Research*, *21*(140), 1–67. https://dl.acm.org/doi/abs/10.5555/3455716.3455856

Rudin, C. (2019). Stop Explaining Black Box Machine Learning Models for High Stakes Decisions and Use Interpretable Models Instead. *Nature Machine Intelligence*, *1*(5), 206–215. DOI: 10.1038/s42256-019-0048-x PMID: 35603010

Tan, H., & Bansal, M. (2019). LXMERT: Learning cross-modality encoder representations from transformers. *Proceedings of EMNLP-IJCNLP*, 5100–5111. DOI: 10.18653/v1/D19-1514

Tu, T., Azizi, S., Driess, D., Mirchandani, S., Toda, K., Mai, P., Chang, J., Onoe, A., Sherber, S., Fletcher, A., Matias, Y., Schroeder, A. M., Adam, H., Tse, D., & Natarajan, V. (2024). Towards generalist biomedical AI. *NEJM AI*, *1*(3). Advance online publication. DOI: 10.1056/AIoa2300138

Zhang, Y., Jiang, H., Miura, Y., Manning, C. D., & Langlotz, C. P. (2023). Contrastive learning of medical visual representations from paired images and text. Proceedings of Machine Learning for Health (ML4H), 2023. https://arxiv.org/abs/2010.00747

Chapter 9 Vision Language Models in Healthcare Through a Multimodal Approach to Medical Imaging and Clinical Applications

Kazi Tanvir
http://orcid.org/0009-0001-0612-6101
American International University-Bangladesh, Bangladesh

Rahul Biswas
http://orcid.org/0009-0009-4459-4756
University of Vaasa, Finland

Dipta Gomes
http://orcid.org/0000-0003-3019-6051
American International University-Bangladesh, Bangladesh

Mahfujur Rahman
http://orcid.org/0000-0002-3245-8767
American International University-Bangladesh, Bangladesh

Noboranjan Dey
http://orcid.org/0009-0007-1991-9198
American International University-Bangladesh, Bangladesh

Md. Reazul Islam
http://orcid.org/0009-0003-7481-5982
University at Albany, State University of New York, USA

ABSTRACT

This chapter explores the emerging role of Vision Language Models (VLMs) in healthcare, focusing on their ability to integrate visual and textual data to improve medical imaging analysis and clinical decision-making. It examines the key components of VLMs, including vision and language models, their fusion techniques, and their applications in tasks like disease detection, report generation, and visual question answering. The chapter also addresses challenges such as data scarcity,

DOI: 10.4018/979-8-3373-7315-7.ch009

ht © 2026, IGI Global Scientific Publishing. Copying or distributing in print or electronic forms without written permission of IGI Global Scientific Publishing is prohibited. Use of this chapter to generative artificial intelligence (AI) technologies is expressly prohibited. The publisher reserves all rights to license its use for generative AI training and machine learning model development.

privacy concerns, and model interpretability. Additionally, it highlights future directions for enhancing model generalization, improving explainability, and ensuring seamless integration into clinical workflows, while emphasizing the importance of ethical considerations and real-world validation for safe deployment in healthcare environments.

1. INTRODUCTION

The evolving landscape of healthcare calls for artificial intelligence systems that do more than simply process one modality of data which are visual scans, textual reports, lab results and then output a decision. Instead, the next wave of tools must integrate what a clinician sees, reads, hears and reasons through (Das Joy et al., 2025). At the heart of this paradigm shift lie vision–language models (VLMs), architectures that jointly learn from imagery and text, and thereby present a viable pathway to unify diagnostic imaging and clinical narratives in a seamless manner. This proposal outlines a chapter that explores how VLMs can be designed, adapted, evaluated and governed within healthcare workflows, ultimately supporting better outcomes and safer deployment.

The central impetus for embracing VLMs is that medical decision-making is inherently multimodal. A radiologist interprets an image in the context of a report, a patient history, lab values and perhaps prior imaging; conversely, a report is enriched and grounded by what the scan data reveals (Sarker et al., 2025). Traditional deep learning systems tend to treat these signals in isolation image models and separate text models. VLMs change this by learning a shared latent space that aligns image regions with textual semantics. In medicine this enables novel capabilities: automatic generation of structured diagnostic reports, visual question answering on patient imagery ("What abnormality is present in the left lower lobe?"), retrieval across modalities (find past cases matching a current presentation), and multimodal risk modelling (image + text). Recent reviews confirm that while many VLMs have been developed in natural-domains, their adaptation for medical imaging and clinical reasoning is advancing rapidly. For example, a 2024 study summarised 18 public medical image–text datasets and 16 recent medical VLM architectures and highlighted key challenges including data scarcity, privacy and evaluation metrics (Hartsock & Rasool, 2024). Another review analysing advancements from 2022 to 2024 found that pre-training on large image–text corpora reduces annotation dependence and improves generalization across downstream tasks (Ryu et al., 2025). Yet, in critical care settings the diagnostic accuracy of open-source VLMs still lags considerably behind proprietary models: one benchmark found open sets achieving up to 40.4% accuracy compared to 68.1% for a strong proprietary model in an emergency-diagnostic task This chapter will therefore seek to bring together multiple strands: the theoretical underpinnings of VLMs, the unique constraints of healthcare data and workflows, the emerging evidence of performance and limitations, and the operational, ethical and governance considerations required for safe deployment. The aim is to provide a valuable resource for researchers, clinicians, data scientists, and healthcare leaders interested in multimodal AI by helping them understand both the progress made and the underlying methods, as well as how to successfully implement these technologies within real-world clinical environments.

Methodologically, the chapter will draw on recent literature (2022–2025) in vision–language modelling, medical imaging, report generation and visual question answering. It will synthesise empirical studies, systematic reviews and benchmark reports, interpret trends, and highlight case studies that demonstrate both success and failure modes. For example, we will examine models like LLaVA-Med, which uses a curriculum learning strategy to fine-tune a vision-language assistant for biomedical image queries (C. Li et al., 2023). We will also examine domain-specific models developed for non-English contexts, such as Qilin-Med-VL which addresses the language gap in multimodal healthcare (J. Liu et al., 2023). One of the important contributions of this work will be an evaluation-driven discussion. While traditional metrics (accuracy, BLEU, ROUGE) remain useful, the chapter will emphasise clinically meaningful evaluation incorporating factual correctness of generated reports, fairness across patient subgroups, algorithmic bias, calibration of risk predictions, and human-in-the-loop validation. The benchmark that found open VLMs under-performing in high-stakes diagnosis underscores the necessity of rigorous evaluation before deployment (Kurz et al., 2025). In addition, the chapter will explore how medical data constraints (privacy, limited annotations, modality heterogeneity) shape model design and selection, and how institutions can mitigate risks through data governance, synthetic augmentation, federated learning and continuous monitoring.

In terms of novelty this chapter fills a key gap by bridging the technical and clinical communities. Many existing works focus either on algorithmic developments or on single-modality applications; fewer have treated vision–language models in medicine from a full-stack perspective by covering training paradigms, adaptation to domain shifts, evaluation frameworks suited to clinical risk, and governance models in healthcare organisations. By linking architecture, data, evaluation, deployment and ethics, the chapter offers a holistic viewpoint that is timely given the rapid progress and the urgency of reliable multimodal systems in healthcare. From a strategic viewpoint, this chapter aims to help transform vision–language models from research curiosities into clinically relevant tools. It provides an actionable roadmap: when should an institution invest in VLM development, when should off-the-shelf models suffice, what evaluation gatekeeping should be in place, how to monitor for drift and unintended consequences, and how to establish a governance framework that aligns with regulatory regimes and ethical norms.

The chapter begins with an introduction to Vision Language Models (VLMs) in healthcare, emphasizing their potential to integrate visual and textual data for enhanced medical decision-making. The subsequent sections cover the core components of VLMs, including vision and language model architectures, followed by discussions on training methodologies and evaluation metrics. Applications of VLMs in medical imaging and diagnostics are explored, highlighting their use in disease classification, report generation, and visual question answering. The chapter then addresses the challenges and limitations of VLMs in healthcare, such as data scarcity, privacy concerns, and model interpretability. Future directions for VLM research, focusing on improving generalization, explainability, and privacy-preserving techniques, are also discussed. Finally, the chapter concludes with a reflection on the transformative potential of VLMs in healthcare, offering a forward-looking perspective on their integration into clinical workflows.

2. A TECHNICAL PERSPECTIVE ON VISION LANGUAGE MODELS (VLMS)

Vision Language Models (VLMs) represent a unified class of artificial intelligence systems capable of understanding and generating information across two modalities which are visual content and natural language. These models combine the representational power of computer vision with the contextual reasoning capabilities of language models, enabling tasks that require joint interpretation of images and text (Hartsock & Rasool, 2024). In the healthcare domain, where diagnostics, clinical documentation, and decision-making often rely on multimodal cues, VLMs have become foundational to next-generation intelligent medical systems. Their importance has grown rapidly due to their ability to automate radiology reporting, support disease classification, generate medical explanations, and enable clinically relevant visual question answering (VQA) systems (Krones et al., 2025).

Healthcare datasets consist of complex imaging modalities such as X-rays, CT scans, MRIs, ultrasound frames, pathology slides, and retinal scans, accompanied by rich textual artifacts including radiology reports, clinical notes, and diagnostic labels. Traditional uni-modal AI models struggle to capture the semantic alignment between these heterogeneous data types. VLMs address this gap by integrating visual representations with textual semantics, allowing the model to learn clinically meaningful associations including linking visual abnormalities in chest X-rays with corresponding diagnostic phrases like "ground-glass opacity" or "consolidation pattern". This multimodal alignment significantly enhances diagnostic accuracy, interpretability, and generalizability across medical tasks (Y. Wang, 2024; Wu, Wang, et al., 2025).

2.1. Core Components of VLMs

2.1.1. Vision Model

The vision subsystem of a VLM is responsible for extracting structural, spatial, and semantic features from medical images. Convolutional Neural Networks (CNNs) such as ResNet, DenseNet, and EfficientNet have historically dominated clinical imaging due to their strong ability to detect subtle visual patterns. Recently, Vision Transformers (ViTs) have gained prominence for their superior attention-based reasoning, especially in high-resolution medical datasets like digital pathology (Y. Wang, 2024). Vision encoders convert pixel-level content into dense embedding vectors that represent pathological regions, anatomical structures, and imaging-specific signatures.

2.1.2. Language Model

Language models enable the interpretation and generation of clinical text. Transformer-based architectures such as BERT, BioBERT, ClinicalBERT, and GPT variants allow models to read radiology reports, understand medical terminology, and generate coherent diagnostic descriptions. These models create embeddings that capture syntax, semantics, and domain-specific medical knowledge, making them highly effective in interpreting structured and unstructured clinical language (C. Zhang et al., 2024).

2.1.3. Fusion of Vision and Language Models

The fusion layer integrates image and text representations into a shared multimodal embedding space. This is typically achieved using cross-modal attention, contrastive learning, or joint embedding architectures (X. Li et al., 2025). In healthcare AI, multimodal fusion links medical image regions with clinical text, helping models associate tumour boundaries with terms like malignant mass or edema (Teoh et al., 2024). Fusion can occur through early fusion of raw features, late fusion of final predictions, or hybrid fusion using attention to align visual and textual tokens. These approaches power advanced medical VLMs, including CLIP-based systems and radiology-focused models like BioViL and MedCLIP (Z. Liu et al., 2025).

2.2. Training Vision Language Models

2.2.1. Datasets

Large-scale multimodal datasets provide the foundation for training VLMs. Generic multimodal datasets such as MS-COCO, Flickr30K, and Visual Genome support general vision–language reasoning (S. Chen et al., 2025).

2.2.2. Model Training Process

Training medical VLMs relies on aligning image–text pairs through objectives such as contrastive learning, masked language modelling, cross-entropy classification, and image-region grounding (Ryu et al., 2025). However, several challenges complicate this process: domain shift, since medical images differ substantially from natural images used in many pre-trained models; sparse and inconsistent textual annotations, as clinical reports vary widely in detail and structure; and high-resolution data demands, because modalities like pathology slides and MRI scans require extensive computational resources for effective training and representation learning (Guan & Liu, 2022).

2.2.3. Transfer Learning

To reduce data requirements in medical VLMs, transfer learning is widely used by leveraging pre-trained vision encoders such as ResNet or ViT trained on ImageNet, and language encoders like BERT or GPT trained on large text corpora. These pre-trained components are then jointly fine-tuned on medical datasets for tasks such as disease classification, report generation, or visual question answering. This strategy significantly accelerates model convergence and provides strong performance even in low-resource clinical environments (Kora et al., 2022; Rahujo et al., 2025).

2.2.4. Evaluation Metrics

Evaluating VLMs in healthcare requires a combination of standard multimodal metrics and clinically focused assessments. Traditional metrics such as accuracy and F1-score are used for classification tasks, while BLEU, ROUGE, and METEOR measure the quality of radiology report generation, and mAP and AUC-ROC assess localisation and binary disease prediction. Beyond these, clinical validation relies on healthcare-specific measures including diagnostic accuracy against radiologist benchmarks, human–AI agreement, VQA accuracy for medical question-answering, and reader-study performance to determine real-world reliability. Together, these metrics ensure that VLMs meet rigorous clinical standards for safety, interpretability, and effectiveness (Z. Li et al., 2025).

A comparison among recent Vision Language Models in Healthcare Applications has been presented in Table 1.

Table 1. Comparison of vision and language models in healthcare applications

Model Type	Example Models	Strengths	Limitations	Common Healthcare Uses
Vision Models	ResNet, EfficientNet, ViT	High diagnostic accuracy; strong spatial reasoning	Limited textual understanding	Disease classification, detection, segmentation
Language Models	BERT, BioBERT, GPT	Strong semantic comprehension; medical text reasoning	No visual understanding	Report generation, clinical text mining
Vision–Language Models	CLIP, BioViL, MedCLIP	Joint image–text reasoning; multimodal alignment	Requires large multimodal datasets	VQA systems, multimodal diagnosis, automated reporting

3. KEY ASPECTS OF VISION LANGUAGE MODELS IN HEALTHCARE

3.1. Medical Imaging and Diagnostics

Medical imaging is one of the most active application areas for vision–language models (VLMs). These models jointly process medical images such as X-rays, magnetic resonance imaging and computed tomography—and their accompanying text, typically radiology reports or clinical notes. By aligning visual patterns with medical language, VLMs can support disease detection, generate draft reports and answer free-text questions about an image, making them powerful tools for diagnostic decision support.

3.1.1. Vision–Language Models for Diagnosing Conditions Through Imaging (X-rays, MRIs, CT scans)

In traditional computer-aided diagnosis, image models are trained only on pixel data and discrete labels. This approach ignores the rich information in narrative reports. Medical VLMs instead learn from paired image–text data. During pre-training, a visual encoder and a language encoder are optimized together so that the representation of an image is close to the representation of its corresponding report in a shared embedding space. After this stage, the visual encoder can be fine-tuned for downstream classification tasks using far fewer labelled examples than standard image-only models (Y. Zhang et al., 2020).

Two influential frameworks illustrate this idea. ConVIRT pre-trains an image encoder on chest X-rays and their reports using a bidirectional contrastive loss, then transfers the encoder to tasks such as lung disease classification and image retrieval (Y. Zhang et al., 2020). It achieves comparable or better accuracy than ImageNet-initialized models while using only around 10 percent of the labelled data (Y. Zhang et al., 2020). MedCLIP extends this strategy to unpaired medical images and texts by decoupling them during training and using a semantic matching loss; this design scales to large datasets and improves zero-shot recognition, where the model can identify new disease labels that were not explicitly seen during fine-tuning (Z. Wang et al., 2022).

Beyond predicting labels, newer multimodal large language models in radiology can generate full reports or respond to questions like "Is there a left-sided pleural effusion?" directly from the image. Surveys show that these systems can assist with triage, preliminary reporting and resident training, although expert verification is still essential (Nam et al., 2025; Yi et al., 2025).

3.1.2. Image–Text Correlation for Improved Disease Detection

The core strength of VLMs lies in learning fine-grained image–text correlations. Radiology reports contain descriptions of anatomical location, shape, extent and uncertainty (for example, "possible right lower-lobe consolidation"). By training contrastive objectives on many image–report pairs, the model discovers which visual patterns correspond to which textual phrases. When a new scan is presented, its embedding is pulled toward the closest textual concepts, allowing the system to recognize abnormalities even when explicit training labels are sparse (Ryu et al., 2025).

Recent surveys of medical VLMs show that stronger image–text alignment consistently improves downstream tasks such as abnormality detection, organ-specific diagnosis and cross-modal retrieval (for example, "find all X-rays similar to this case"). Recent surveys note that cross-modal alignment in medical vision–language models enable image–text retrieval and can support basic interpretability, for example by linking visual findings to semantically similar report phrases and past cases (Jiang et al., 2021; Ryu et al., 2025).

Figure 1. Flow diagram for multimodal vision–language modelling

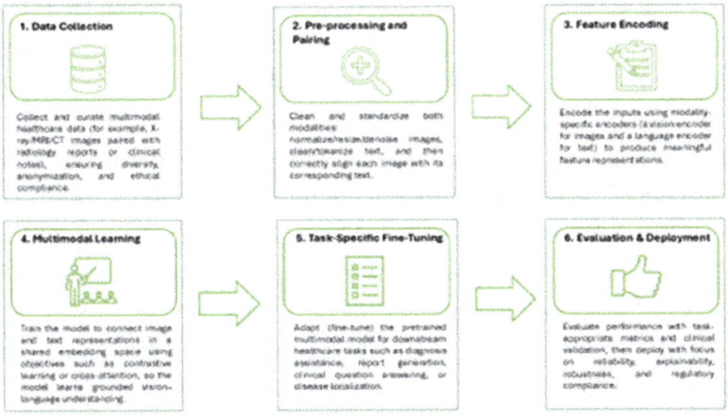

Figure 1 presents a research-oriented flow diagram for multimodal Vision–Language modeling, illustrating the complete pipeline from data collection to deployment. It shows how medical images and textual data are pre-processed, encoded, and jointly learned through multimodal training before being adapted to specific healthcare tasks. Finally, the framework emphasizes systematic evaluation and deployment with a focus on accuracy, explainability, robustness, and regulatory compliance.

3.2. Radiology Report Generation

Radiology report generation is a natural fit for vision–language models (VLMs) because the task already combines images and text. Instead of only predicting labels (for example, "pneumonia: yes/no"), VLMs learn to map an input image to a full narrative report that includes findings, impressions and sometimes recommendations. (Hartsock & Rasool, 2024) review medical vision–language models for report generation and visual question answering, while (Mamdouh et al., 2025) show that recent report-generation systems can speed up reporting, reduce radiologists' workload, and produce more consistent reports. (Z. Wang et al., 2022) introduce LLM-RG4, a high-performing radiology report generation framework. In practice, such systems are expected to assist, not replace, radiologists, who remain responsible for final report approval.

3.2.1. How VLMs automate and enhance report generation

Technically, most systems consist of a visual encoder and a language model decoder. During training, paired image–report data teach the model to align visual features with textual tokens so that the decoder can "translate" image embeddings into coherent sentences. Some models are end-to-end generators, while others use retrieval-augmented generation, first retrieving similar past cases and then adapting their reports. This architecture allows VLMs to automatically draft reports that cover standard sections, highlight key abnormalities and maintain consistent style across cases (Hartsock & Rasool, 2024).

From a workflow perspective, VLMs are usually deployed as assistive tools. The model generates a first draft that the radiologist edits instead of starting from a blank page. Studies report that this "human-in-the-loop" setup can shorten reporting time, reduce repetitive documentation and help junior radiologists produce reports that are closer in quality to senior experts (Hartsock & Rasool, 2024).

(Tanno et al., 2025) fine-tuned a large vision–language foundation model into "Flamingo-CXR", a system that generates full reports for chest radiographs. In a reader study with board-certified radiologists across intensive-care and outpatient settings, many AI-generated reports were rated as equivalent or preferable to the original clinical reports, especially for studies without major abnormalities (Tanno et al., 2025). When used in an assistive mode—radiologists editing the AI draft—report quality remained comparable to expert-only reports while potentially reducing workload. This case shows that VLM-based systems can safely act as drafting tools for high-volume chest X-ray reporting when radiologists remain in the loop.

(Lei et al., 2024)) proposed AutoRG-Brain, the first grounded brain MRI report generation system. The model first segments brain structures and anomaly regions, then generates region-wise textual findings guided by these pixel-level masks, using the RadGenome-Brain MRI dataset. In clinical-style evaluations, AutoRG-Brain helped junior radiologists produce reports that were closer to senior experts' assessments, indicating its usefulness as both a productivity and training aid (Lei et al., 2024). This case illustrates how VLMs can link detailed spatial information in MRI to structured narrative reports for complex neuroimaging studies.

3.3. Clinical Decision-Making Support

Vision–language models (VLMs) and multimodal large language models extend traditional clinical decision support systems (CDSS) by jointly analysing images, free-text notes and structured data such as vital signs or laboratory results. Instead of outputting a single prediction, these systems can summarize the case, rank likely diagnoses and suggest investigations or treatments with short explanations. Recent surveys report growing interest in embedding Vision–Language Models into Clinical Decision Support Systems (CDSS) to provide explainable, multimodal insights that support clinical decision-making processes.

3.3.1. Vision–Language Models in CDSS

In a VLM-enabled CDSS, medical images (for example, radiology or pathology) are encoded by a visual backbone, while clinical notes, problem lists and guideline snippets are processed by a language model. A fusion layer aligns these representations and a retrieval component can bring in additional evidence from guidelines or literature before the model generates a recommendation. This architecture allows the system to reason across modalities, such as linking "new enhancing brain lesion on MRI" with prior chemotherapy history and suggesting appropriate work-up. Reviews of medical multimodal models report that this kind of architecture is being explored for triage, diagnostic support and therapy selection in multiple specialties (Jiang et al., 2021).

3.3.2. Applications in Oncology, Cardiology and Neurology

In precision oncology, (Lammert et al., 2024) introduced MEREDITH, an expert-guided large language model that uses retrieval-augmented generation to integrate pathology reports, molecular profiles and guideline text. For complex cancer cases, MEREDITH produced treatment options that showed high overlap with tumour-board decisions, illustrating how VLM-style systems can help clinicians navigate rapidly expanding evidence while keeping humans in control (Lammert et al., 2024).

In cardiology, multimodal artificial intelligence models combine imaging (for example, echocardiography, cardiac magnetic resonance imaging), electrocardiograms and clinical risk factors to stratify cardiovascular risk more accurately than single-modality models. (Yang et al., 2025) review systems that fuse retinal images, cardiac signals and clinical data to predict heart-attack risk, supporting tailored prevention and follow-up schedules.

In neurology, (Jiang et al., 2021) proposed an attention-based fusion network that uses electronic health record (EHR) variables to guide how a convolutional neural network focuses on brain magnetic resonance imaging. The model predicted outcomes for intracerebral hemorrhage and Alzheimer's disease more accurately than image-only or EHR-only baselines, showing that multimodal reasoning can directly influence treatment-intensity decisions and rehabilitation planning (Jiang et al., 2021).

3.4. Multimodal Data for Enhanced Diagnosis

3.4.1. Combining Visual and Textual Data to Improve Diagnostic Accuracy

Clinicians naturally combine visual findings with narrative history and laboratory data when making diagnoses. Multimodal machine-learning models try to emulate this process by fusing imaging with EHR information. A systematic review by (S.-C. Huang et al., 2020) found that deep-learning models that combined medical imaging with EHR data consistently outperformed single-modality models for tasks such as disease detection, prognosis and readmission prediction. Attention-based and transformer-based fusion architectures further improve performance and interpretability by learning which modality is most informative for a given prediction.

A concrete example is the integration of brain imaging with clinical text for neuro-critical care. (Jiang et al., 2021) fused brain magnetic resonance imaging with EHR variables such as age, blood pressure and Glasgow Coma Scale using a multimodal attention module. The network learned to focus on different brain regions depending on the patient's clinical state and achieved higher accuracy in predicting neurological outcome than either image-only or EHR-only models, providing a more holistic view of the patient (Jiang et al., 2021). Such approaches can easily be extended to full VLMs by replacing structured EHR fields with free-text notes and enabling the model to output both a label and a natural-language explanation. (Xiao et al., 2023) argue that these multimodal large language models are a natural next step for diagnosis, as they can process radiological images, discharge summaries and guideline passages within a single framework.

Overall, evidence from fusion studies and emerging VLM-based systems suggests that combining radiological images with clinical text improves diagnostic accuracy, yields richer explanations and better reflects real clinical reasoning. At the same time, authors emphasize the need for external validation, bias analysis and careful governance before such models are widely adopted in routine practice (S.-C. Huang et al., 2020; Xiao et al., 2023).

3.5. Patient Engagement and Communication

Patient engagement depends heavily on how clearly information is explained. Many patients struggle to understand imaging results, complex terminology or why a particular treatment has been recommended. Recent work on large language models and multimodal large language models shows that these systems can simplify medical jargon, summarize reports and answer follow-up questions in conversational language, which can strengthen trust and shared decision-making (AlSaad et al.,

2024; Bradshaw et al., 2025). Vision–language models (VLMs) extend this idea by allowing patients to ask questions not only about text but also about their own medical images.

3.5.1. VLMs and Visual Question Answering Systems for Patient Queries

Medical visual question answering (Med-VQA) is a vision–language task where the system receives a medical image together with a natural-language question and must return a plausible answer, such as "Is there a fracture?" or "Where is the tumour located?" (Lin et al., 2023). Surveys of Med-VQA emphasize that, beyond supporting clinicians, mature systems could directly assist patients in interpreting their images and understanding what clinicians see (Lin et al., 2023).

Several datasets have been created to model realistic questions. VQA-RAD, for example, contains radiology images paired with questions originally posed by clinicians (Lau et al., 2018). In a patient-facing scenario, a VLM-based VQA system could be integrated into a secure portal or mobile application. After a scan and radiology report are completed, the patient could upload the key image and ask questions such as "Where is the problem you mentioned?", "Is this finding serious?" or "Why do I need a follow-up CT in six months?" The model would highlight the relevant region on the image and generate an answer in plain language, possibly in multiple languages, while linking back to the official report. Recent reviews show that medical vision–language models already support visual question answering for clinicians (Hartsock & Rasool, 2024; Ryu et al., 2025). Safe deployment therefore requires strict validation, transparent communication of model limits and a design in which VLMs supplement rather than replace clinician–patient conversations.

4. ILLUSTRATING THE TECHNICAL COMPONENTS OF VLMS

4.1. Model Architectures

4.1.1. Vision Model: Convolutional Neural Networks (CNNs)

Convolutional Neural Networks (CNNs) constitute the image-processing backbone of VLMs. CNNs are fundamental building blocks of computer vision applications and can automatically learn hierarchical features from raw pixel inputs. These convolutional networks convolve spatial filters with image data to model spatial patterns like edges, textures, and shapes at multiple levels of abstraction. Subsequently, the detected feature descriptors can be used for classification, segmentation, or detection (Busch et al., 2024).

In medical imaging, CNNs can be adapted to identify complex diagnostic patterns in images such as X-rays, MRIs, and CT scans and are often used to detect anomalies, including tumors and fractures. For instance, models such as ResNet and EfficientNet, which employ residual connections and efficient layers, achieve better performance while reducing computational cost (Lee et al., 2024).

4.1.2. Language Model: Transformer-based Models

For text data, models based on transformer architectures, such as BERT (Bidirectional Encoder Representations from Transformers) and GPT (Generative Pre-trained Transformer), have driven a paradigm shift in natural language understanding. Such transduction models employ induced attentional mechanisms to capture long-distance dependencies among words, thereby enabling effective context understanding in text sequences (Yi et al., 2025) A Survey on Multimodal Large Language Models in Radiology for Report Generation and Visual Question Answering. Pre-trained on large amounts of text, BERT performs well on a variety of natural language processing tasks (e.g., question answering and text classification) by modeling bi-directional context. GPT, however, is a generative model that predicts the next word in a sequence and is therefore better suited to text generation. These transformer models were increasingly used to analyze medical reports, patient histories, and clinical notes that inform decision-making.

4.1.3. Multimodal Fusion

Multimodal Vision-Language Models (VLMs) integrate vision and language within a single model, enabling it to understand both visual and textual content. The three main classes of fusion are early, late, and hybrid.

- Early Fusion is achieved by combining the feature representations of two modalities at early layers without much processing, to support joint learning for both inputs. This strategy may, in some cases, be less flexible, as the model must combine the two modalities from the outset.
- Late Fusion, however, treats each modality separately using distinct pipelines and fusing their outputs at some point. This approach preserves the features of each modality but may ignore intermodal interactions.
- Hybrid Fusion seeks to overcome the limitations of these two approaches by permitting a certain extent of interactions with other modalities in intermediate layers, while keeping their separate processing in others.

Finally, cross-modal attention mechanisms, such as those in ViLBERT and related models, enable the model to attend to relevant regions in both the image and text. Such attention helps match image features to their corresponding textual components, thereby enhancing the model's understanding of derived combinatorial data (Z. Li et al., 2025).

4.2. Data Preprocessing for VLMs

4.2.1. Image Preprocessing

In medical image analysis, proper image preprocessing is an important step in enhancing CNN performance. Popular preprocessing methods also include resizing (to match the model's input dimension) and normalization (scaling pixel values to [0, 1], though other scaling ranges, such as [-1, 1], have also been used). Data Augmentation Data augmentation is a popular way for artificially increasing the size of a set by transforming each sample, for instance, horizontally flipping images or slightly rotating them to improve the model's generalization performance on unseen data (Yi et al., 2025).

4.2.2. Text Preprocessing

Text Preprocessing. For the textual part (or simply text preprocessing), we begin by tokenizing the sentence, that is, splitting it into individual words or subwords. Stopword removal is another crucial step that filters out common, non-informative words (e.g., 'the' or 'and') from the analysis. Embedding generation methods, such as Word2Vec and GloVe, are used to learn to map words to continuous vectors that capture semantic relationships, enabling the model to understand how a word is used in context (Yi et al., 2025).

4.2.3. Handling Imbalanced Data

In many medical datasets, particularly for rare diseases or conditions, such data imbalance is prevalent. To address this problem, several methods, such as oversampling the minority class or under sampling the majority class, can be used. Alternatively, the class weight of the loss can be adjusted during training, so that the model places greater emphasis on underrepresented classes and performs better on rare cases (Buess et al., 2025).

4.3. Multimodal Alignment

4.3.1. Aligning Visual Features with Textual Descriptions

VLMs aim to fuse document images and text data, a computational process formulated as a mapping that combines image and text information for training or learning. This alignment enables the model to compare features across modalities effectively. For example, "a broken femur" in text and an X-ray image are both mapped to a common vector space, allowing the model to correlate visual features with textual terms.

Models such as CLIP (Contrastive Language-Image Pretraining) and VisualBERT are designed to perform exactly this. For instance, CLIP effectively pairs images with their corresponding text by learning from a large-scale image-text dataset. VisualBERT and ViLBERT are extensions of BERT that incorporate visual information via natural language; thus, they are suitable for applications such as medical diagnosis and clinical decision-making, where understanding both modalities is required (Z. Li et al., 2025).

4.4. End-to-End Training Pipeline

4.4.1. Dataset Creation and Model Selection

An end-to-end training pipeline for a VLM is typically constructed by first collecting a multimodal dataset comprising medical images and their corresponding textual annotations. Training the model to learn correspondences between visual features and their textual descriptions requires these datasets. Model selection is critical; we can use different architectures for image and text. For example, while processing visual data, CNNs are generally used, whereas transformer models such as BERT or GPT are used for textual data (Yi et al., 2025).

4.4.2. Loss Functions and Optimization

For classification, a common loss is cross-entropy, which penalizes misclassification. Hey Google, I am bored. This loss is minimized during model training. The loss function in such models (like CLIP) is a kind of specialized contrastive loss function: it tries to learn embeddings so that the positive pairs of image and text are closer in the embedding space compared to negative pairs.

4.4.3. Transfer Learning and Fine-Tuning

One of the big advantages of VLMs is their capability to use transfer learning, where a model that has already been pre-trained on large data can be fine-tuned in domain-specific tasks. In healthcare, by transferring and finetuning models such as CLIP on medical datasets, we are able to capture relevant features and patterns on the concept of healthcare, which can ultimately enhance performance for tasks such as disease classification or medical image captioning (Z. Li et al., 2025).

Table 2. Common models for VLM applications in medical imaging.

Model	Description	Applications in Healthcare
CLIP	A vision-language model that aligns image and text via contrastive learning.	Disease classification, image-text alignment
ViLBERT	An extension of BERT to process multimodal data, also using text and images at the same time.	Medical image captioning, clinical decision support
VisualBERT	A vision and language model learned jointly from both modalities.	Medical image analysis, diagnostic assistance

Table 2 summarizes key models used in Vision-Language Model (VLM) applications for medical imaging, highlighting their capabilities and primary uses in healthcare. These models are essential for improving automated disease detection and assisting healthcare professionals by processing and analyzing both medical images and clinical texts.

Figure 2. Workflow of a vision-language model for disease classification

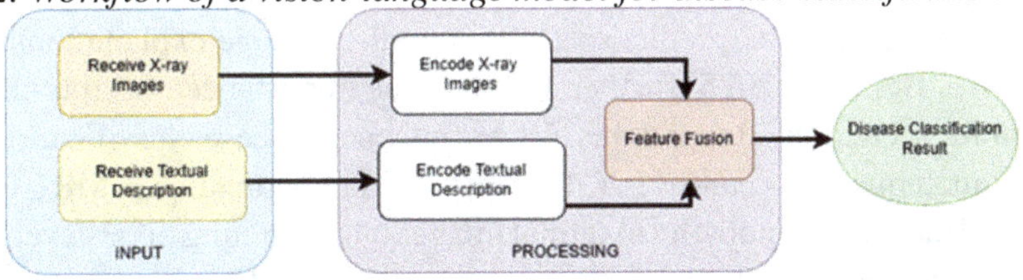

Figure 2 shows the flow of a VLM for disease classification. The system takes X-ray images and their text descriptions as input. These two inputs are handled independently: the X-ray images are fed through a CNN encoder, and the text descriptions are processed by a language model (such as BERT or GPT). The encoded image and text representation pairs are then integrated in the Feature Fusion stage. This fusion enables the model to combine visual and text information, yielding a final

Disease Classification Result that can assist doctors in identifying and classifying potential diseases in X-ray images.

5. VISION LANGUAGE MODELS FOR MEDICAL IMAGING

Medical imaging encompassing X-rays, CT scans, MRI, ultrasound, and digital pathology is central to modern diagnostics (Abhisheka et al., 2023). Traditional automated imaging models often struggle with ambiguous patterns, limited context, or multimodal clinical reasoning. VLMs overcome these limitations by integrating visual signals with textual knowledge, enabling context-rich diagnostic interpretation. Through multimodal fusion, VLMs can localise abnormalities, interpret medical context, generate descriptive clinical findings, and answer visual questions, providing a foundation for AI-augmented radiology workflows (Tong et al., 2025).

5.1. Applications in Radiology

VLMs can convert raw medical images into structured radiology reports by fusing image embeddings with medical language modelling, helping reduce reporting workload, minimise inconsistencies, and detect subtle abnormalities. Recent studies demonstrate that multimodal alignment between images and clinical text significantly enhances report generation and medical VQA performance, showing that VLMs trained on paired radiology datasets can produce clinically coherent descriptions while maintaining high diagnostic relevance (Mir et al., 2025). A domain-adapted example is pneumonia detection from chest X-rays, where the model identifies features such as consolidation, ground-glass opacities, pleural effusion, and air bronchograms, generating both diagnostic predictions and natural-language explanations; (Bai et al., 2024; Wu, He, et al., 2025) further highlight the importance of rigorous clinical evaluation for such tools. Beyond this, VLMs enhance disease classification across modalities including lung cancer in CT, cardiovascular anomalies in MRI, fractures in X-ray, and diabetic retinopathy in retinal images by combining pixel-level patterns with textual medical knowledge. Recent work, such as that by (Urooj et al., 2025), shows that modern large-model adaptation techniques significantly improve multimodal performance across diverse clinical datasets. Some Recent advancements of Disease Classification using VLMs has been presented in Table 3.

Table 3. Examples of disease classification using VLMs

Disease Area	Imaging Modality	VLM Capability	Example Outcome
Cancer	CT, MRI, pathology	Tumour detection and captioning	Identifies malignant lesions with explanation
Cardiovascular	MRI, ECG-image pairs	Structural abnormality detection	Detects ventricular hypertrophy
Ophthalmology	Retinal fundus	DR severity grading	Detects proliferative DR
Orthopaedics	X-ray	Fracture detection	Identifies fractures with text justification

5.2. Visual Question Answering (VQA) in Medical Imaging

Medical VQA enables clinicians to query images using natural-language prompts—for example, "Is there fluid in the left lung?" or "Where is the tumour located?"—with systems generating evidence-grounded answers through fine-grained cross-modal alignment, as demonstrated by (Lin et al., 2023). In ophthalmology, VLM-based VQA supports retinal screening by answering questions about optic-disc cupping, haemorrhages, or macular oedema (X. Chen et al., 2024). When integrated into hospital PACS, decision-support platforms, or EHR systems, VLMs offer real-time diagnostic assistance, automated report drafting, reduced errors through multimodal verification, and better continuity across imaging and textual documentation (Solomon et al., 2023). EHR-integrated deployments further enhance clinical decision-making by linking imaging findings with historical diagnoses, treatments, and progression patterns, as highlighted by (Wu, He, et al., 2025).

6. VISION LANGUAGE MODELS FOR BIOMEDICAL APPLICATIONS

Vision Language Models (VLMs) have emerged as a transformative paradigm in biomedical artificial intelligence by enabling joint reasoning over visual and textual data. Unlike unimodal deep learning approaches, VLMs integrate heterogeneous biomedical information such as medical images, genomic data, and clinical narratives within a unified representation space, thereby supporting more comprehensive and explainable decision-making. Recent advances between 2023 and 2025 have demonstrated the applicability of VLMs across biomedical image analysis, drug discovery, genomics, medical text mining, and real-world clinical systems (Guan et al., 2025; Ryu et al., 2025; Warner et al., 2024).

6.1. Biomedical Image Analysis

Biomedical image analysis represents one of the most mature and impactful application domains of VLMs. By learning fine-grained alignments between medical images and corresponding textual descriptions, VLMs facilitate advanced reasoning tasks such as disease classification, lesion localization, visual question answering (VQA), and report generation.

6.1.1. Histopathology, CT, and MRI Analysis

Recent studies have demonstrated that domain-specific VLMs significantly outperform conventional convolutional neural networks in pathology image understanding. (Lu et al., 2024) introduced a visual-language foundation model trained on large-scale histopathology slides paired with expert annotations, enabling robust tumor grading and subtyping in computational pathology. Similarly, PathologyVLM proposed by (Dai et al., 2025) leverages curated pathology image-text datasets and two-stage multimodal training to achieve state-of-the-art performance in pathology VQA tasks.

In radiology, VLMs have been successfully extended to volumetric imaging. Med3DVLM integrates three-dimensional CT and MRI data with radiology reports, addressing the challenge of aligning spatial features with clinical language (Xin et al., 2025). This approach enables multi-task learning across image-text retrieval, report generation, and diagnostic question answering, demonstrating the scalability of VLMs beyond 2D imaging.

6.1.2. Case Study: Cancer Detection

VLMs have shown strong potential in cancer detection across imaging modalities. In breast cancer screening, multimodal foundation models trained on mammograms and textual findings demonstrate improved sensitivity and interpretability compared to image-only systems (S. Zhang et al., 2025). Similarly, dermatological applications leverage image-text pairs from dermoscopy images and clinical notes to enhance skin cancer classification, particularly in low-data and long-tail disease settings (Z. Huang et al., 2023).

Ophthalmology provides another compelling case study. EyeCLIP, a large-scale visual-language foundation model, integrates multimodal ophthalmic images with partial clinical text to achieve robust disease classification and zero-shot generalization (Shi et al., 2024, 2025). These results highlight the ability of VLMs to generalize across imaging devices, disease categories, and patient populations. Table 4 presents a structured overview of representative VLM-based VQA techniques in radiology and biomedical imaging.

Table 4. VLM-based techniques for visual question answering in radiology

Model	Imaging Modality	Task	Key Contribution
PathologyVLM (Dai et al., 2025)	Histopathology	VQA	Domain-specific alignment for pathology reasoning
Med3DVLM (Xin et al., 2025)	CT, MRI	VQA, Report Generation	Efficient 3D image-text fusion
EyeCLIP (Shi et al., 2025)	Fundus, OCT	VQA, Classification	Multimodal ophthalmic foundation model
UMIT (Yu et al., 2025)	X-ray, CT, PET	Multi-task VQA	Unified multimodal instruction tuning

6.2. Drug Discovery and Development

Beyond imaging, VLMs are increasingly applied to drug discovery and biomedical research by jointly modelling molecular structures, biomedical images, and scientific literature.

6.2.1. Predicting Molecular Structures and Drug–Target Interactions

Multimodal biomedical foundation models trained on large-scale image-text pairs enable semantic understanding of molecular diagrams, protein structures, and pharmacological descriptions. (S. Zhang et al., 2025) demonstrated that multimodal models trained on millions of biomedical image-text pairs can support drug–target interaction prediction and chemical property inference. These models benefit from textual context derived from experimental reports, enhancing interpretability in early-stage drug screening.

6.2.2. Case Study: Drug Efficacy and Safety Prediction

Medical text mining combined with visual representations of molecular graphs allows VLMs to extract adverse drug reactions and predict side effects from heterogeneous sources. Survey studies indicate that such multimodal approaches outperform text-only bioinformatics pipelines in identifying drug efficacy patterns and safety signals (Sun et al., 2025; Warner et al., 2024). Table 5 summarizes key biomedical and pharmaceutical applications of VLMs.

Table 5. Applications of vision language models in drug discovery and biomedical research

Application Area	Data Modalities	Outcome
Drug-target prediction (Zhang et al., 2025)	Molecular images + text	Improved binding inference
Adverse effect mining (Sun et al., 2025)	Literature + visuals	Side-effect detection
Biomedical QA (Thapa et al., 2024)	Figures + abstracts	Knowledge discovery

6.3. Genomics and Personalized Medicine

VLMs also support precision medicine by integrating genomic data with medical imaging and clinical narratives. Multimodal foundation models can correlate genetic markers with phenotypic manifestations observed in imaging, enabling individualized risk stratification and treatment planning.

Recent ophthalmology studies demonstrate how multimodal vision-language frameworks integrate retinal imaging with patient metadata to predict disease progression and treatment response (Jin et al., 2026; Qiu et al., 2024). These approaches illustrate the feasibility of personalized diagnostic pipelines that adapt to patient-specific characteristics.

Moreover, VLM-based instruction-tuned systems such as UMIT facilitate multilingual and cross-institutional deployment, enhancing accessibility to personalized care in global healthcare settings (Yu et al., 2025).

6.4. Medical Text Mining and Analysis

Medical literature and clinical documentation constitute vast unstructured data sources. VLMs extend traditional natural language processing by grounding textual insights in visual evidence.

Multimodal large language models such as MedPLIB enable pixel-level grounding and fine-grained visual reasoning guided by textual prompts, supporting advanced biomedical question answering and image region interpretation (Z. Huang et al., 2023). These capabilities allow researchers to identify novel biomarkers by linking imaging phenotypes with textual descriptions extracted from PubMed and clinical trial reports.

Systematic reviews confirm that VLM-based text-image mining improves evidence synthesis, hypothesis generation, and clinical knowledge discovery compared to unimodal approaches (Ryu et al., 2025; Sun et al., 2025).

6.5. Clinical Applications and Healthcare Integration

In real-world clinical environments, VLMs enable multi-source data fusion by combining imaging, electronic health records (EHRs), and clinical notes. Vision-language systems have been successfully deployed for automated radiology report generation and outcome prediction, as demonstrated in CT pulmonary angiography studies (Zhong et al., 2025). Clinical Applications of VLMs has been presented in Figure 3 and 4.

Figure 3. VLM-driven radiology report generation from chest X-ray images

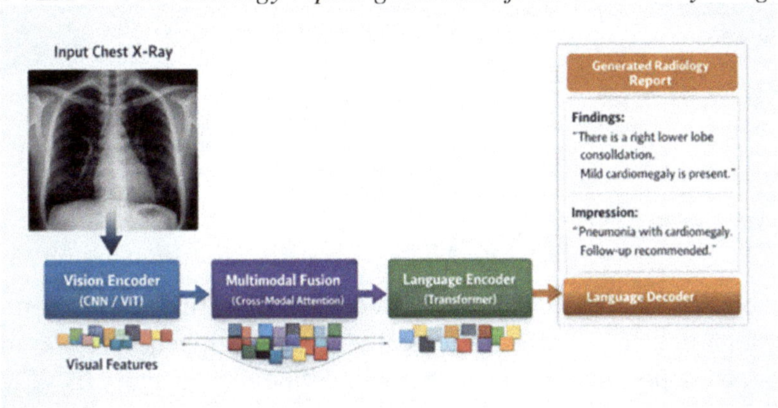

Advanced architectures such as Abn-BLIP improve abnormality detection and structured reporting by aligning pathological findings with language representations, reducing diagnostic omissions (Zhong et al., 2025). These systems support clinician workflows and enhance explainability in AI-assisted diagnosis.

Narrative reviews further highlight the role of VLMs in real-time clinical trial monitoring and decision support by integrating multimodal patient data streams (Guan et al., 2025; Simon et al., 2024). Image 5 illustrates an example of VLM-driven radiology report generation from chest X-ray images. Image 6 depicts the integration of VLMs within EHR systems, showcasing multimodal data fusion for clinical decision support.

Vision Language Models represent a foundational shift in biomedical artificial intelligence by enabling holistic reasoning across visual, textual, and structured data. From pathology and radiology to drug discovery and personalized medicine, recent high-impact studies demonstrate that VLMs improve diagnostic accuracy, interpretability, and clinical utility. As datasets, architectures, and regulatory frameworks mature, VLMs are poised to become integral components of next-generation biomedical and healthcare systems.

Figure 4. Integration of VLMs within EHR systems

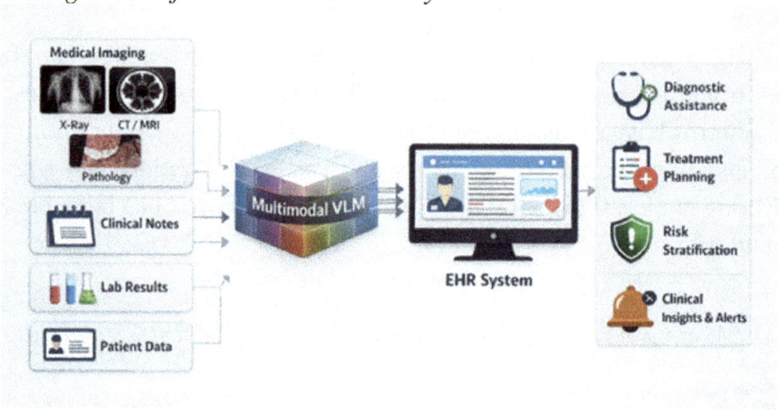

7. FUTURE DIRECTIONS

The evolution of Vision Language Models (VLMs) in healthcare presents a dynamic and promising frontier in medical artificial intelligence. However, several challenges and opportunities remain that will define the trajectory of VLMs in the coming years.

7.1. Enhanced Model Generalization Across Medical Domains

While current VLMs demonstrate considerable success in specific imaging modalities such as radiology and pathology, there is a critical need to extend these models to a broader range of medical domains. Future research should focus on improving the generalization capabilities of VLMs across different specialties (e.g., cardiology, neurology) and integrating them into multi-specialty environments. Achieving robust cross-domain performance will require large-scale, diverse multimodal datasets that incorporate not only imaging but also patient records, genomic data, and electronic health records (EHRs) (Wu, He, et al., 2025).

7.2. Addressing Data Scarcity and Privacy Concerns

A significant challenge in training VLMs for medical applications lies in data scarcity, especially in rare diseases or small population groups. Future advancements could include exploring synthetic data generation, federated learning, and multi-center collaborations to overcome data limitations while ensuring compliance with privacy regulations such as HIPAA. Privacy-preserving techniques such as differential privacy and federated learning will be pivotal in enabling VLMs to learn from decentralized data without compromising patient confidentiality.

7.3. Multimodal Model Interpretability and Explainability

For the widespread clinical adoption of VLMs, their interpretability is paramount. Future work should prioritize the development of models that not only provide predictions but also explain their reasoning processes, linking specific image features with clinical terms in a manner that is understandable to healthcare professionals. Enhancing explainability will build trust in AI systems, especially when these systems make high-stakes decisions in clinical environments.

7.4. Integration with Clinical Workflows

Successful integration of VLMs into clinical workflows will require a seamless interface between AI systems and healthcare practitioners. Future research must explore practical deployment strategies that facilitate the use of VLMs in real-time decision-making while ensuring they align with existing clinical systems like EHRs and PACS. Additionally, understanding the role of VLMs in human-in-the-loop (HITL) settings will be crucial, where clinicians actively supervise and validate the AI's outputs.

7.5. Long-term Validation and Continuous Monitoring

As VLMs are deployed in clinical environments, continuous monitoring and periodic validation are essential to ensure they remain effective and safe. Future work should focus on developing frameworks for ongoing evaluation, focusing not only on technical metrics (e.g., accuracy, precision) but also on clinical metrics such as diagnostic confidence, patient outcomes, and cost-effectiveness. Moreover, real-world testing across diverse healthcare settings will help fine-tune VLMs for optimal performance.

8. CONCLUSION

Vision Language Models (VLMs) represent a revolutionary step in the integration of artificial intelligence with healthcare, combining the strengths of both visual and textual data to address complex diagnostic and clinical challenges. As explored throughout this chapter, VLMs have shown tremendous potential in automating and augmenting medical imaging tasks such as disease detection, report generation, and clinical decision support. These models are also paving the way for more comprehensive diagnostic systems that combine radiological imaging, clinical notes, and patient history into a unified decision-making tool.

Despite the rapid advancements in VLMs, several hurdles remain. Challenges such as data scarcity, privacy concerns, model interpretability, and the seamless integration of these technologies into clinical workflows need to be addressed. Future research should focus on improving model generalization across medical domains, enhancing explainability to build clinician trust, and ensuring that privacy-preserving techniques are effectively implemented in line with regulatory standards.

Moreover, the long-term success of VLMs will depend on their ability to evolve with the clinical landscape. Ongoing evaluation, coupled with ethical frameworks that address bias and fairness, will be essential for safe and equitable deployment. VLMs have the potential to transform healthcare by enabling more accurate diagnostics, reducing clinician workload, and ultimately improving patient outcomes. As this technology matures, it will play an integral role in advancing personalized and precision medicine, offering a glimpse into the future of intelligent healthcare systems.

REFERENCES

Abhisheka, B., Biswas, S. K., Purkayastha, B., Das, D., & Escargueil, A. (2023). Recent trend in medical imaging modalities and their applications in disease diagnosis: A review. *Multimedia Tools and Applications*, *83*(14), 43035–43070. DOI: 10.1007/s11042-023-17326-1

AlSaad, R., Abd-alrazaq, A., Boughorbel, S., Ahmed, A., Renault, M.-A., Damseh, R., & Sheikh, J. (2024). Multimodal Large Language Models in Health Care: Applications, Challenges, and Future Outlook. *Journal of Medical Internet Research*, *26*, e59505. DOI: 10.2196/59505 PMID: 39321458

Bai, H., Dai, Y., Hsu, W.-C., Imami, M., Jiao, Z., Jones, C., Loizou, N., Peng, J., Sair, H., Shen, J., Wang, Y., Wu, J., & Zhang, P. (2024). Enhancing vision-language models for medical imaging: Bridging the 3D gap with innovative slice selection. *Advances in Neural Information Processing Systems*, *37*, 99947–99964. DOI: 10.52202/079017-3171

Bradshaw, T. J., Tie, X., Warner, J., Hu, J., Li, Q., & Li, X. (2025). Large Language Models and Large Multimodal Models in Medical Imaging: A Primer for Physicians. *Journal of Nuclear Medicine*, *66*(2), 173–182. DOI: 10.2967/jnumed.124.268072 PMID: 39819692

Buess, L., Keicher, M., Navab, N., Maier, A., & Tayebi Arasteh, S. (2025). From large language models to multimodal AI: A scoping review on the potential of generative AI in medicine. *Biomedical Engineering Letters*, *15*(5), 845–863. DOI: 10.1007/s13534-025-00497-1 PMID: 40917142

Busch, F., Hoffmann, L., Dos Santos, D. P., Makowski, M. R., Saba, L., Prucker, P., Hadamitzky, M., Navab, N., Kather, J. N., Truhn, D., Cuocolo, R., Adams, L. C., & Bressem, K. K. (2024). Large language models for structured reporting in radiology: Past, present, and future. *European Radiology*, *35*(5), 2589–2602. DOI: 10.1007/s00330-024-11107-6 PMID: 39438330

Chen, S., Wu, Z., Zhang, K., Li, C., Zhang, B., Ma, F., Yu, F. R., & Li, Q. (2025). Exploring Embodied Multimodal Large Models: Development, datasets, and future directions. *Information Fusion*, *122*, 103198. DOI: 10.1016/j.inffus.2025.103198

Chen, X., Chen, R., Xu, P., Zhang, W., Shang, X., He, M., & Shi, D. (2024). *Visual Question Answering in Ophthalmology: A Progressive and Practical Perspective* (Version 1). arXiv. DOI: 10.48550/ARXIV.2410.16662

Dai, D., Zhang, Y., Yang, Q., Xu, L., Shen, X., Xia, S., & Wang, G. (2025). Pathologyvlm: A large vision-language model for pathology image understanding. *Artificial Intelligence Review*, *58*(6), 186. DOI: 10.1007/s10462-025-11190-1

Das Joy, S., Dey, N., & Islam, Md. R., Mahmud, M. A., Rahman, M., Tanvir, K., & Gomes, D. (2025). Synthetic Healthcare Data in Generation, Validation, and Integration for Ethical and Scalable Health Innovation: In M. Ahmad (Ed.), *Advances in Synthetic Healthcare Data* (pp. 65–108). IGI Global Scientific Publishing. DOI: 10.4018/979-8-3373-5641-9.ch003

Guan, H., Chen, X., Shen, C., Zhu, X., Xu, H., & Li, C. (2025). Z Visual-language foundation models for medical and clinical diagnosis and treatments. *The Visual Computer*, *41*(15), 12399–12410. DOI: 10.1007/s00371-025-04067-5

Guan, H., & Liu, M. (2022). Domain Adaptation for Medical Image Analysis: A Survey. *IEEE Transactions on Bio-Medical Engineering*, *69*(3), 1173–1185. DOI: 10.1109/TBME.2021.3117407 PMID: 34606445

Hartsock, I., & Rasool, G. (2024). Vision-language models for medical report generation and visual question answering: A review. *Frontiers in Artificial Intelligence*, *7*, 1430984. DOI: 10.3389/frai.2024.1430984 PMID: 39628839

Huang, S.-C., Pareek, A., Seyyedi, S., Banerjee, I., & Lungren, M. P. (2020). Fusion of medical imaging and electronic health records using deep learning: A systematic review and implementation guidelines. *NPJ Digital Medicine*, *3*(1), 136. DOI: 10.1038/s41746-020-00341-z PMID: 33083571

Huang, Z., Bianchi, F., Yuksekgonul, M., Montine, T. J., & Zou, J. (2023). A visual–language foundation model for pathology image analysis using medical Twitter. *Nature Medicine*, *29*(9), 2307–2316. DOI: 10.1038/s41591-023-02504-3 PMID: 37592105

Jiang, C., Chen, Y., Chang, J., Feng, M., Wang, R., & Yao, J. (2021). *Fusion of medical imaging and electronic health records with attention and multi-head machanisms* (Version 1). arXiv. DOI: 10.48550/ARXIV.2112.11710

Jin, K., Yu, T., Ying, G., Ge, Z., Li, K. Z., Zhou, Y., Shi, D., Wang, M., Goktas, P., & Grzybowski, A. (2026). A systematic review of vision and vision-language foundation models in ophthalmology. *Advances in Ophthalmology Practice and Research*, *6*(1), 8–19. DOI: 10.1016/j.aopr.2025.10.004 PMID: 41532028

Kora, P., Ooi, C. P., Faust, O., Raghavendra, U., Gudigar, A., Chan, W. Y., Meenakshi, K., Swaraja, K., Plawiak, P., & Rajendra Acharya, U. (2022). Transfer learning techniques for medical image analysis: A review. *Biocybernetics and Biomedical Engineering*, *42*(1), 79–107. DOI: 10.1016/j.bbe.2021.11.004

Krones, F., Marikkar, U., Parsons, G., Szmul, A., & Mahdi, A. (2025). Review of multimodal machine learning approaches in healthcare. *Information Fusion*, *114*, 102690. DOI: 10.1016/j.inffus.2024.102690 PMID: 41799790

Kurz, C. F., Merzhevich, T., Eskofier, B. M., Kather, J. N., & Gmeiner, B. (2025). Benchmarking vision-language models for diagnostics in emergency and critical care settings. *NPJ Digital Medicine*, *8*(1), 423. DOI: 10.1038/s41746-025-01837-2 PMID: 40640347

Lammert, J., Dreyer, T., Mathes, S., Kuligin, L., Borm, K. J., Schatz, U. A., Kiechle, M., Lörsch, A. M., Jung, J., Lange, S., Pfarr, N., Durner, A., Schwamborn, K., Winter, C., Ferber, D., Kather, J. N., Mogler, C., Illert, A. L., & Tschochohei, M. (2024). Expert-Guided Large Language Models for Clinical Decision Support in Precision Oncology. *JCO Precision Oncology*, *8*(8), e2400478. DOI: 10.1200/PO-24-00478 PMID: 39475661

Lau, J. J., Gayen, S., Ben Abacha, A., & Demner-Fushman, D. (2018). A dataset of clinically generated visual questions and answers about radiology images. *Scientific Data*, *5*(1), 180251. DOI: 10.1038/sdata.2018.251 PMID: 30457565

Lee, T., Tu, H., Wong, C. H., Zheng, W., Zhou, Y., Mai, Y., Roberts, J. S., Yasunaga, M., Yao, H., Xie, C., & Liang, P. (2024). *VHELM: A Holistic Evaluation of Vision Language Models* (Version 2). arXiv. DOI: 10.52202/079017-4464

Lei, J., Zhang, X., Wu, C., Dai, L., Zhang, Y., Zhang, Y., Wang, Y., Xie, W., & Li, Y. (2024). *AutoRG-Brain: Grounded Report Generation for Brain MRI* (Version 3). arXiv. DOI: 10.48550/ARXIV.2407.16684

Li, C., Wong, C., Zhang, S., Usuyama, N., Liu, H., Yang, J., Naumann, T., Poon, H., & Gao, J. (2023). *LLaVA-Med: Training a Large Language-and-Vision Assistant for Biomedicine in One Day* (Version 1). arXiv. DOI: 10.48550/ARXIV.2306.00890

Li, X., Li, L., Jiang, Y., Wang, H., Qiao, X., Feng, T., Luo, H., & Zhao, Y. (2025). Vision-Language Models in medical image analysis: From simple fusion to general large models. *Information Fusion*, *118*, 102995. DOI: 10.1016/j.inffus.2025.102995

Li, Z., Wu, X., Du, H., Liu, F., Nghiem, H., & Shi, G. (2025). *A Survey of State of the Art Large Vision Language Models: Alignment, Benchmark, Evaluations and Challenges*. DOI: 10.1109/CVPRW67362.2025.00147

Lin, Z., Zhang, D., Tao, Q., Shi, D., Haffari, G., Wu, Q., He, M., & Ge, Z. (2023). Medical visual question answering: A survey. *Artificial Intelligence in Medicine*, *143*, 102611. DOI: 10.1016/j.artmed.2023.102611 PMID: 37673579

Liu, J., Wang, Z., Ye, Q., Chong, D., Zhou, P., & Hua, Y. (2023). *Qilin-Med-VL: Towards Chinese Large Vision-Language Model for General Healthcare* (Version 2). arXiv. DOI: 10.48550/ARXIV.2310.17956

Liu, Z., Yin, Z., Mi, Z., Guo, B., & Zheng, Z. (2025). A Comparative Analysis of Three Data Fusion Methods and Construction of the Fusion Method Selection Paradigm. *Mathematics*, *13*(8), 1218. DOI: 10.3390/math13081218

Lu, M. Y., Chen, B., Williamson, D. F. K., Chen, R. J., Liang, I., Ding, T., Jaume, G., Odintsov, I., Le, L. P., Gerber, G., Parwani, A. V., Zhang, A., & Mahmood, F. (2024). A visual-language foundation model for computational pathology. *Nature Medicine*, *30*(3), 863–874. DOI: 10.1038/s41591-024-02856-4 PMID: 38504017

Mamdouh, D., Attia, M., Osama, M., Mohamed, N., Lotfy, A., Arafa, T., Rashed, E. A., & Khoriba, G. (2025). Advancements in Radiology Report Generation: A Comprehensive Analysis. *Bioengineering (Basel, Switzerland)*, *12*(7), 693. DOI: 10.3390/bioengineering12070693 PMID: 40722385

Mir, A. N., Rizvi, D. R., & Nissar, I. (2025). Enhancing medical image report generation using a self-boosting multimodal alignment framework. *Health Information Science and Systems*, *13*(1), 58. DOI: 10.1007/s13755-025-00378-y PMID: 41018682

Nam, Y., Kim, D. Y., Kyung, S., Seo, J., Song, J. M., Kwon, J., Kim, J., Jo, W., Park, H., Sung, J., Park, S., Kwon, H., Kwon, T., Kim, K., & Kim, N. (2025). Multimodal Large Language Models in Medical Imaging: Current State and Future Directions. *Korean Journal of Radiology*, *26*(10), 900. DOI: 10.3348/kjr.2025.0599 PMID: 41015856

Qiu, J., Wu, J., Wei, H., Shi, P., Zhang, M., Sun, Y., Li, L., Liu, H., Liu, H., Hou, S., Zhao, Y., Shi, X., Xian, J., Qu, X., Zhu, S., Pan, L., Chen, X., Zhang, X., Jiang, S., & Yuan, W. (2024). Development and Validation of a Multimodal Multitask Vision Foundation Model for Generalist Ophthalmic Artificial Intelligence. *NEJM AI*, *1*(12). Advance online publication. DOI: 10.1056/AIoa2300221

Rahujo, A., Atif, D., Inam, S. A., Khan, A. A., & Ullah, S. (2025). A survey on the applications of transfer learning to enhance the performance of large language models in healthcare systems. *Discover Artificial Intelligence*, *5*(1), 90. DOI: 10.1007/s44163-025-00339-0

Ryu, J. S., Kang, H., Chu, Y., & Yang, S. (2025). Vision-language foundation models for medical imaging: A review of current practices and innovations. *Biomedical Engineering Letters*, *15*(5), 809–830. DOI: 10.1007/s13534-025-00484-6 PMID: 40917147

Sarker, D., Sadi, M. T. H., Gomes, D., & Hasan, Md. M. (2025). Securing Patient Privacy and Data Protection by Federated Learning in AI-Driven Healthcare: In N. K. Mun, C.-S. Shieh, D. Ather, A. Panwar, & V. Jain (Eds.), *Advances in Computational Intelligence and Robotics* (pp. 317–352). IGI Global Scientific Publishing. DOI: 10.4018/979-8-3373-3306-9.ch012

Shi, D., Zhang, W., Yang, J., Huang, S., Chen, X., Xu, P., Jin, K., Lin, S., Wei, J., Yusufu, M., Liu, S., Zhang, Q., Ge, Z., Xu, X., & He, M. (2025). A multimodal visual–language foundation model for computational ophthalmology. *NPJ Digital Medicine*, *8*(1), 381. DOI: 10.1038/s41746-025-01772-2 PMID: 40542189

Shi, D., Zhang, W., Yang, J., Huang, S., Chen, X., Yusufu, M., Jin, K., Lin, S., Liu, S., Zhang, Q., & He, M. (2024, September). *EyeCLIP: A visual-language foundation model for multi-modal ophthalmic image analysis*. arXiv. https://doi.org//arXiv.2409.06644DOI: 10.48550

Simon, B. D., Ozyoruk, K. B., Gelikman, D. G., Harmon, S. A., & Türkbey, B. (2024). *The future of multimodal artificial intelligence models for integrating imaging and clinical metadata: A narrative review*. Diagnostic and Interventional Radiology., DOI: 10.4274/dir.2024.242631

Solomon, J., Dauber-Decker, K., Richardson, S., Levy, S., Khan, S., Coleman, B., Persaud, R., Chelico, J., King, D., Spyropoulos, A., & McGinn, T. (2023). Integrating Clinical Decision Support Into Electronic Health Record Systems Using a Novel Platform (EvidencePoint): Developmental Study. *JMIR Formative Research*, *7*, e44065. DOI: 10.2196/44065 PMID: 37856193

Sun, Y., Wen, X., Zhang, Y., Jin, L., Yang, C., Zhang, Q., Jiang, M., Xu, Z., Guo, W., Su, J., & Jiang, X. (2025). Visual-language foundation models in medical imaging: A systematic review and meta-analysis of diagnostic and analytical applications. *Computer Methods and Programs in Biomedicine*, *268*, 108870. DOI: 10.1016/j.cmpb.2025.108870 PMID: 40424873

Tanno, R., Barrett, D. G. T., Sellergren, A., Ghaisas, S., Dathathri, S., See, A., Welbl, J., Lau, C., Tu, T., Azizi, S., Singhal, K., Schaekermann, M., May, R., Lee, R., Man, S., Mahdavi, S., Ahmed, Z., Matias, Y., Barral, J., & Ktena, I. (2025). Collaboration between clinicians and vision–language models in radiology report generation. *Nature Medicine*, *31*(2), 599–608. DOI: 10.1038/s41591-024-03302-1 PMID: 39511432

Teoh, J. R., Dong, J., Zuo, X., Lai, K. W., Hasikin, K., & Wu, X. (2024). Advancing healthcare through multimodal data fusion: A comprehensive review of techniques and applications. *PeerJ. Computer Science*, *10*, e2298. DOI: 10.7717/peerj-cs.2298 PMID: 39650483

Tong, R., Xu, T., Ju, X., & Wang, L. (2025). Progress in Medical AI: Reviewing Large LanguageModels and Multimodal Systems for Diagonosis. *AI Med*, *1*(1), 1–2. DOI: 10.71423/aimed.20250105 PMID: 40918416

Urooj, B., Fayaz, M., Ali, S., Dang, L. M., & Kim, K. W. (2025). Large Language Models in Medical Image Analysis: A Systematic Survey and Future Directions. *Bioengineering (Basel, Switzerland)*, *12*(8), 818. DOI: 10.3390/bioengineering12080818 PMID: 40868331

Wang, Y. (2024). Emotional Dependence Path of Artificial Intelligence Chatbot Based on Structural Equation Modeling. *Procedia Computer Science*, *247*, 1089–1094. DOI: 10.1016/j.procs.2024.10.131

Wang, Z., Wu, Z., Agarwal, D., & Sun, J. (2022). *MedCLIP: Contrastive Learning from Unpaired Medical Images and Text* (Version 1). arXiv. DOI: 10.18653/v1/2022.emnlp-main.256

Warner, E., Lee, J., Hsu, W., Syeda-Mahmood, T., Kahn, C. E., Gevaert, O., & Rao, A. (2024). Multimodal Machine Learning in Image-Based and Clinical Biomedicine: Survey and Prospects. *International Journal of Computer Vision*, *132*(9), 3753–3769. DOI: 10.1007/s11263-024-02032-8 PMID: 39211895

Wu, J., He, K., Mao, R., Shang, X., & Cambria, E. (2025). Harnessing the potential of multimodal EHR data: A comprehensive survey of clinical predictive modeling for intelligent healthcare. *Information Fusion*, *123*, 103283. DOI: 10.1016/j.inffus.2025.103283

Wu, J., Wang, Y., Zhong, Z., Liao, W., Trayanova, N., Jiao, Z., & Bai, H. X. (2025). Vision-language foundation model for 3D medical imaging. *Npj Artificial Intelligence*, *1*(1), 17. DOI: 10.1038/s44387-025-00015-9

Xiao, J., Pisutsin, P., & Feroskhan, M. (2023). Collaborative Target Search With a Visual Drone Swarm: An Adaptive Curriculum Embedded Multistage Reinforcement Learning Approach. *IEEE Transactions on Neural Networks and Learning Systems*, •••, 1–15. DOI: 10.1109/TNNLS.2023.3331370 PMID: 37983144

Xin, Y., Ates, G. C., Gong, K., & Shao, W. (2025, December). *Med3DVLM: An Efficient Vision-Language Model for 3D Medical Image Analysis*. arXiv. https://doi.org//arXiv.2503.20047DOI: 10.48550

Yang, X., Li, Y., Wang, J., Jia, Y., Yi, Z., & Chen, M. (2025). Utilizing multimodal artificial intelligence to advance cardiovascular diseases. *Precision Clinical Medicine*, *8*(3), pbaf016. Advance online publication. DOI: 10.1093/pcmedi/pbaf016 PMID: 40799363

Yi, Z., Xiao, T., & Albert, M. V. (2025). A Survey on Multimodal Large Language Models in Radiology for Report Generation and Visual Question Answering. *Information (Basel)*, *16*(2), 136. DOI: 10.3390/info16020136

Yu, H., Yi, S., Niu, K., Zhuo, M., & Li, B. (2025, March). *UMIT: Unifying Medical Imaging Tasks via Vision-Language Models*. arXiv. https://doi.org//arXiv.2503.15892DOI: 10.48550

Zhang, C., Peng, B., Sun, X., Niu, Q., Liu, J., Chen, K., Li, M., Feng, P., Bi, Z., Liu, M., Zhang, Y., Song, X., Fei, C., Yin, C. H., Yan, L. K., He, H., & Wang, T. (2024). *From Word Vectors to Multimodal Embeddings: Techniques, Applications, and Future Directions For Large Language Models* (Version 3). arXiv. DOI: 10.48550/ARXIV.2411.05036

Zhang, S., Xu, Y., Usuyama, N., Xu, H., Bagga, J., Tinn, R., Preston, S., Rao, R., Wei, M., Valluri, N., Wong, C., Tupini, A., Wang, Y., Mazzola, M., Shukla, S., Liden, L., Gao, J., Crabtree, A., Piening, B., & Poon, H. (2025). A Multimodal Biomedical Foundation Model Trained from Fifteen Million Image–Text Pairs. *NEJM AI*, *2*(1). Advance online publication. DOI: 10.1056/AIoa2400640

Zhang, Y., Jiang, H., Miura, Y., Manning, C. D., & Langlotz, C. P. (2020). *Contrastive Learning of Medical Visual Representations from Paired Images and Text* (Version 2). arXiv. DOI: 10.48550/ARXIV.2010.00747

Zhong, Z., Wang, Y., Bi, L., Ma, Z., Ahn, S. H., Mullin, C. J., Greineder, C. F., Atalay, M. K., Collins, S., Baird, G. L., Lin, C. T., Stayman, W., Kolb, T. M., Kamel, I., Bai, H. X., & Jiao, Z. (2025, November). *Abn-BLIP: Abnormality-aligned Bootstrapping Language-Image Pre-training for Pulmonary Embolism Diagnosis and Report Generation from CTPA*. arXiv. https://doi.org//arXiv.2503.02034DOI: 10.48550

Chapter 10

Vision–Language Models for Medical Imaging

S. S. Kumar
http://orcid.org/0000-0002-7988-2768
Noorul Islam Centre for Higher Education, India

R. S. Vinod Kumar
Noorul Islam Centre for Higher Education, India

ABSTRACT

Vision–Language Models (VLMs) have emerged as a powerful paradigm for medical imaging by jointly learning from visual data and clinical language. Unlike traditional vision-only approaches, VLMs integrate medical images with radiology reports, clinical notes, and textual prompts, enabling richer semantic understanding, improved generalization, and enhanced interpretability. This chapter presents a comprehensive overview of VLMs for medical imaging, covering their motivation, fundamental architectures, training data requirements, optimization strategies, and evaluation methodologies. A detailed taxonomy of medical VLMs is discussed, including contrastive, generative, and foundation-based models. The chapter further explores key applications such as diagnosis, segmentation, report generation, visual question answering, and clinical decision support. Critical challenges and future research directions toward robust, human-centered, and clinically validated multimodal AI systems are outlined.

1. INTRODUCTION

Medical imaging plays a central role in contemporary healthcare, supporting disease screening, diagnosis, treatment planning, and longitudinal patient monitoring.

DOI: 10.4018/979-8-3373-7315-7.ch010

ght © 2026, IGI Global Scientific Publishing. Copying or distributing in print or electronic forms without written permission of IGI Global Scientific Publishing is prohibited. Use of this chapter to generative artificial intelligence (AI) technologies is expressly prohibited. The publisher reserves all rights to license its use for generative AI training and machine learning model development.

Imaging modalities such as X-ray, computed tomography (CT), magnetic resonance imaging (MRI), ultrasound, fundus imaging, and digital pathology provide rich visual evidence of anatomical structures and pathological changes. Over the past decade, deep learning has significantly advanced automated medical image analysis, enabling strong performance in tasks such as classification, detection, and segmentation.

Despite these advances, most conventional medical image analysis models operate in a single-modality setting and rely exclusively on visual information extracted from images. In real clinical practice, however, medical decision-making is inherently multimodal. Clinicians interpret images together with radiology reports, pathology narratives, clinical notes, electronic health records, and prior examinations. Textual information conveys high-level semantic context, including anatomical localization, disease progression, uncertainty expressions, and differential diagnoses, which cannot be reliably inferred from images alone.

This gap between vision-only models and the multimodal nature of clinical reasoning limits the clinical usability, interpretability, and generalization ability of traditional medical AI systems. VLMs address this limitation by jointly modeling visual and textual data within a unified learning framework. Originally developed in the broader computer vision and natural language processing communities, VLMs learn aligned representations between images and text through large-scale pretraining on image–text pairs, enabling cross-modal understanding, reasoning, and generation (Bordes et al., 2024).

Recent progress in foundation models and large language models (LLMs) has further accelerated the adoption of VLMs in medical imaging. Contrastive learning-based VLMs learn modality-agnostic embeddings that support zero-shot and few-shot learning, while generative VLMs integrate powerful language decoders capable of producing structured medical reports and answering clinically meaningful questions (Lin et al., 2025). Hybrid architectures that connect pretrained vision encoders with large language models through lightweight fusion modules have demonstrated strong adaptability across diverse medical imaging tasks with limited task-specific supervision.

The medical domain presents several challenges that make Vision–Language learning particularly attractive. Annotated medical datasets are scarce due to privacy concerns, high annotation costs, and the requirement for expert knowledge. Moreover, medical imaging tasks demand high reliability, transparency, and explainability. By applying weakly supervised image–text pairs such as radiology images and reports, medical VLMs reduce dependence on dense annotations while simultaneously improving interpretability through language-based explanations (Wang et al., 2025).

Consequently, VLMs are being explored across a wide range of medical imaging applications, including image classification, organ and lesion segmentation, medical report generation, visual question answering, image–text retrieval, and clinical decision support (Yiyao et al., 2025). Rather than serving as isolated task-specific solutions, medical VLMs represent a shift toward general-purpose multimodal medical AI systems that more closely align with human clinical reasoning and communication.

This chapter provides a comprehensive overview of VLMs for medical imaging, focusing on their motivations, fundamental architectures, training strategies, datasets, applications, and challenges. By synthesizing insights from recent foundational and medical-domain studies, the chapter aims to clarify the role of VLMs in medical image analysis and highlight their potential impact on the next generation of intelligent healthcare systems.

2. MOTIVATION FOR VISION–LANGUAGE LEARNING IN MEDICINE

Medical practice is fundamentally multimodal. Clinical decision-making rarely relies on a single source of information; instead, it emerges from the joint interpretation of medical images, textual reports, patient history, laboratory results, and domain knowledge accumulated through clinical experience. For instance, a radiologist interpreting a CT scan simultaneously considers prior reports, symptom descriptions, and known disease patterns, while a pathologist examines histopathology slides in conjunction with textual annotations and diagnostic guidelines. This intrinsic multimodality of healthcare motivates the need for artificial intelligence systems that can reason across both visual and linguistic modalities.

Figure 1 illustrates the conceptual difference between traditional vision-only medical imaging models and VLMs that jointly reason over images and clinical text.

Figure 1. Comparison between vision-only medical imaging models and VLMs

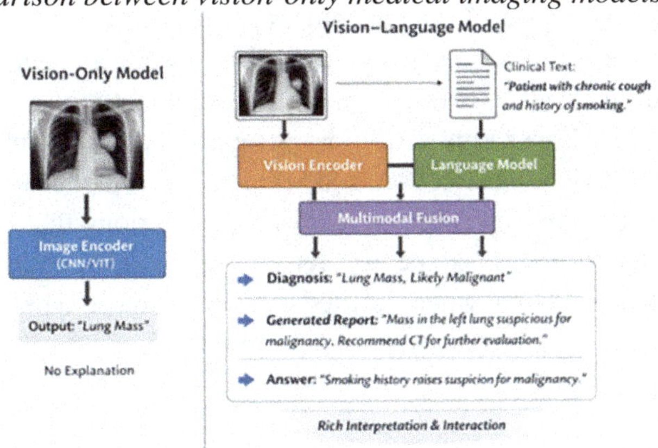

2.1 Limitations of Vision-Only Medical Imaging Models

Conventional deep learning models for medical imaging have predominantly focused on visual data alone. Although convolutional neural networks (CNNs) and vision transformers (ViTs) have achieved remarkable performance in tasks such as classification, detection, and segmentation, they exhibit several inherent limitations. First, vision-only models often struggle with generalization across datasets, scanners, institutions, and patient populations, as they lack access to semantic and contextual cues provided by language (Xiang et al., 2025). Second, these models typically require large, densely annotated datasets, which are difficult and expensive to obtain in the medical domain. Third, their predictions are often opaque, providing limited insight into the reasoning process behind a decision, which restricts clinical trust and adoption.

Moreover, many medical imaging tasks involve ambiguous or subtle visual patterns that are difficult to interpret without linguistic context. Radiology reports frequently include uncertainty expressions, differential diagnoses, and longitudinal comparisons, reflecting the nuanced nature of clinical reasoning. Vision-only models are not designed to capture such semantic richness, leading to brittle performance in complex real-world scenarios.

2.2 Language as a Source of Clinical Knowledge and Supervision

Language plays a critical role in medicine by encoding expert knowledge, clinical guidelines, and diagnostic reasoning. Medical reports, textbooks, and clinical notes provide structured and unstructured descriptions of anatomy, pathology, and disease progression. VLMs exploit this linguistic information as an additional source of supervision, enabling models to associate visual patterns with clinically meaningful concepts rather than low-level image features alone (Bordes et al., 2024).

From a learning perspective, language offers several advantages. Textual descriptions are often easier to obtain than pixel-level annotations and can be reused across multiple tasks. For example, a radiology report implicitly contains information relevant to classification, localization, and severity assessment. By aligning images with reports, VLMs can learn transferable representations that support multiple downstream tasks without task-specific retraining. This capability is particularly valuable in medical imaging, where labeled data are scarce and heterogeneous (Ryu et al., 2025).

2.3 Addressing Data Scarcity and Generalization Challenges

Data scarcity is a persistent challenge in medical AI due to privacy constraints, ethical considerations, and the high cost of expert annotation. VLMs help mitigate this issue by employing weakly supervised image–text pairs, such as image–report datasets, which are more widely available than pixel-level labels. Contrastive pre-training on such data enables models to learn robust cross-modal representations that generalize across diseases, imaging modalities, and institutions.

In addition, VLMs support zero-shot and few-shot learning by enabling inference through natural language prompts. Instead of training a new model for each disease or task, clinicians can specify textual descriptions of conditions or anatomical structures, allowing the model to adapt dynamically. This flexibility is especially beneficial for rare diseases and emerging clinical scenarios where annotated data are limited or unavailable.

2.4 Interpretability, Transparency, and Clinical Trust

Interpretability is a key requirement for deploying AI systems in healthcare. Clinicians must understand and trust model outputs, particularly in high-stakes diagnostic settings. VLMs enhance interpretability by producing language-based explanations, such as textual rationales, generated reports, or answers to natural language questions. These outputs align more closely with clinical communication practices than numeric scores or heatmaps alone.

Furthermore, language grounding encourages models to reason at a semantic level, linking visual evidence to diagnostic terms and clinical findings. This explicit association between image regions and textual concepts facilitates error analysis, model auditing, and regulatory evaluation. As a result, VLMs offer a pathway toward more transparent and accountable medical AI systems (Wang et al., 2025).

2.5 Enabling New Clinical Applications

Beyond improving existing tasks, VLMs enable entirely new forms of interaction with medical images. Applications such as medical visual question answering allow clinicians to query images using natural language, supporting interactive exploration and education. Automated report generation reduces documentation burden and promotes consistency in clinical reporting. Language-guided segmentation and retrieval enable flexible, user-driven analysis without retraining task-specific models.

Taken together, these motivations highlight why Vision–Language learning is particularly well suited to medical imaging. By aligning visual perception with clinical language, VLMs move medical AI closer to human-like reasoning, offering scalable, interpretable, and generalizable solutions that better reflect real-world clinical practice.

3. FUNDAMENTALS OF VLMS

VLMs are multimodal learning frameworks designed to jointly process visual and textual information and to learn shared semantic representations across these modalities. Unlike traditional pipelines that treat images and text as independent inputs, VLMs explicitly model cross-modal interactions, enabling reasoning, alignment, and generation that more closely resemble human perception and communication. This section introduces the fundamental building blocks, learning objectives, and architectural paradigms that underpin modern VLMs, with particular emphasis on their relevance to medical imaging.

3.1 Core Components of VLMs

Most VLMs are composed of three principal components: a vision encoder, a language encoder or decoder, and a multimodal fusion mechanism.

Vision Encoder. The vision encoder is responsible for extracting informative representations from images. In medical VLMs, commonly used vision encoders include CNNs and ViTs. CNN-based encoders are effective at capturing local textures and fine-grained spatial details, which are important for detecting lesions or subtle pathological patterns. Vision transformers, on the other hand, divide images into patches and model long-range dependencies using self-attention, making them well suited for capturing global anatomical context and complex spatial relationships.

Language Encoder or Decoder. The language component processes textual inputs such as radiology reports, clinical notes, questions, or prompts. Transformer-based language models are typically used due to their strong contextual modeling capabilities. In contrastive VLMs, the language encoder maps text into a shared embedding space with images, whereas in generative VLMs, a language decoder generates free-form text conditioned on visual representations. In medical applications, the language model implicitly encodes clinical terminology, diagnostic reasoning patterns, and reporting conventions.

Multimodal Fusion Module. The fusion module integrates visual and textual representations. This integration can be achieved through simple projection into a shared embedding space, cross-attention mechanisms that allow one modality to attend to the other, or query-based adapters that selectively extract visual information relevant to language queries. Effective fusion is critical in medical imaging, where fine-grained alignment between image regions and clinical concepts is required.

The fundamental components and information flow within a Vision–Language Model are depicted in Figure 2.

Figure 2. General architecture of a vision–language model, showing the interaction between vision encoders, language models, and multimodal fusion mechanisms used in medical imaging tasks

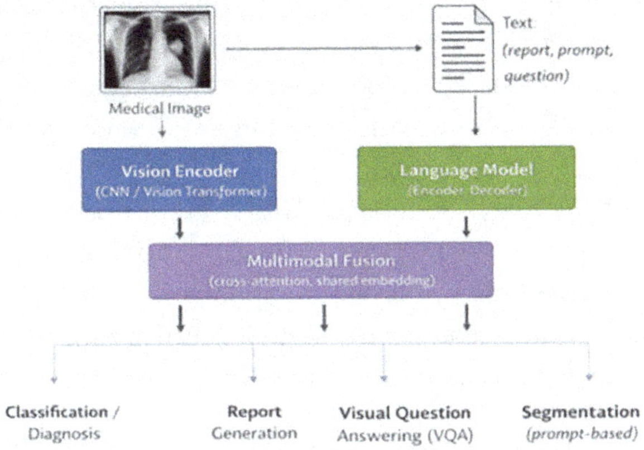

3.2 Attention Mechanisms and Cross-Modal Interaction

Attention mechanisms form the backbone of modern VLMs. Self-attention allows models to capture relationships within a single modality, such as dependencies between words in a sentence or interactions between image patches. Cross-attention extends this concept across modalities, enabling textual tokens to attend to visual features or vice versa.

In medical VLMs, cross-attention facilitates clinically meaningful grounding by associating localized visual findings with descriptive terms. For example, a phrase such as "consolidation in the right lower lobe" can be linked to specific regions in a chest radiograph. This explicit cross-modal interaction supports interpretability, improves alignment, and enhances downstream performance in tasks such as report generation and visual question answering.

3.3 Learning Objectives and Training Paradigms

VLMs employ a variety of learning objectives to align visual and textual modalities:

- **Contrastive Learning.** Contrastive objectives train models to pull matched image–text pairs closer in embedding space while pushing mismatched pairs apart. This paradigm is widely used in medical VLMs due to its scalability and ability to leverage weakly labeled image–report pairs. Contrastive pretraining yields modality-agnostic representations that generalize well across tasks and support zero-shot inference (Wang et al., 2022).
- **Masked Modeling.** Masked language modeling or masked image modeling tasks require the model to predict missing tokens or image patches based on contextual information. These objectives encourage deeper semantic understanding within and across modalities and are often combined with contrastive learning (Hondru et al., 2025).
- **Generative Objectives.** Generative VLMs are trained to produce text conditioned on images or to generate images from text. In medical imaging, text generation is particularly important for applications such as automated report generation and clinical summarization. Generative objectives enable models to capture reporting style, clinical phrasing, and structured narratives.

3.4 Architectural Paradigms of VLMs

Based on how vision and language components are connected, VLM architectures can be broadly categorized into three paradigms.

Dual-Encoder Architectures. Dual-encoder models process images and text independently and project them into a shared embedding space. Similarity between embeddings is used for alignment and retrieval. These architectures are computationally efficient and well suited for large-scale pretraining and zero-shot tasks but provide limited fine-grained interaction.

Encoder–Decoder Architectures. Encoder–decoder models use a vision encoder and a language decoder connected through cross-attention. This design supports rich multimodal interaction and is commonly used in generative tasks such as report generation and visual question answering. However, it is computationally more expensive than dual-encoder designs.

Hybrid and Adapter-Based Architectures. Recent medical VLMs adopt hybrid designs that connect pretrained vision encoders and large language models through lightweight adapters or query-based modules. This approach preserves the strengths of large foundation models while enabling parameter-efficient adaptation to medical imaging tasks.

3.5 From General VLMs to Medical VLMs

While many foundational VLMs are pretrained on natural image–text data, direct application to medical imaging is hindered by domain gaps in visual appearance and language usage. Medical VLMs address this issue through domain-specific pretraining, fine-tuning, or prompt-based adaptation using medical datasets. By incorporating clinical language and medical imagery, these models learn representations that are more aligned with healthcare tasks and clinical reasoning patterns.

In summary, the fundamentals of VLMs lie in their ability to jointly encode, align, and reason over visual and textual information. Through carefully designed architectures, attention mechanisms, and learning objectives, VLMs provide a flexible and powerful foundation for multimodal medical image analysis, setting the stage for the applications and challenges discussed in subsequent sections.

4. TAXONOMY OF VLMS IN MEDICAL IMAGING

The fast development of VLMs has led to a wide variety of architectures and learning strategies specific to various medical imaging tasks. To comprehend the manner in which current models are constructed, the way they vary in their functionality and complexity, and which models can be chosen or modified to serve a particular clinical use, a clear taxonomy is necessary. In this section, medical VLMs are grouped together according to their architectural design and learning paradigm and the extent of integration of both vision and language elements.

Figure 3 presents a high-level taxonomy of VLMs used in medical imaging based on architectural design and learning paradigm.

Figure 3. Taxonomy of VLMs in medical imaging, categorizing models into contrastive, generative, and foundation-based architectures

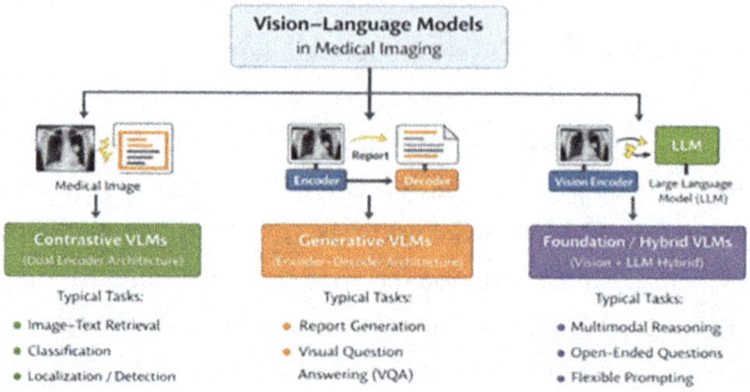

4.1 Contrastive VLMs

One of the oldest and most influential types of VLMs are the contrastive ones. Such models are usually designed in form of dual-encoder where images and text are processed by a vision encoder and a language encoder respectively. Both modalities are projected into the same embedding space by the encoders and the training is directed by an objective of contrastive classification that maximizes similarity between image-text pairs which are matched and minimizes similarity between mismatched pairs.

Contrastive VLMs are typically trained on paired data sets of medical images and radiology reports. Such a weekly supervised setting enables models to operate on massive amounts of clinical data without annotations to be too dense. After training, these models can also facilitate both zero-shot and few-shot inference, by comparing image embeddings with textual disease descriptions or prompts, which makes them especially useful in rare diseases and data-scarcity scenarios.

However, contrastive VLMs do not support fine-grained cross-modal interaction, as images and text do not directly interact when making inference. Consequently, they excel in retrieval and classification but not in tasks that need a lot of detailed reasoning or language generation e.g. report synthesis or interactive question answering.

4.2 Generative VLMs

Generative VLMs extend beyond embedding alignment by explicitly modeling the conditional generation of language from visual inputs. These models typically adopt an encoder–decoder architecture, where a vision encoder extracts image features and a language decoder generates text through cross-attention to visual representations. Generative VLMs are central to applications such as automated medical report generation, clinical summarization, and visual question answering.

In the medical domain, generative VLMs learn not only visual–semantic alignment but also reporting style, clinical phrasing, and structured narrative patterns commonly used in radiology and pathology. This makes them well suited for clinical workflows that require natural language outputs. Nevertheless, generative models are computationally expensive and may produce hallucinated or clinically incorrect statements if not carefully constrained and evaluated, highlighting the importance of domain-specific fine-tuning and validation.

4.3 Hybrid and Foundation VLMs

More recent models are called hybrid or foundation VLMs, which use large pretrained vision encoders and large language models (LLMs). Rather than learning vision and language features together in one place, these models join pretrained backbones together with lightweight fusion modules, like adapters or query-based transformers. The design relies on the generalization capability of foundation models and allows being easily adapted to medical imaging tasks.

In medical imaging, foundation VLMs are highly multi-tasked, where classification, segmentation guidance, report generation and visual question answering can be deployed all together under the same unified framework. The parameter-efficient fine-tuning methods also decrease the computational expenses, which ensures that these models are more feasible to implement in research and practice. Their complexity and scale, however, present challenges regarding interpretability, resource needs and regulatory compliance.

4.4 Task-Oriented Taxonomy of Medical VLMs

Beyond architectural design, medical VLMs can also be categorized based on their primary clinical application:

- **Classification-Oriented VLMs**, which focus on disease identification and severity assessment using language-guided prompts.
- **Segmentation-Oriented VLMs**, where language is used to guide or refine anatomical or lesion segmentation.
- **Report Generation and VQA Models**, which emphasize natural language generation and interactive reasoning.
- **Retrieval and Decision Support Models**, which align images with textual knowledge bases to assist clinical decision-making.

This task-oriented perspective highlights how the same underpinning VLM architecture can be modified to a wide range of medical goals, by modifying training strategy, prompting, or fine-tuning.

4.5 Comparison with Traditional Multimodal Fusion Approaches

The conventional multimodal medical imaging tools usually depend on late fusion or hand-designed feature concatenation which constrain the ability to scale and provide generalization. In comparison, VLMs are trained as a single representation by end-to-end training, which allows them to be transferred across tasks and modalities freely. The transition between basic fusion and large VLMs is a paradigm shift in terms of how multimodal medical information is being modeled and used. To provide a structured overview of the diverse design philosophies adopted in medical VLMs, Table 1 summarizes the main architectural categories, their key characteristics, strengths, limitations, and typical clinical applications.

Table 1. Taxonomy of VLMs in medical imaging

Category	Architecture	Key Characteristics	Strengths	Limitations	Typical Applications
Contrastive VLMs	Dual-encoder	Shared embedding space, contrastive loss	Scalable, zero-/few-shot learning	Limited fine-grained interaction	Classification, retrieval
Generative VLMs	Encoder–decoder	Cross-attention, text generation	Rich explanations, reporting	Hallucination risk, high cost	Report generation, VQA
Foundation / Hybrid VLMs	Pretrained vision + LLM	Adapter or query-based fusion	Multi-task, parameter-efficient	Complex, resource intensive	General-purpose medical AI

Altogether, this taxonomy shows that medical imaging VLMs can fall between the extremes of lightweight contrastive models and huge foundation systems. The comprehension of these categories will give a systematic approach to choosing the right models, determining the gaps in the research as well as the subsequent future evolution of multimodal medical AI.

5. TRAINING DATA AND PREPROCESSING

Effective VLMs rely on training data and preprocessing strategies, particularly in the medical field, where data availability, quality, and ethical limitations are very different when compared to natural image-text learning. The success of medical VLMs is not limited to model architecture, but also the curation, cleaning, alignment, and preparation of multimodal data to various training phases. This section gives more discussion on data source, preprocessing pipelines and design considerations that are important in constructing robust and clinically reliable medical VLMs. Table 2 summarizes the key types of data that are used to train medical VLMs, the accompanying challenges, and their preprocessing needs.

Table 2. Training data types and preprocessing considerations

Data Type	Examples	Key Challenges	Typical Preprocessing Steps
Image–report pairs	X-ray–report, CT–report	Noise, weak labels	Section parsing, de-identification
Pathology images	Whole-slide images	Large size, multi-scale	Patch extraction, magnification
VQA datasets	Image–Q&A	Limited scale	Prompt normalization
Clinical text	Guidelines, notes	Abbreviations, negation	Terminology normalization

5.1 Nature of Medical Vision–Language Data

Medical Vision-Language learning is based on the paired visual and textual information that are similar to actual clinical processes. Medical data is usually institution-specific, domain-sensitive and tightly regulated by privacy laws, unlike web-scale natural data sets. Common forms of medical vision–language data include:

- **Radiology image–report pairs**, where modalities such as chest X-ray, CT, and MRI are aligned with free-text radiology reports. These reports encapsulate diagnostic impressions, findings, uncertainty expressions, and anatomical localization, making them a rich but noisy source of supervision.
- **Pathology images with diagnostic descriptions**, including whole-slide images paired with pathology summaries or synoptic reports, which support fine-grained tissue-level reasoning.
- **Medical visual question answering (VQA) datasets**, consisting of clinician-annotated question–answer pairs grounded in medical images, enabling interactive and explainable reasoning.
- **Educational and knowledge-based text**, such as clinical guidelines, textbooks, and ontologies, which are sometimes integrated to enhance the linguistic and semantic coverage of the language component.

Medical datasets are smaller but richer in semantic content compared to natural-domain datasets, so they must be handled with care to ensure that they are as useful as possible with multimodal learning.

5.2 Weak Supervision and Label Efficiency

One of the prime reasons behind Vision-Language learning in medicine is the lack of high-quality annotations. The dense labels, e.g. pixel-wise segmentation masks or detailed diagnostic labels, can only be computed by expert clinicians and are expensive to acquire. Medical VLMs overcome this difficulty by employing weak supervision using image-text pairs, with the textual reports used as indirect labels. Even though the reports might be incomplete, ambiguous or stylistically divergent, they give useful semantic clues that guide the representation learning.

The contrastive and generative training goals enable VLMs to learn meaningful associations between text and images even when there is noise. This label-efficient learning paradigm minimizes the need to use tedious annotations and this paradigm has the potential to scale across institutions and modalities.

5.3 Synthetic Data Generation and Augmentation

Synthetic data generation has become a significant part of medical VLM training in order to further alleviate data scarcity. It is possible to use large language models to generate pseudo-reports, clinical queries or structured prompts based on labels that already exist, or use vision models to generate coarse visual annotations or region proposals. The synthetic samples increase the coverage of training and enhance robustness in a case where real data are scarce.

Moreover, medical images are augmented by using conventional methods of data augmentation, such as geometric transformations, intensity perturbations, and modality-specific augmentations. But in contrast to natural images, medical augmentations have to maintain anatomical and pathological plausibility. Excessive augmentation can bring in clinically invalid pattern and reduce the reliability of models.

5.4 Preprocessing of Clinical Text

Clinical text is quite different to general-language corpora. It is marked by the use of abbreviations, short notations, negations, uncertainty words, and institution-specific styles of reporting. Text preprocessing is thus necessary in order to minimize noise and enhance alignment between images and text. Typical preprocessing steps include:

- De-identification and removal of personally identifiable information to ensure patient privacy
- Section parsing of reports into standardized components such as findings and impressions
- Normalization of abbreviations and synonyms using medical vocabularies and ontologies
- Explicit handling of negation and uncertainty expressions common in clinical narratives

These can be used to ensure that models bring attention to clinically relevant semantics instead of textual artifacts that occur incidentally, and these improvements contribute to both alignment and downstream performance.

5.5 Image Preprocessing Across Medical Modalities

Medical images have high variability in terms of modalities, resolutions, and acquisition schemes. The preprocessing pipelines should, therefore, be aware of the modality. Intensity normalization, spatial resizing, patch extraction, and modality-specific transformations are some of the common practices. An example is that CT images are usually windowed to highlight the range of tissue of interest, whereas digital pathology images may be imaged at a variety of magnifications to highlight cellular and contextual features.

Regular image preprocessing is important to facilitate consistent training and convergence of multimodal alignment, especially between the data from various institutions or scanners.

5.6 Pretraining Versus Task-Specific Fine-Tuning

Medical VLMs are usually trained in multi-stage paradigm that has different data requirements:

Pretraining stage: It focuses on the data scale and diversity. General multimodal representations are learned using large sets of image-text pairs that are weakly correlated. Common noise-tolerant objectives and automated filtering are used at this point.

Fine-tuning phase: Gives attention to the quality of data and clinical usefulness. Smaller datasets that have been carefully selected are adapted to a particular task, like report generation, segmentation guidance or visual question answering.

With this division, models enjoy the advantage of wide multimodal coverage and task-specific accuracy and reliability.

5.7 Ethical, Privacy, and Bias Considerations

The selection of training data has tremendous effects on fairness, safety, and reliability. Medical data tends to be biased based on demographics, institutions, or modality, which can be magnified by big data models. The responsible data curation thus involves the use of careful auditing, balanced sampling and bias conscious evaluation protocols.

The issue of privacy protection is also essential. Rigorous de-identification, secure data management, and federated or decentralized training systems are some of the methods that are actively being examined in order to allow collaborative model creation, without requiring direct data transfer. These ethical and regulatory issues should be tackled in order to make the medical VLMs safe and effective in clinical practice.

Overall, the success of medical VLMs is based on training data and preprocessing strategies. By combining weakly supervised multimodal data, careful preprocessing, synthetic augmentation, and ethically informed data governance, VLMs can achieve scalable, generalizable, and clinically meaningful performance.

6. MODEL TRAINING AND OPTIMIZATION

Model training and optimization determine how effectively VLMs learn cross-modal representations and how reliably they perform in high-stakes medical applications. Unlike conventional deep learning pipelines, medical VLM training involves multiple stages, diverse learning objectives, and careful trade-offs between performance, computational cost, and clinical safety. This section elaborates on the principal training paradigms, optimization strategies, and practical considerations for developing robust medical VLMs.

6.1 Multi-Stage Training Paradigm

Most medical VLMs follow a multi-stage training strategy, rather than a single end-to-end optimization process. This paradigm reflects the need to balance large-scale representation learning with task-specific clinical adaptation.

- **Pretraining Stage**: Models are trained on large collections of image–text pairs using weak supervision. The goal is to learn general multimodal representations that align visual features with linguistic concepts across modalities and diseases. Noise tolerance and scalability are prioritized at this stage.

- **Intermediate or Alignment Stage**: Some models introduce an explicit alignment phase, where cross-modal grounding is refined using curated datasets, region-level supervision, or structured report parsing.
- **Task-Specific Fine-Tuning Stage**: Models are adapted to downstream tasks such as classification, segmentation guidance, report generation, or visual question answering using high-quality, domain-specific datasets.

This staged approach improves generalization while maintaining clinical relevance and stability.

The multi-stage training pipeline commonly adopted for medical VLMs is illustrated in Figure 4.

Figure 4. Multi-stage training and optimization pipeline for medical VLMs, highlighting pretraining, alignment, fine-tuning, and deployment stages

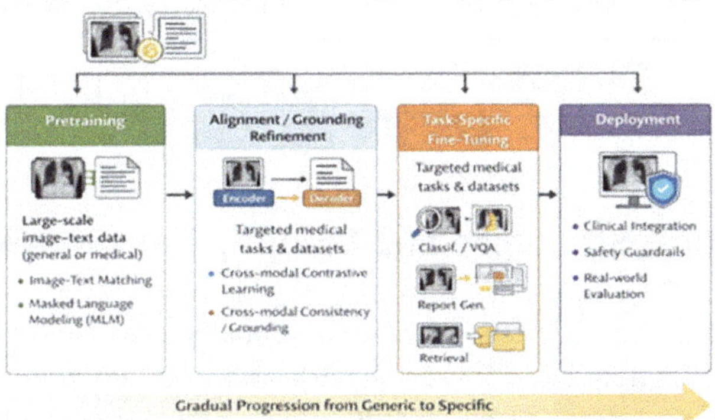

6.2 Training Objectives for Medical VLMs

Medical VLMs employ a combination of complementary training objectives:

- **Contrastive Learning Objectives**: These objectives encourage matched image–text pairs to have similar embeddings while separating mismatched pairs. Contrastive learning is highly scalable and well suited for weakly labeled medical data, enabling zero-shot and few-shot inference.
- **Generative Learning Objectives**: Generative training optimizes the conditional likelihood of text given images or vice versa. This objective is essential for report generation and visual question answering, as it captures clinical language structure and narrative flow.

- **Masked Modeling Objectives**: Masked language or image modeling tasks promote deeper contextual understanding and are often combined with contrastive or generative objectives to enhance robustness.

The choice and combination of objectives depend on the target clinical application and available data. Table 3 provides a concise comparison of the primary training objectives used in medical VLMs and highlights their relevance to different clinical tasks.

Table 3. Training objectives and their medical relevance

Objective	Description	Benefits	Primary Use Cases
Contrastive learning	Aligns image–text embeddings	Robust, scalable	Zero-shot diagnosis, retrieval
Generative learning	Text generation from images	Interpretability	Report generation, VQA
Masked modeling	Predicts missing tokens/ patches	Contextual understanding	Pretraining robustness

6.3 Optimization Strategies and Stability Considerations

The large multimodal models are computationally expensive to train and also sensitive to optimization decisions. Medical VLMs need learning rates and batch size, and optimizer settings to be carefully tuned to achieve stable convergence. Training stability has been demonstrated to be enhanced by curriculum learning strategies that expose them gradually to more complex tasks or higher quality data.

Common regularization methods include dropout, weight decay, and early stopping which are used to reduce overfitting especially when finetuning on small medical datasets. The decoding constraints and temperature control are applied in the generative models to minimize the hallucinations and the outputs that are clinically plausible.

6.4 Parameter-Efficient Fine-Tuning

With the magnitude of the modern foundation models, it is not always feasible to update all the parameters during medical adaptation. Parameters-efficient fine-tuning (PEFT) methods have thus been at the centre of VLM optimization in medicine.

These are adapter modules, low-rank parameter updates and prompt-based tuning methods.

PEFT allows the effective adjustment to new tasks and new institutions without losing the overall knowledge, acquired during pretraining. The strategy makes computational cost lower, reduces chances of catastrophic forgetting, and has been used in clinical environments that are resource-constrained.

6.5 Cross-Modal Grounding and Alignment Refinement

Precise grounding of visual areas and linguistic concepts play an important role in medical imaging. The use of training methods based on region-level supervision, bounding boxes, or attention regularization can assist the models to match textual words with particular anatomical structures or pathological phenomenon. More refinement is done through negative sampling and contrastive hard mining, which prevents spurious correlations. Better grounding increases interpretability and clinically meaningful reasoning especially where localization or explanation of tasks is needed.

6.6 Evaluation-Aware Training and Safety Constraints

In contrast to the natural-domain applications, medical AI systems should comply with the strict safety and reliability standards. Increasingly pipelines are being trained with evaluation-conscious objectives, in which models are also optimized to be accurate, robust, consistent, and aware of uncertainty. Ensemble training, confidence calibration and human-in-the-loop refinement are some of the techniques that are investigated to enhance reliability.

Moreover, generative medical VLMs require hallucination-aware training and a general decoding approach because wrong textual words can have severe clinical implications.

6.7 Computational Efficiency and Deployment Considerations

Medical institutions usually have limited computational resources and thus efficiency becomes a factor to consider. The most popular methods of decreasing memory footprint and latency are model compression, mixed-precision training and inference optimization model. Components can also be updated or replaced separately with the use of modular architectures, which makes them easy to maintain and comply with regulations.

In short, medical imaging VLMs can be trained and optimized effectively only with the help of a delicate balance between scalability, accuracy, interpretability, and safety. Through multi-stage training, suitable learning goals, parameter-efficient adaptation, and evaluation-aware optimization, medical VLMs can be developed as robust and clinically viable multi-modal systems that can be used to support a broad spectrum of healthcare tasks.

7. APPLICATIONS OF VLMS IN MEDICAL IMAGING

VLMs operate by learning a unified semantic representation that connects medical images with clinical language. At the core of every application, a vision encoder extracts spatial and contextual features from medical images, while a language encoder processes textual inputs such as disease descriptions, clinical prompts, or questions. These representations are aligned within a shared embedding space or fused through cross-attention mechanisms. Depending on the clinical task, this alignment is used to perform semantic matching, spatial localization, generative reasoning, or interactive inference. The following subsections describe how VLMs function across major medical imaging applications.

The major application areas enabled by VLMs in medical imaging are summarized in Figure 5.

Figure 5. Key applications of VLMs in medical imaging, ranging from diagnosis and segmentation to report generation, retrieval, and clinical decision support

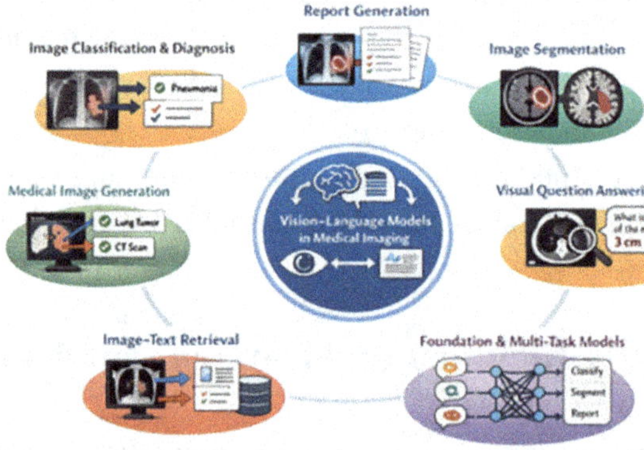

7.1 Medical Image Classification and Diagnosis

In medical image classification, the goal is to infer disease presence, type, or severity from medical images. In a Vision–Language framework, the working process begins with image acquisition and preprocessing, followed by feature extraction using a vision encoder that captures anatomical structures, textures, and pathological patterns. Simultaneously, disease descriptions or diagnostic prompts are encoded into semantic representations using a language model.

Rather than mapping images to fixed categorical labels, the model projects both image and text embeddings into a common semantic space. Diagnostic inference is performed by computing similarity scores between the image embedding and multiple disease-related text embeddings. The disease description that exhibits the strongest semantic alignment with the image is selected as the predicted diagnosis. This prompt-driven reasoning enables flexible classification, supports rare and unseen diseases, and allows diagnostic decisions to be explained through language-based similarity.

7.2 Medical Image Segmentation

Medical image segmentation requires precise delineation of anatomical structures or pathological regions at pixel or voxel resolution. In Vision–Language Models, segmentation is reformulated as a language-guided localization task. The medical image is encoded to produce spatial feature maps that preserve anatomical layout, while textual inputs describing the target region—such as organ names, lesion attributes, or spatial relations—are encoded separately.

Cross-modal attention mechanisms align linguistic tokens with corresponding image regions, allowing the model to identify areas of interest. Based on this alignment, the segmentation module generates masks that highlight regions consistent with the textual description. This approach allows segmentation targets to be specified dynamically using natural language, enabling zero-shot and open-vocabulary segmentation while reducing dependence on exhaustive manual annotations.

7.3 Medical Image Report Generation

Medical report generation involves converting complex visual information into structured clinical narratives. In a Vision–Language Model, this process starts with extracting multi-scale visual features from the medical image, capturing both global context and localized abnormalities. These features are then provided to a language decoder through cross-attention layers.

During text generation, the decoder attends selectively to relevant image regions at each word generation step, ensuring that textual descriptions are grounded in visual evidence. The model generates clinically coherent sentences that describe findings, impressions, and recommendations in a structured manner. Additional constraints, such as report sectioning or diagnostic context, can be incorporated to enhance accuracy and reduce unsupported statements. The result is an interpretable report that reflects both visual content and clinical reasoning.

7.4 Medical Visual Question Answering (VQA)

Medical Visual Question Answering enables interactive reasoning over medical images through natural language questions. The working process begins by encoding the medical image and the input question independently. The question encoding captures semantic intent, including clinical focus and expected answer type, while the image encoding represents visual context.

Cross-modal fusion aligns question-related concepts with corresponding visual regions, allowing the model to focus on relevant anatomical or pathological areas. The fused representation is then used to generate or select an appropriate answer. This process supports both factual responses and explanatory answers, enabling transparent and interactive clinical inquiry that aids education, diagnosis, and decision support.

7.5 Image–Text Retrieval and Clinical Case Search

Image–text retrieval supports clinical case search by enabling cross-modal matching between images and textual queries. During training, images and text are jointly embedded into a shared semantic space. At inference time, a query, either an image or a text description, is encoded and compared against stored embeddings using similarity measures.

This process retrieves clinically similar cases based on both visual appearance and semantic meaning, supporting case-based reasoning, comparative diagnosis, and learning from historical examples. Retrieval also serves as a foundational capability for large-scale multimodal learning and clinical knowledge discovery.

7.6 Medical Image Generation and Data Augmentation

Medical image generation uses language inputs to control the synthesis of realistic medical images. In Vision–Language frameworks, textual embeddings specifying disease type, anatomical location, or severity condition the image generation process. The model learns to map semantic descriptions to corresponding visual patterns through generative modeling.

Generated images can be used for data augmentation, simulation, and privacy-preserving training. This process helps address data scarcity and class imbalance while allowing controlled exploration of disease variations, thereby improving robustness and generalization of downstream medical imaging models.

7.7 Medical Foundation Models and General Large Models

Medical foundation models aim to unify multiple medical imaging tasks within a single Vision–Language architecture. These models integrate a vision encoder with a large language model and rely on instruction-based prompts to define task behavior. The same model can perform classification, segmentation, report generation, VQA, or retrieval depending on the prompt provided.

The working process is prompt-driven rather than architecture-specific, enabling flexible multi-task reasoning. While this unification improves scalability and usability, it also requires careful control mechanisms to ensure reliability, efficiency, and clinical safety across diverse tasks.

Across all applications, Vision–Language Models operate by grounding visual understanding in linguistic context. By aligning image features with clinical language, these models transform medical image analysis into a semantic reasoning process. This unified working mechanism enables flexible task adaptation, improved interpretability, and scalable deployment, positioning Vision–Language Models as a foundational technology for future medical imaging systems.

An overview of the key application areas of VLMs in medical imaging, along with their clinical benefits and associated risks, is presented in Table 4.

Table 4. Applications of VLMs in medical imaging

Application	Role of Language	Clinical Benefit	Key Risks
Classification	Disease prompts	Flexibility, rare diseases	Bias
Segmentation	Textual region description	Prompt-based generalization	Ambiguity
Report generation	Structured narrative	Reduced workload	Hallucinations
VQA	Interactive queries	Education, decision support	Misinterpretation

8. EVALUATION METRICS AND BENCHMARKS

To determine the effectiveness, reliability and clinical preparedness of VLMs in medical imaging, rigorous evaluation is necessary. In contrast to traditional vision-based models, medical VLMs need to be tested at the levels of visual and linguistic representations and their cross-modality. In addition, assessment in the medical field should consider clinical correctness, safety, interpretability, and robustness, which extend beyond the usual machine learning measures. This section gives a detailed description of the evaluation metrics, benchmark tasks and emerging best practices in medical imaging.

8.1 Evaluation Dimensions for Medical VLMs

The performance of medical VLMs can be assessed along multiple complementary dimensions:

- **Visual understanding**, which measures how accurately the model interprets medical images.
- **Language understanding and generation**, which evaluates the correctness and clinical relevance of textual outputs.
- **Cross-modal alignment**, which examines how well visual evidence is grounded in language and vice versa.
- **Clinical validity and safety**, which determine whether model outputs are reliable and acceptable in healthcare settings.

A comprehensive evaluation framework must consider all these dimensions simultaneously.

8.2 Metrics for Image-Centric Tasks

For image-centric tasks such as classification, detection, and segmentation, medical VLMs are often evaluated using established computer vision metrics:

- **Classification metrics**, including accuracy, sensitivity, specificity, area under the receiver operating characteristic curve (AUC), and F1-score, are used to assess disease recognition performance.
- **Segmentation metrics**, such as Dice similarity coefficient, Jaccard index (IoU), and Hausdorff distance, quantify the overlap and boundary accuracy between predicted and ground-truth masks.
- **Localization and detection metrics**, including mean average precision (mAP), are applied when region-level predictions are involved.

While these metrics remain essential, they do not fully capture the multimodal reasoning capabilities of VLMs.

8.3 Metrics for Language Generation and Understanding

For language-centric tasks such as medical report generation and visual question answering, evaluation relies on natural language processing metrics:

- **Lexical overlap metrics**, including BLEU, ROUGE, and METEOR, measure similarity between generated text and reference reports.
- **Semantic similarity metrics**, such as BERTScore, assess meaning-level alignment and are more robust to paraphrasing.
- **Task-specific accuracy**, particularly in VQA, evaluates whether generated answers are clinically correct.

However, purely automatic text metrics may correlate weakly with clinical usefulness. As a result, they are often supplemented with domain-specific evaluation tools and expert review.

8.4 Cross-Modal Alignment and Grounding Evaluation

A defining feature of VLMs is their ability to align visual and textual information. Evaluating this capability requires specialized metrics and protocols:

- **Image–text retrieval metrics**, such as recall@K and mean reciprocal rank, assess how well models associate images with corresponding textual descriptions.
- **Grounding and attention-based evaluations** analyze whether textual terms correspond to appropriate image regions, often using region-level annotations or saliency analysis.

Effective alignment evaluation is particularly important in medical imaging, where incorrect grounding may lead to misleading clinical explanations.

8.5 Benchmark Datasets for Medical VLMs

Several benchmark datasets have been developed to evaluate VLMs in the medical domain. These benchmarks span multiple modalities and tasks, including:

- Image–report datasets for report generation and retrieval
- Medical VQA benchmarks for interactive reasoning
- Multi-task datasets combining classification, segmentation, and language understanding

Benchmark diversity is critical, as performance on a single dataset may not generalize across institutions or imaging modalities. Cross-dataset evaluation is therefore encouraged to assess robustness and generalization.

8.6 Human Evaluation and Clinical Validation

Considering the shortcomings of automated metrics, human assessment is a core part of medical VLM evaluation. Clinical correctness, usefulness, coherence, and safety are the criteria used by expert clinicians to review outputs. Human-in-the-loop testing is especially significant to applications involving report generation and decision support systems, where the presence of subtle errors can be disastrous.

Clinical validation trials such as retrospective and prospective studies are becoming more commonly accepted requirements prior to real-world adoption. These types of studies do not only examine the accuracy of a model but also the integration of workflow and its effects in clinical decision-making.

To summarize the commonly used evaluation metrics across different medical Vision–Language tasks, Table 5 outlines the metrics employed for image analysis, language generation, retrieval, and clinical validation.

Table 5. Evaluation metrics for medical VLMs

Task Type	Metrics	Notes
Classification	Accuracy, AUC, F1	Disease imbalance sensitive
Segmentation	Dice, IoU, Hausdorff	Boundary accuracy important
Language generation	BLEU, ROUGE, BERTScore	Weak clinical correlation
Retrieval	Recall@K, MRR	Measures alignment
Clinical validation	Expert review	Gold standard

9. CHALLENGES, ETHICAL ISSUES, AND LIMITATIONS

However, even though VLMs in medical imaging are rapidly advancing, there are a number of underlying issues that prevent their extensive use in clinical practice. One of the main concerns is the lack of diversity, variety and possible bias of medical training data. Most datasets are based on individual institutions or devices and homogenous populations, and thus have lesser generalizability across hospitals, scanners, and population groups. Large VLMs can exacerbate biases based on age, ethnicity and representation of rare diseases, especially when institutional practices or subjective interpretation of clinical text, such as radiology reports, is used to represent the clinical text. The solution to these problems lies in proper curation of data, multi-institutional data gathering, bias auditing, and protocols to ensure fairness.

The other significant shortcoming of medical VLMs is their reliability and interpretability. Generative VLMs have hallucinatory tendencies, and can generate fluent but incorrect or unfounded textual outputs that can lead to false diagnoses or irresponsible clinical advice. Although using language makes things more transparent, internal processes of decisions tend to be black-box, and generated rationales or attention maps do not necessarily accurately reflect the real model rationales. Clinical reliability thus requires explicit vision-language grounding, conservative decoding algorithms, uncertainty estimation, and human-in-the-loop validation particularly in the case of report generation and clinical decision support.

Medical VLMs are also limited by privacy, regulatory compliance, computational cost and workflow integration. Sensitive patient data training presents issues with data leakage and confidentiality despite the de-identification of the data, and the strict healthcare regulations restrict inter-institutional data exchange. VLMs on a large scale also require a lot of computational resources that pose accessibility and sustainability problems, especially with real-time or on-premise clinical applications. Also, the implementation of VLMs into daily clinical practices will provoke concerns about accountability and responsibility as AI outputs may affect medical decisions. As a result, VLMs should be implemented as the support systems under the supervision of clinicians, with the aid of regular supervision, post deployment assessment, and explicit governance guidelines. These limitations should be clearly identified and met to realize the safe, ethical, and effective use of VLMs in healthcare.

The major challenges facing medical VLMs and their corresponding future research directions are summarized in Table 6.

Table 6. Key challenges and future research directions

Challenge	Impact	Future Direction
Data scarcity & bias	Poor generalization	Multi-institutional pretraining
Hallucination	Clinical risk	Faithful grounding
Interpretability	Trust issues	Clinically meaningful explanations
Privacy	Regulatory barriers	Federated learning
Computational cost	Limited deployment	Parameter-efficient models

10. FUTURE RESEARCH DIRECTIONS

Medical imaging VLM are still in an early and fast developing phase, and there is a lot of potential to develop their robustness, generalization, and clinical applicability. One of the most important future directions is the creation of large-scale domain-specific multimodal pretraining strategies adapted to medical data. The existing models usually use small institutional datasets or transfer learning on natural-image corpora which restricts generalization and creates a bias. Extending the concept of pretraining to a variety of imaging modalities, institutions, as well as patient groups, in addition to structured clinical records, time history, and laboratory data, can support more multimodal representations that more closely represent real-world clinical reasoning.

Improvement of cross-modal grounding, reliability and robustness is another critical research challenge. Even though modern VLMs produce fluent and informative texts, it is an open question whether textual answers are accurately based on visual evidence. The future studies need to focus on region-wise oversight, systematic report matching, causal reasoning, and grounding-conscious assessment guidelines to minimize hallucinations and enhance interpretability. Meanwhile, robustness-sensitive training strategies, including domain adaptation, continual learning, and explicit uncertainty modeling, are necessary to deploy safely when the distribution shifts with changes in scanners, acquisition protocols, and patient demographics, especially in the rare or ambiguous clinical setting.

The next generation medical VLM will even be influenced by privacy preservation, computational efficiency, and human-centered design. Legal and ethical limitations can be overcome by privacy-saving models like federated learning and secure optimization that can facilitate collaboration of multiple institutions without necessarily sharing data. Meanwhile, the parameter-efficient architectures and sustainable training methods are required to minimize the computational and environmental costs. Finally, the development of general purpose, clinically validated medical AI systems will need workflow-sensitive model development, human-in-the-loop testing, benchmarking standards, and close interactions between AI researchers, clinicians, and regulatory agencies. These issues will be critical to the process of converting the VLM research prototypes into trusted tools that can have a substantive effect on healthcare delivery.

11. CONCLUSION

VLMs have emerged as a powerful and unifying paradigm for medical imaging by bridging the long-standing gap between visual perception and clinical language understanding. By jointly modeling medical images and textual information, VLMs move beyond traditional vision-only approaches and align more closely with real-world clinical reasoning. This chapter has presented a comprehensive overview of VLMs in the medical domain, covering their motivation, fundamental architectures, training strategies, applications, evaluation methodologies, and associated challenges. The integration of language into medical image analysis enables richer semantic representations, improved generalization, and enhanced interpretability, supporting applications such as language-guided diagnosis, segmentation, report generation, visual question answering, and clinical decision support.

Despite their significant promise, VLMs face important limitations, including data scarcity and bias, hallucination risks in generative outputs, interpretability challenges, privacy and regulatory constraints, and substantial computational demands. Addressing these challenges requires careful model design, ethical data governance, and close collaboration among AI researchers, clinicians, and regulatory authorities. Looking forward, advances in domain-specific multimodal pretraining, faithful cross-modal grounding, robustness and uncertainty awareness, privacy-preserving learning, and human-centered system design will be essential for translating VLMs into clinically trusted tools. With rigorous validation and responsible deployment, VLMs have the potential to evolve into general-purpose medical AI systems that augment clinician expertise, reduce workload, and ultimately improve patient care.

REFERENCES

Bordes, F., Pang, R. Y., Ajay, A., Li, A. C., Bardes, A., Petryk, S., . . . Chandra, V. (2024). An introduction to vision-language modeling. *arXiv preprint arXiv:2405.17247*.

Hondru, V., Croitoru, F. A., Minaee, S., Ionescu, R. T., & Sebe, N. (2025). Masked Image Modeling: A Survey. *International Journal of Computer Vision*, *133*(10), 7154–7200. DOI: 10.1007/s11263-025-02524-1

Lin, H., Xu, C., & Qin, J. (2025). Taming Vision-Language Models for Medical Image Analysis: A Comprehensive Review. 10.48550/arXiv.2506.18378.

Ryu, J. S., Kang, H., Chu, Y., & Yang, S. (2025). Vision-language foundation models for medical imaging: A review of current practices and innovations. *Biomedical Engineering Letters*, *15*(5), 809–830. DOI: 10.1007/s13534-025-00484-6 PMID: 40917147

Wang, P., Lu, W., Lu, C., Zhou, R., Li, M., & Qin, L. (2025). Large Language Model for Medical Images: A Survey of Taxonomy, Systematic Review, and Future Trends. *Big Data Min. Anal.*, *8*(2), 496–517. DOI: 10.26599/BDMA.2024.9020090

Wang, Z., Wu, Z., Agarwal, D., & Sun, J. (2022, December). Medclip: Contrastive learning from unpaired medical images and text. In *Proceedings of the 2022 Conference on Empirical Methods in Natural Language Processing* (pp. 3876-3887). DOI: 10.18653/v1/2022.emnlp-main.256

Compilation of References

Abdelrahman, A. Y. M. (2025). Deep Learning-Based Brain Tumor Diagnosis on Smartphones Using Optimized MobileNetV2 Models. *Journal of Information Technology*, *5*(13), 1–13. DOI: 10.70619/vol5iss13pp1-13-698

Abhisheka, B., Biswas, S. K., Purkayastha, B., Das, D., & Escargueil, A. (2023). Recent trend in medical imaging modalities and their applications in disease diagnosis: A review. *Multimedia Tools and Applications*, *83*(14), 43035–43070. DOI: 10.1007/s11042-023-17326-1

Acharya, A., Shrestha, S., Chen, A., Conte, J., Avramovic, S., Sikdar, S., Anastasopoulos, A., & Das, S. (2024). Clinical risk prediction using language models: Benefits and considerations. *Journal of the American Medical Informatics Association : JAMIA*, *31*(9), 1856–1864. DOI: 10.1093/jamia/ocae030 PMID: 38412328

Agarwal, M., van der Pol, C. B., Patlas, M. N., Udare, A., Chung, A. D., & Rubino, J. (2021). Optimizing the radiologist work environment: Actionable tips to improve workplace satisfaction, efficiency, and minimize burnout. *La Radiologia Medica*, *126*(10), 1255–1257. DOI: 10.1007/s11547-021-01397-x PMID: 34269963

Ahmed, Y. K., & Naji, A. N. (2025). Smart feature extraction using deep learning for early diagnosis of chronic diseases in next-generation medical decision support systems. *Network Modeling and Analysis in Health Informatics and Bioinformatics*, *14*(1), 140. DOI: 10.1007/s13721-025-00641-y

Al Rahhal, M. M., Bazi, Y., Elgibreen, H., & Zuair, M. (2023). Vision-language models for zero-shot classification of remote sensing images. *Applied Sciences (Basel, Switzerland)*, *13*(22), 12462. DOI: 10.3390/app132212462

Alabdulqader, E. A., Umer, M., Alnowaiser, K., Wang, H., Alarfaj, A. A., & Ashraf, I. (2024). Image Processing-based Resource-Efficient Transfer Learning Approach for Cancer Detection Employing Local Binary Pattern Features. *Mobile Networks and Applications*, 1–17.

Alayrac, J.-B., Donahue, J., Luc, P., Miech, A., Barr, I., Hasson, Y., Lenci, K., Dzabraev, A., & Zisserman, A. (2022). Flamingo: A visual language model for few-shot learning. *Advances in Neural Information Processing Systems, 35*, 23716–23736. DOI: 10.52202/068431-1723

Alexander, A. M., Fitzgibbons, L. M., Kunz, H. E., Ortiz Correa, Z. K., Nair, K. S., Port, J., & Lanza, I. R. (2025). Intermuscular adipose tissue in healthy human aging—Effects of exercise training and implications to metabolic health. *Journal of Applied Physiology (Bethesda, Md.), 139*(5), 1300–1308. DOI: 10.1152/japplphysiol.00719.2025 PMID: 41115067

Aljawarneh, S. A., & Al-Quraan, R. (2023). Pneumonia detection using enhanced convolutional neural network model on chest x-ray images. *Big Data*. PMID: 37074075

Al-Qaness, M. A., Zhu, J., Al-Alimi, D., Dahou, A., Alsamhi, S. H., Elaziz, M. A., & Ewees, A. A. (2024). Chest x-ray images for lung disease detection using Deep Learning techniques: A Comprehensive survey. *Archives of Computational Methods in Engineering, 31*(6), 3267–3301. DOI: 10.1007/s11831-024-10081-y

AlSaad, R., Abd-alrazaq, A., Boughorbel, S., Ahmed, A., Renault, M.-A., Damseh, R., & Sheikh, J. (2024). Multimodal Large Language Models in Health Care: Applications, Challenges, and Future Outlook. *Journal of Medical Internet Research, 26*, e59505. DOI: 10.2196/59505 PMID: 39321458

Alsentzer, E., Murphy, J. R., Boag, W., Weng, W. H., Jin, D., Naumann, T., & McDermott, M. B. A. (2019). Publicly available clinical BERT embeddings. *Proceedings of the 2nd Clinical Natural Language Processing Workshop*, 72–78. Minneapolis, Minnesota, USA. Association for Computational Linguistics. DOI: 10.18653/v1/W19-1909

Alshanketi, F., Alharbi, A., Kuruvilla, M., Mahzoon, V., Siddiqui, S. T., Rana, N., & Tahir, A. (2024). *Pneumonia Detection from Chest X-Ray Images Using Deep Learning and Transfer Learning for Imbalanced Datasets*. Deleted Journal., DOI: 10.1007/s10278-024-01334-0

An, Q., Chen, W., & Shao, W. (2024). A Deep Convolutional Neural Network for Pneumonia Detection in X-ray Images with Attention Ensemble. *Diagnostics (Basel), 14*(4), 390. DOI: 10.3390/diagnostics14040390 PMID: 38396430

Antol, S., Agrawal, A., Lu, J., Mitchell, M., Batra, D., Zitnick, C. L., & Parikh, D. (2015). VQA: Visual question answering. *Proceedings of the IEEE International Conference on Computer Vision*, 2425–2433. DOI: 10.1109/ICCV.2015.279

Ardic, N., & Dinc, R. (2025). Emerging trends in multi-modal artificial intelligence for clinical decision support: A narrative review. *Health Informatics Journal, 31*(3), 14604582251366141. DOI: 10.1177/14604582251366141 PMID: 40808352

Arunachalam, P., Usharani, R., Thirumal, S., Swarnalatha, A. P., & Maheswari, B. U. (2024). *Study on AI-Powered Advanced Drug Discovery for Enhancing Privacy and Innovation in Healthcare*. Igi Global., DOI: 10.4018/979-8-3693-3212-2.ch003

Ashrafee, M. I., Sourav, K. B., Dolna, M. K., & Haque, S. (2023). *Pneumonia Disease detection using the convolutional neural network* (Doctoral dissertation, Brac University).

Awadalla, A., Gao, I., Gardner, J., Hessel, J., Hanafy, Y., Zhu, W., Marathe, K., Bitton, Y., Gadre, S., Sagawa, S., Jitsev, J., Kornblith, S., Koh, P. W., Ilharco, G., Wortsman, M., & Schmidt, L. OpenFlamingo. (2023). An open-source framework for training large autore-gressive vision-language models, URL https://arxiv.org/abs/2308.01390. arXiv:2308.01390.

Bae, S., Kyung, D., Ryu, J., Cho, E., Lee, G., Kweon, S., & Choi, E. (2023). Ehrxqa: A multi-modal question answering dataset for electronic health records with chest x-ray images. *Advances in Neural Information Processing Systems, 36*, 3867–3880. DOI: 10.52202/075280-0170

Bai, H., Dai, Y., Hsu, W.-C., Imami, M., Jiao, Z., Jones, C., Loizou, N., Peng, J., Sair, H., Shen, J., Wang, Y., Wu, J., & Zhang, P. (2024). Enhancing vision-language models for medical imaging: Bridging the 3D gap with innovative slice selection. *Advances in Neural Information Processing Systems, 37*, 99947–99964. DOI: 10.52202/079017-3171

Bannur, S., Hyland, S., Liu, Q., Perez-Garcia, F., Bhatt, M., Castro, D. C., Boecking, B., Sharma, H., Mehra, S., Rosman, H., & Alvarez-Valle, J. (2023). Learning to exploit temporal structure for biomedical vision–language processing. *Proceedings of the IEEE/CVF Conference on Computer Vision and Pattern Recognition*, 15016–15027. DOI: 10.1109/CVPR52729.2023.01442

Bareja, R., Carrillo-Perez, F., Zheng, Y., Pizurica, M., Nandi, T. N., Shen, J., . . . Gevaert, O. (2025). Evaluating Vision and Pathology Foundation Models for Computational Pathology: A Comprehensive Benchmark Study. medRxiv, 2025-05. DOI: 10.1101/2025.05.08.25327250

Bauer, U. (2021). Ripser: Efficient computation of Vietoris–Rips persistence barcodes. *Journal of Applied and Computational Topology, 5*(3), 391–423. DOI: 10.1007/s41468-021-00071-5

Berger, A. H., ... (2024). Topologically Faithful Multi-class Segmentation in Medical Imaging. In MICCAI 2024 (Lecture Notes in Computer Science). https://doi.org/DOI: 10.1007/978-3-031-72111-3_68

Bhuria, R., & Gupta, S. (2024, November). Innovative AI Solutions for Pneumonia Detection: Exploring DenseNet-161 in Medical Imaging. In 2024 5th International Conference on Data Intelligence and Cognitive Informatics (ICDICI) (pp. 638-643). IEEE.

Boecking, B., (2022). Making the Most of Text Semantics to Improve Biomedical Vision-Language Processing. In Avidan, S., Brostow, G., Cissé, M., Farinella, G. M., & Hassner, T. (Eds.), Lecture Notes in Computer Science: Vol. 13696. *Computer Vision – ECCV 2022. ECCV 2022*. Springer., DOI: 10.1007/978-3-031-20059-5_1

Bordes, F., Pang, R. Y., Ajay, A., Li, A. C., Bardes, A., Petryk, S., . . . Chandra, V. (2024). An introduction to vision-language modeling. *arXiv preprint arXiv:2405.17247.*

Bordes, F., Pang, R. Y., Ajay, A., Li, A. C., Bardes, A., Petryk, S., et al. (2024). An introduction to vision-language modeling. arXiv preprint

Bradshaw, T. J., Tie, X., Warner, J., Hu, J., Li, Q., & Li, X. (2025). Large Language Models and Large Multimodal Models in Medical Imaging: A Primer for Physicians. *Journal of Nuclear Medicine*, *66*(2), 173–182. DOI: 10.2967/jnumed.124.268072 PMID: 39819692

Buess, L., Keicher, M., Navab, N., Maier, A., & Tayebi Arasteh, S. (2025). From large language models to multimodal AI: A scoping review on the potential of generative AI in medicine. *Biomedical Engineering Letters*, *15*(5), 845–863. DOI: 10.1007/s13534-025-00497-1 PMID: 40917142

Busch, F., Hoffmann, L., Dos Santos, D. P., Makowski, M. R., Saba, L., Prucker, P., Hadamitzky, M., Navab, N., Kather, J. N., Truhn, D., Cuocolo, R., Adams, L. C., & Bressem, K. K. (2024). Large language models for structured reporting in radiology: Past, present, and future. *European Radiology*, *35*(5), 2589–2602. DOI: 10.1007/s00330-024-11107-6 PMID: 39438330

Bustos, A., Pertusa, A., Salinas, J.-M., & de la Iglesia-Vayá, M. (2020). PadChest: A large chest x-ray image dataset with multi-label annotated reports. *Medical Image Analysis*, *66*, 101797. Advance online publication. DOI: 10.1016/j.media.2020.101797 PMID: 32877839

Cai, T.. (2023). Aligning large multimodal models with radiology knowledge. arXiv:2309.05683. https://arxiv.org/abs/2309.05683

Çallı, E., Sogancioglu, E., Van Ginneken, B., Van Leeuwen, K. G., & Murphy, K. (2021). Deep learning for chest X-ray analysis: A survey. *Medical Image Analysis*, *72*, 102125.

Campanella, G., Hanna, M. G., Geneslaw, L., Miraflor, A., Werneck Krauss Silva, V., Busam, K. J., Brogi, E., Reuter, V. E., Klimstra, D. S., & Fuchs, T. J. (2019). Clinical-grade computational pathology using weakly supervised deep learning on whole slide images. *Nature Medicine*, *25*(8), 1301–1309. DOI: 10.1038/s41591-019-0508-1 PMID: 31308507

Cao, W., Zhang, J., Xia, Y., Mok, T. C., Li, Z., Ye, X., & Zhang, L. (2024). Bootstrapping chest ct image understanding by distilling knowledge from x-ray expert models. In *Proceedings of the IEEE/CVF Conference on Computer Vision and Pattern Recognition* (pp. 11238-11247). DOI: 10.1109/CVPR52733.2024.01068

Carroll, A. N., Storms, L. A., Malempati, C., Shanavas, R. V., & Badarudeen, S. (2024). Generative Artificial Intelligence and Prompt Engineering: A Primer for Orthopaedic Surgeons. *JBJS Reviews*, *12*(10). Advance online publication. DOI: 10.2106/JBJS.RVW.24.00122 PMID: 39361780

Cascella, M., Semeraro, F., Montomoli, J., Bellini, V., Piazza, O., & Bignami, E. (2024). The Breakthrough of Large Language Models Release for Medical Applications: 1-Year Timeline and Perspectives. *Journal of Medical Systems*, *48*(1), 22. Advance online publication. DOI: 10.1007/s10916-024-02045-3 PMID: 38366043

Chazal, F., & Michel, B. (2021). An introduction to topological data analysis: Fundamental and practical aspects for data scientists. *Frontiers in Artificial Intelligence*, *4*, 667963. DOI: 10.3389/frai.2021.667963 PMID: 34661095

Chen, S., & Wang, Y. (2021). Approximation algorithms for 1-Wasserstein distance between persistence diagrams. In 19th International Symposium on Experimental Algorithms (SEA 2021) (LIPIcs, Vol. 190, Article 14). Schloss Dagstuhl – Leibniz-Zentrum für Informatik. https://doi.org/DOI: 10.4230/LIPIcs.SEA.2021.14

Chen, X., Chen, R., Xu, P., Zhang, W., Shang, X., He, M., & Shi, D. (2024). *Visual Question Answering in Ophthalmology: A Progressive and Practical Perspective* (Version 1). arXiv. DOI: 10.48550/ARXIV.2410.16662

Chen, Z., Varma, M., Delbrouck, J.-B., Paschali, M., Blankemeier, L., Van Veen, D., Valanarasu, J. M. J., Youssef, A., Cohen, J. P., Reis, E. P., & Langlotz, C. P. (2024). CheXagent: Towards a foundation model for chest x-ray analysis. arXiv preprint. https://doi.org//arXiv.2401.12208DOI: 10.48550

Chen, J., Duan, H., Zhang, X., Gao, B., Grau, V., & Han, J. (2025). From Gaze to Insight: Bridging Human Visual Attention and Vision Language Model Explanation for Weakly-Supervised Medical Image Segmentation. *IEEE Transactions on Medical Imaging, PP, 1*. Advance online publication. DOI: 10.1109/TMI.2025.3616598 PMID: 41052168

Chen, S., Wu, Z., Zhang, K., Li, C., Zhang, B., Ma, F., Yu, F. R., & Li, Q. (2025). Exploring Embodied Multimodal Large Models: Development, datasets, and future directions. *Information Fusion*, *122*, 103198. DOI: 10.1016/j.inffus.2025.103198

Chukwu, S. C., Rafii, M. Y., Ramlee, S. I., Ismail, S. I., Oladosu, Y., Okporie, E., Onyishi, G., Utobo, E., Ekwu, L., Swaray, S., & Jalloh, M. (2019). Marker-assisted selection and gene pyramiding for resistance to bacterial leaf blight disease of rice (Oryza sativa L.). *Biotechnology, Biotechnological Equipment*, *33*(1), 440–455. DOI: 10.1080/13102818.2019.1584054

Clough, J. R., Byrne, N., Oksuz, I., Zimmer, V. A., Schnabel, J. A., & King, A. P. (2020). A topological loss function for deep learning-based image segmentation using persistent homology. *IEEE Transactions on Pattern Analysis and Machine Intelligence*, *44*(12), 8766–8778. DOI: 10.1109/TPAMI.2020.3013679 PMID: 32886606

Conduah, A. K., Ofoe, S., & Siaw-Marfo, D. (2025). Data privacy in healthcare: Global challenges and solutions. *Digital Health*, *11*, 20552076251343959. Advance online publication. DOI: 10.1177/20552076251343959 PMID: 40475296

Dai, D., Zhang, Y., Yang, Q., Xu, L., Shen, X., Xia, S., & Wang, G. (2025). Pathologyvlm: A large vision-language model for pathology image understanding. *Artificial Intelligence Review*, *58*(6), 186. DOI: 10.1007/s10462-025-11190-1

Dai, W., Li, J., Li, D., Tiong, A. M. H., Zhao, J., Wang, W., Li, B., Fung, P. N., & Hoi, S. C. H. (2023). InstructBLIP: Towards general-purpose vision-language models with instruction tuning. *Advances in Neural Information Processing Systems*, *36*, 49250–49267. DOI: 10.52202/075280-2142

Dangi, R. R., Sharma, A., & Vageriya, V. (2025). Transforming healthcare in low-resource settings with artificial intelligence: Recent developments and outcomes. *Public Health Nursing*, *42*(2), 1017–1030. DOI: 10.1111/phn.13500 PMID: 39629887

Das Joy, S., Dey, N., & Islam, Md. R., Mahmud, M. A., Rahman, M., Tanvir, K., & Gomes, D. (2025). Synthetic Healthcare Data in Generation, Validation, and Integration for Ethical and Scalable Health Innovation: In M. Ahmad (Ed.), *Advances in Synthetic Healthcare Data* (pp. 65–108). IGI Global Scientific Publishing. DOI: 10.4018/979-8-3373-5641-9.ch003

Das, D. C., & Akter, M. S.Debashis Chandra DasMst Shahana Akter. (2025). AI-Powered Multimodal Diagnostics in Modern Healthcare: A Shift Toward Integrative Intelligence. *Asia Pacific Journal of Medical Innovations*, *2*(3), 47–57. DOI: 10.70818/apjmi.v02i03.027

Davis, S. E., Lasko, T. A., Chen, G., Siew, E. D., & Matheny, M. E. (2022). Open questions and research gaps for monitoring and updating AI-enabled tools in clinical settings. *Frontiers in Digital Health*, *4*, 958284. DOI: 10.3389/fdgth.2022.958284 PMID: 36120717

Dernbach, S., Michel, A., Agarwal, K., Brissette, C., Gupta, G., & Choudhury, S. (2024). Thinking Fast and Laterally: Multi-Agentic Approach for Reasoning about Uncertain Emerging Events. arXiv preprint arXiv:2412.07977.

Devlin, J., Chang, M., Lee, K., & Toutanova, K. (2019). BERT: Pre-training of Deep Bidirectional Transformers for Language Understanding. *North American Chapter of the Association for Computational Linguistics*. 4171–4186. DOI: 10.18653/v1/N19-1423

Dey, N., Schlemper, J., Salehi, S. S. M., Zhou, B., Gerig, G., & Sofka, M. (2022). ContraReg: Contrastive learning of multi-modality unsupervised deformable image registration. In Medical Image Computing and Computer Assisted Intervention (MICCAI). https://doi.org/DOI: 10.1007/978-3-031-16446-0_7

Dombrowski, M., Prenner, A., & Kainz, B. (2024). Bias assessment and data drift detection in medical image analysis: A survey. arXiv preprint arXiv:2409.17800.

Domínguez-Rodríguez, S., Liz-López, H., Panizo-LLedot, A., Ballesteros, Á., Dagan, R., Greenberg, D., Gutiérrez, L., Rojo, P., Otheo, E., Galán, J. C., Villanueva, S., García, S., Mosquera, P., Tagarro, A., Moraleda, C., & Camacho, D. (2023). Testing the performance, adequacy, and applicability of an artificial intelligence model for pediatric pneumonia diagnosis. *Computer Methods and Programs in Biomedicine*, *242*, 107765. DOI: 10.1016/j.cmpb.2023.107765 PMID: 37704545

Dosovitskiy, A., Beyer, L., Kolesnikov, A., Weissenborn, D., Zhai, X., Unterthiner, T., Dehghani, M., Minderer, M., Heigold, G., Gelly, S., Uszkoreit, J., & Houlsby, N. (2021). An image is worth 16x16 words: Transformers for image recognition at scale. *International Conference on Learning Representations (ICLR)*. DOI: 10.48550/arXiv.2010.11929

Duan, J., Zhang, M., Song, M., Xu, X., & Lu, H. (2025). Eye Tracking-Enhanced Deep Learning for Medical Image Analysis: A Systematic Review on Data Efficiency, Interpretability, and Multimodal Integration. *Bioengineering (Basel, Switzerland)*, *12*(9), 954. DOI: 10.3390/bioengineering12090954 PMID: 41007199

Edirisinghe, D., Nimalsiri, W., Hennayake, M., Meedeniya, D., & Lim, G. (2025). [-Ray Report Generation Using Abnormality Guided Vision Language Model. IEEE Access.]. *Chest*, •••, X.

Elendu, C., Amaechi, D. C., Elendu, T. C., Jingwa, K. A., Okoye, O. K., John Okah, M., Ladele, J. A., Farah, A. H., & Alimi, H. A. (2023). Ethical implications of AI and robotics in healthcare. *Revista de Medicina (São Paulo)*, *102*(50), e36671. DOI: 10.1097/MD.0000000000036671 PMID: 38115340

Elshan, E., Binzer, B., & Winkler, T. J. (2025). From Software Users to Software Creators: An Exploration of the Core Characteristics of the Citizen Developer Role and the Related Re-and Upskilling Programs: From Software Users to Software Creators.... *Business & Information Systems Engineering*, *67*(1), 31–53. DOI: 10.1007/s12599-024-00915-1

Fang, M., Wang, Z., Pan, S., Feng, X., Zhao, Y., Hou, D., Wu, L., Xie, X., Zhang, X.-Y., Tian, J., & Dong, D. (2025). Large models in medical imaging: Advances and prospects. *Chinese Medical Journal*, *138*(14), 1647–1664. DOI: 10.1097/CM9.0000000000003699 PMID: 40539307

FDA. (2021). Artificial intelligence/machine learning (AI/ML)-based software as a medical device (SaMD) action plan. U.S. Food and Drug Administration. https://www.fda.gov/medical-devices/software-medical-device-samd/artificial-intelligence-and-machine-learning-software-medical-device

Food and Drug Administration (FDA). (2021). *Good Machine Learning Practice for Medical Device Development: Guiding Principles.*

Food and Drug Administration. (2025). Artificial intelligence-enabled device software functions: Lifecycle management and marketing submission recommendations (Docket No. FDA-2024-D-4488). U.S. Department of Health and Human Services. https://www.fda.gov/media/184856/download

Fu, G., El Jurdi, R., Chougar, L., Dormont, D., Valabregue, R., Lehéricy, S., & Colliot, O.The ICEBERG Study Group. (2024). Projected pooling loss for red nucleus segmentation with soft topology constraints. *Journal of Medical Imaging (Bellingham, Wash.)*, *11*(4), 044002. DOI: 10.1117/1.JMI.11.4.044002 PMID: 38988992

Gadzicki, K., Khamsehashari, R., & Zetzsche, C. (2020). Early vs. late fusion in multimodal convolutional neural networks. *Proceedings of the 2020 IEEE 23rd International Conference on Information Fusion (FUSION)*, 1–7. DOI: 10.23919/FUSION45008.2020.9190246

George, S., Naveen, G., Saifullah, S., & Joe, I. P. (2022, June). An efficient neural network model for pneumonia detection. In 2022 International Conference on Computing, Communication, Security and Intelligent Systems (IC3SIS) (pp. 1-7). IEEE. DOI: 10.1109/IC3SIS54991.2022.9885488

Ghadekar, P., Gupta, N., Samgir, S., Umbare, S., Rathod, K., Deshpande, N., & Chaudhari, L. (2025). *Transparent Clinical Support Through Cross-Modal Fusion and Aligned Explanations*. Springer Science Business Media Llc. DOI: 10.21203/rs.3.rs-6636328/v1

Godbin, A. B., & Jasmine, S. G. (2024, July). Pediatric Pneumonia Detection in Chest X-ray Images: A Deep Feature Analysis Approach Enhanced with LightGBM. In *2024 IEEE International Conference on Electronics, Computing and Communication Technologies (CONECCT)* (pp. 1-6). IEEE. DOI: 10.1109/CONECCT62155.2024.10677083

Goddard, K., Roudsari, A., & Wyatt, J. C. (2012). Automation bias: A systematic review of frequency, effect mediators, and mitigators. *Journal of the American Medical Informatics Association: JAMIA*, *19*(1), 121–127. DOI: 10.1136/amiajnl-2011-000089 PMID: 21685142

Gridach, M., Nanavati, J., Abidine, K. Z. E., Mendes, L., & Mack, C. (2025). Agentic ai for scientific discovery: A survey of progress, challenges, and future directions. arXiv preprint arXiv:2503.08979.

Groh, M., Harris, C., Soenksen, L., Lau, F., Han, R., Kim, A., Koochek, A., & Manrai, A. K. (2021). Evaluating deep neural networks trained on clinical images in dermatology with the Fitzpatrick 17k dataset. *Proceedings of the IEEE/CVF Conference on Computer Vision and Pattern Recognition Workshops*, 1820–1828. DOI: 10.1109/CVPRW53098.2021.00201

Gu, P., et al. (2025). TopoImages: Incorporating Local Topology Encoding into Deep Learning Models. https://doi.org/.DOI: 10.1145/3746027.3755546

Guan, H., Chen, X., Shen, C., Zhu, X., Xu, H., & Li, C. (2025). Z Visual-language foundation models for medical and clinical diagnosis and treatments. *The Visual Computer*, *41*(15), 12399–12410. DOI: 10.1007/s00371-025-04067-5

Guan, H., & Liu, M. (2022). Domain Adaptation for Medical Image Analysis: A Survey. *IEEE Transactions on Bio-Medical Engineering*, *69*(3), 1173–1185. DOI: 10.1109/TBME.2021.3117407 PMID: 34606445

Guerrero-Tamayo, A., Oleagordia-Ruiz, I., & Garcia-Zapirain, B. (2025). Vision-language zero-shot models for radiographic image classification: A systematic review. *Machine Learning with Applications*, •••, 100826.

Güler, O., & Polat, K. (2022). Classification performance of deep transfer learning methods for pneumonia detection from chest x-ray images. *Journal of Artificial Intelligence and Systems*, *4*(1), 107–126.

Gu, X., Chen, Y., & Tong, W. (2024). KARAN: Mitigating Feature Heterogeneity and Noise for Efficient and Accurate Multimodal Medical Image Segmentation. *Electronics (Basel)*, *13*(23), 4594. DOI: 10.3390/electronics13234594

Hamidieh, K., Zhang, H., Gerych, W., Hartvigsen, T., & Ghassemi, M. (2024). Identifying implicit social biases in vision-language models. vol. 7, In *Proceedings of the AAAI/ACM conference on AI, ethics, and society* (pp. 547–561). Conference paper. DOI: 10.1609/aies.v7i1.31657

Ha, P. N., Doucet, A., & Tran, G. S. (2023, February). Vision Transformer for Pneumonia Classification in X-ray Images. In *Proceedings of the 2023 8th International Conference on Intelligent Information Technology* (pp. 185-192). DOI: 10.1145/3591569.3591602

Hartsock, I., & Rasool, G. (2024). Vision-language models for medical report generation and visual question answering: A review. *Frontiers in Artificial Intelligence*, *7*, 1430984. Advance online publication. DOI: 10.3389/frai.2024.1430984 PMID: 39628839

Hartung, T. (2025). AI, agentic models and lab automation for scientific discovery–the beginning of scAInce. *Frontiers in Artificial Intelligence*, *8*, 1649155. DOI: 10.3389/frai.2025.1649155 PMID: 40951330

Hasan, M. R., Ullah, S. M. A., & Islam, S. M. R. (2024). Recent advancement of deep learning techniques for pneumonia prediction from chest X-ray image. *Medica-Report*, *7*, 100106. DOI: 10.1016/j.hmedic.2024.100106

Hasan, M. T., & Ahmed, I. (2025). AI-DRIVEN ANOMALY DETECTION FOR DATA LOSS PREVENTION AND SECURITY ASSURANCE IN ELECTRONIC HEALTH RECORDS. *Review of Applied Science and Technology*, *04*(03), 35–67. DOI: 10.63125/dzyr0648

Hersche, M., Moor-Smith, S., Hofmann, T., & Rahimi, A. (2025). Soft-Masked Diffusion Language Models. arXiv preprint arXiv:2510.17206.

Hilling, D. E., Ihaddouchen, I., Buijsman, S., Townsend, R., Gommers, D., & Van Genderen, M. E. (2025). The imperative of diversity and equity for the adoption of responsible AI in healthcare. *Frontiers in Artificial Intelligence*, *8*, 1577529. Advance online publication. DOI: 10.3389/frai.2025.1577529 PMID: 40309720

Hondru, V., Croitoru, F. A., Minaee, S., Ionescu, R. T., & Sebe, N. (2025). Masked Image Modeling: A Survey. *International Journal of Computer Vision*, *133*(10), 7154–7200. DOI: 10.1007/s11263-025-02524-1

Hossain, M., Mahabub, S., Masum, A., & Jahan, I. (2024). Natural Language Processing (NLP) in Analyzing Electronic Health Records for Better Decision Making. *Journal of Computer Science and Technology Studies*, *6*(5), 216–228. DOI: 10.32996/jcsts.2024.6.5.18

Huang, C., Jiang, A., Feng, J., Zhang, Y., Wang, X., & Wang, Y. (2024). Adapting visual-language models for generalizable anomaly detection in medical images. In *Proceedings of the IEEE/CVF conference on computer vision and pattern recognition* (pp. 11375–11385). Conference paper. DOI: 10.1109/CVPR52733.2024.01081

Huang, L., Koutra, D., Kulkarni, A., Prioleau, T., Wu, Q., Yan, Y., . . . Zhou, D. (2025, May). Towards Agentic AI for Science: Hypothesis Generation, Comprehension, Quantification, and Validation. In Companion Proceedings of the ACM on Web Conference 2025 (pp. 1639-1642).

Huang, S. C., Jensen, M., Yeung-Levy, S., Lungren, M. P., Poon, H., & Chaudhari, A. S. (2025). A systematic review and implementation guidelines of multimodal foundation models in medical imaging. *Research Square*, rs-3. DOI: 10.21203/rs.3.rs-5537908/v1

Huang, S.-C., Pareek, A., Seyyedi, S., Banerjee, I., & Lungren, M. P. (2020). Fusion of medical imaging and electronic health records using deep learning: A systematic review and implementation guidelines. *NPJ Digital Medicine*, *3*(1), 136. DOI: 10.1038/s41746-020-00341-z PMID: 33083571

Huang, S.-C., Shen, L., Lungren, M. P., & Yeung, S. (2021). GLoRIA: A multimodal global-local representation learning framework for label-efficient medical image recognition. *Proceedings of the IEEE/CVF International Conference on Computer Vision*, 3942–3951. DOI: 10.1109/ICCV48922.2021.00391

Huang, S., Tan, J., & Liang, J. (2024). A survey on medical vision-language models: Datasets, methods, and evaluation. arXiv:2406.06580. https://arxiv.org/abs/2406.06580

Huang, Y., Gillis-Smith, G., & Huang, Z. (2020). Clinical natural language processing in 2020: Challenges and opportunities. *Journal of Biomedical Informatics, 112*, 103656. Advance online publication. DOI: 10.1016/j.jbi.2020.103656

Huang, Z., Bianchi, F., Yuksekgonul, M., Montine, T. J., & Zou, J. (2023). A visual–language foundation model for pathology image analysis using medical Twitter. *Nature Medicine*, *29*(9), 2307–2316. DOI: 10.1038/s41591-023-02504-3 PMID: 37592105

Irvin, J., Rajpurkar, P., Ko, M., Yu, Y., Ciurea-Ilcus, S., Chute, C., Marklund, H., Haghgoo, B., Ball, R., Shpanskaya, K., Seekins, J., Mong, D. A., Halabi, S. S., Sandberg, J. K., Jones, R., Larson, D. B., Langlotz, C. P., Patel, B. N., Lungren, M. P., & Ng, A. Y. (2019, July). Chexpert: A large chest radiograph dataset with uncertainty labels and expert comparison. *Proceedings of the AAAI Conference on Artificial Intelligence*, *33*(01), 590–597. DOI: 10.1609/aaai.v33i01.3301590

Jain, S., Agrawal, A., Saporta, A., Truong, S. Q., Nguyen Duong, D., Bui, T., Chambon, P., Lungren, M., Ng, A., Langlotz, C., & Rajpurkar, P. (2021). RadGraph: Extracting Clinical Entities and Relations from Radiology Reports (version 1.0.0). *PhysioNet*. RRID:SCR_007345.

Jain, S., & Wallace, B. C. (2019). Attention is not explanation. *Proceedings of the 2019 Conference of the North American Chapter of the Association for Computational Linguistics: Human Language Technologies*, 1, 3543–3556. DOI: 10.18653/v1/N19-1357

Jalnnavar, A., Kanakareddi, S. G., Handur, V. S., Chikaraddi, A., & Giraddi, S. (2023, September). Disease Prediction Model Using Deep Transfer Learning. In International Conference on Intelligent Computing Systems and Applications (pp. 13-29). Singapore: Springer Nature Singapore.

Jia, C., Yang, Y., & Xia, Y.. (2021). Scaling up visual and vision-language representation learning with noisy text supervision. In *International Conference on Machine Learning (PMLR)*, pp. 4904-4916.

Jia, C., Yang, Y., Xia, Y., Chen, Y.-T., Parekh, Z., Pham, H., Le, Q., Sung, Y.-H., Li, Z., & Duerig, T. (2021). Scaling up visual and vision-language representation learning with noisy text supervision. *Proceedings of the 38th International Conference on Machine Learning*, 139, 4904–4916. DOI: 10.48550/arXiv.2102.05918

Jiang, C., Chen, Y., Chang, J., Feng, M., Wang, R., & Yao, J. (2021). *Fusion of medical imaging and electronic health records with attention and multi-head machanisms* (Version 1). arXiv. DOI: 10.48550/ARXIV.2112.11710

Jin, K., Yu, T., Ying, G., Ge, Z., Li, K. Z., Zhou, Y., Shi, D., Wang, M., Goktas, P., & Grzybowski, A. (2026). A systematic review of vision and vision-language foundation models in ophthalmology. *Advances in Ophthalmology Practice and Research*, *6*(1), 8–19. DOI: 10.1016/j.aopr.2025.10.004 PMID: 41532028

Johnson, A. E. W., Pollard, T. J., Berkowitz, S. J., Greenbaum, N. R., Lungren, M. P., Deng, C., . . . Horng, S. (2019). MIMIC-CXR: A large publicly available database of labeled chest radiographs. CoRR. *arXiv preprint arXiv:1901.07042*.

Johnson, A. E. W., Pollard, T. J., Berkowitz, S. J., Greenbaum, N. R., Lungren, M. P., Deng, C.-Y., Mark, R. G., & Horng, S. (2019). MIMIC-CXR, a de-identified publicly available database of chest radiographs with free-text reports. *Scientific Data*, *6*(1), 317. Advance online publication. DOI: 10.1038/s41597-019-0322-0 PMID: 31831740

Kaabachi, B., Despraz, J., Meurers, T., Otte, K., Halilovic, M., Kulynych, B., Prasser, F., & Raisaro, J. L. (2025). A scoping review of privacy and utility metrics in medical synthetic data. npj. *Digital Medicine*, *8*(1), 60. DOI: 10.1038/s41746-024-01359-3 PMID: 39870798

Kamrul, S. M., Jobair, H. F. M., Bofan, H., Cheng, J. Q., & Huanying, G. (2025). Multimodal Models in Healthcare: Methods, Challenges, and Future Directions for Enhanced Clinical Decision Support. *Information (Basel)*, *16*(11), 971. DOI: 10.3390/info16110971

Kao, J. P., & Kao, H. T. (2025). Large Language Models in radiology: A technical and clinical perspective. *European Journal of Radiology Artificial Intelligence*, *2*, 100021. DOI: 10.1016/j.ejrai.2025.100021

Kermany, D., Zhang, K., & Goldbaum, M. (2018). Labeled optical coherence tomography (oct) and chest x-ray images for classification *Mendeley Data*, v2 https://doi.org/https://nihcc.app.box.com/v/ChestXray-NIHCCDOI: 10.17632/rscbjbr9sj

Kharbas, V. K., Raghu, N., & Choudhury, P. (2024). Enhancing rule-based methods for pulmonary effusion diagnosis. In *Proceedings of the 2024 15th International Conference on Computing Communication and Networking Technologies (ICCCNT)* (pp. 1–5). IEEE. DOI: 10.1109/ICCCNT61001.2024.10724858

Khoriba, G., Nouman, M., & Rashed, E. A. (2025). Large language models in medical image understanding. In: Cutting-edge artificial intelligence advances and implications in real-world applications. CRC Press, p. 32 Pages. DOI: 10.1201/9781032632483-7

Kim, H., Lee, S.-Y., You, S. C., Huh, S., Kim, J.-E., Kim, S.-T., Ko, D.-R., Kim, J. H., Lee, J. H., Lim, J. S., Park, M. S., & Lee, K. Y. (2025). A Bilingual On-Premises AI Agent for Clinical Drafting: Implementation Report of Seamless Electronic Health Records Integration in the Y-KNOT Project. *JMIR Medical Informatics*, *13*(8), v13i8e76848. Advance online publication. DOI: 10.2196/76848 PMID: 41284981

Kora, P., Ooi, C. P., Faust, O., Raghavendra, U., Gudigar, A., Chan, W. Y., Meenakshi, K., Swaraja, K., Plawiak, P., & Rajendra Acharya, U. (2022). Transfer learning techniques for medical image analysis: A review. *Biocybernetics and Biomedical Engineering*, *42*(1), 79–107. DOI: 10.1016/j.bbe.2021.11.004

Kore, A., Bavil, E. A., Subasri, V., Abdalla, M., Fine, B., Dolatabadi, E., & Abdalla, M. (2024). Empirical data drift detection experiments on real-world medical imaging data. Nature Communications, 15, (Article number associated with DOI). https://doi.org/.DOI: 10.1038/s41467-024-46142-w

Krones, F., Marikkar, U., Parsons, G., Szmul, A., & Mahdi, A. (2025). Review of multimodal machine learning approaches in healthcare. *Information Fusion*, *114*, 102690. DOI: 10.1016/j.inffus.2024.102690 PMID: 41799790

Kumar, R., Sporn, K., Gowda, C., Paladugu, P., Alnemri, A., Khanna, A., & Zaman, N. (2025). *Integrating Multi-Modal Predictive Modeling*. Imaging Biomarkers, and EHR-Linked Decision Support Systems in Spine-Focused Biomedical Informatics.

Kurz, C. F., Merzhevich, T., Eskofier, B. M., Kather, J. N., & Gmeiner, B. (2025). Benchmarking vision-language models for diagnostics in emergency and critical care settings. *NPJ Digital Medicine*, *8*(1), 423. DOI: 10.1038/s41746-025-01837-2 PMID: 40640347

Kurz, C. F., Merzhevich, T., Eskofier, B. M., Kather, J. N., & Gmeiner, B. (2025). Benchmarking vision-language models for diagnostics in emergency and critical care settings. npj. *Digital Medicine*, *8*(1), 423. PMID: 40640347

Lamaakal, I., Maleh, Y., El Makkaoui, K., Ouahbi, I., Pławiak, P., Alfarraj, O., Almousa, M., & Abd El-Latif, A. A. (2025). Tiny Language Models for Automation and Control: Overview, Potential Applications, and Future Research Directions. *Sensors (Basel)*, *25*(5), 1318. DOI: 10.3390/s25051318 PMID: 40096098

Lammert, J., Dreyer, T., Mathes, S., Kuligin, L., Borm, K. J., Schatz, U. A., Kiechle, M., Lörsch, A. M., Jung, J., Lange, S., Pfarr, N., Durner, A., Schwamborn, K., Winter, C., Ferber, D., Kather, J. N., Mogler, C., Illert, A. L., & Tschochohei, M. (2024). Expert-Guided Large Language Models for Clinical Decision Support in Precision Oncology. *JCO Precision Oncology*, *8*(8), e2400478. DOI: 10.1200/PO-24-00478 PMID: 39475661

Lau, J. J., Gayen, S., Ben Abacha, A., & Demner-Fushman, D. (2018). A dataset of clinically generated visual questions and answers about radiology images. *Scientific Data*, *5*(1), 180251. DOI: 10.1038/sdata.2018.251 PMID: 30457565

Lee, T., Tu, H., Wong, C. H., Zheng, W., Zhou, Y., Mai, Y., Roberts, J. S., Yasunaga, M., Yao, H., Xie, C., & Liang, P. (2024). *VHELM: A Holistic Evaluation of Vision Language Models* (Version 2). arXiv. DOI: 10.52202/079017-4464

Lee, S., Youn, J., Kim, H., Kim, M., & Yoon, S. H. (2025). CXR-LLAVA: A multimodal large language model for interpreting chest X-ray images. *European Radiology*, *35*(7), 4374–4386. DOI: 10.1007/s00330-024-11339-6 PMID: 39812665

Lei, J., Zhang, X., Wu, C., Dai, L., Zhang, Y., Zhang, Y., Wang, Y., Xie, W., & Li, Y. (2024). *AutoRG-Brain: Grounded Report Generation for Brain MRI* (Version 3). arXiv. DOI: 10.48550/ARXIV.2407.16684

Lettner, J., Królikowska, A., Ramadanov, N., Oleksy, Ł., Hakam, H. T., Becker, R., & Prill, R. (2024). Evaluating the Reliability of MyotonPro in Assessing Muscle Properties: A Systematic Review of Diagnostic Test Accuracy. *Medicina (Kaunas, Lithuania)*, *60*(6), 851. DOI: 10.3390/medicina60060851 PMID: 38929468

Levenson, R. M., Singh, Y., Rieck, B., Hathaway, Q. A., Farrelly, C., Rozenblit, J., Prasanna, P., Erickson, B., Choudhary, A., Carlsson, G., & Sarkar, D. (2024). Advancing precision medicine: Algebraic topology and differential geometry in radiology and computational pathology. *Laboratory Investigation*, *104*(6), 102060. DOI: 10.1016/j.labinv.2024.102060 PMID: 38626875

Li, C., Wong, C., Zhang, S., Usuyama, N., Liu, H., Yang, J., Naumann, T., Poon, H., & Gao, J. (2023). *LLaVA-Med: Training a Large Language-and-Vision Assistant for Biomedicine in One Day* (Version 1). arXiv. DOI: 10.48550/ARXIV.2306.00890

Li, C., Wong, C., Zhang, S., Usuyama, N., Liu, H., Yang, J., Naumann, T., Poon, H., & Gao, J. (2023). LLaVA-Med: Training a large language-and-vision assistant for biomedicine in one day. *Advances in Neural Information Processing Systems*, *36*, 28541–28564. DOI: 10.48550/arXiv.2306.00890

Li, C., Wong, C., Zhang, S., Usuyama, N., Liu, H., Yang, J., Naumann, T., Poon, H., & Gao, J. (2023). LLaVA-Med: Training a large language-and-vision assistant for biomedicine in one day. *In Proceedings of the 37th International Conference on Neural Information Processing Systems (NIPS '23).* Curran Associates Inc., Red Hook, NY, USA, *Article 1240,* 28541–28564.

Li, J., Li, D., Xiong, C., & Hoi, S. (2022). BLIP: Bootstrapping language-image pre-training for unified vision-language understanding and generation. *Proceedings of the 39th International Conference on Machine Learning*, 162, 12888–12900. DOI: 10.48550/arXiv.2201.12086

Lin, H., Xu, C., & Qin, J. (2025). Taming Vision-Language Models for Medical Image Analysis: A Comprehensive Review. 10.48550/arXiv.2506.18378.

Lin, Z., Zhang, D., Tao, Q., Shi, D., Haffari, G., Wu, Q., He, M., & Ge, Z. (2023). Medical visual question answering: A survey. *Artificial Intelligence in Medicine*, *143*, 102611. DOI: 10.1016/j.artmed.2023.102611 PMID: 37673579

Liu, J., Wang, Z., Ye, Q., Chong, D., Zhou, P., & Hua, Y. (2023). *Qilin-Med-VL: Towards Chinese Large Vision-Language Model for General Healthcare* (Version 2). arXiv. DOI: 10.48550/ARXIV.2310.17956

Liu, Z., Li, H., Lu, J., Ma, G., Hong, X., Iacca, G., . . . Wang, L. (2025). Nature's Insight: A Novel Framework and Comprehensive Analysis of Agentic Reasoning Through the Lens of Neuroscience. arXiv preprint arXiv:2505.05515.

Liu, A., Guo, Y., Yong, J.-H., & Xu, F. (2024). Multi-grained radiology report generation with sentence-level image-language contrastive learning. *IEEE Transactions on Medical Imaging*, *43*(7), 2657–2669. Advance online publication. DOI: 10.1109/TMI.2024.3372638 PMID: 38437149

Liu, B., Lu, D., Wei, D., Wu, X., Wang, Y., Zhang, Y., & Zheng, Y. (2023). Improving medical vision-language contrastive pretraining with semantics-aware triage. *IEEE Transactions on Medical Imaging*, *42*(12), 3579–3589. DOI: 10.1109/TMI.2023.3294980 PMID: 37440389

Liu, B., Lu, Z., & Wang, Y. (2024). Towards medical vision-language contrastive pre-training via study-oriented semantic exploration. In *Proceedings of the 32nd ACM International Conference on Multimedia (MM '24)*. https://doi.org/DOI: 10.1145/3664647.3681531

Liu, C., Tian, Y., Chen, W., Song, Y., & Zhang, Y. (2024, March). Bootstrapping large language models for radiology report generation. *Proceedings of the AAAI Conference on Artificial Intelligence*, *38*(17), 18635–18643. DOI: 10.1609/aaai.v38i17.29826

Liu, H., Li, C., Wu, Q., & Lee, Y. J. (2023). Visual instruction tuning. *Advances in Neural Information Processing Systems*, *36*, 34892–34916. DOI: 10.48550/arXiv.2304.08485

Liu, X., Rivera, S. C., Moher, D., Calvert, M. J., & Denniston, A. K.Spirit-AI and CONSORT-AI Working Group. (2020). Reporting guidelines for clinical trials evaluating artificial intelligence interventions are needed. *Nature Medicine*, *26*, 1364–1366. DOI: 10.1038/s41591-020-1034-x PMID: 32908283

Liu, Z., Yin, Z., Mi, Z., Guo, B., & Zheng, Z. (2025). A Comparative Analysis of Three Data Fusion Methods and Construction of the Fusion Method Selection Paradigm. *Mathematics*, *13*(8), 1218. DOI: 10.3390/math13081218

Li, X., Li, L., Jiang, Y., Wang, H., Qiao, X., Feng, T., Luo, H., & Zhao, Y. (2025). Vision-Language Models in medical image analysis: From simple fusion to general large models. *Information Fusion*, *118*, 102995. DOI: 10.1016/j.inffus.2025.102995

Li, Y., Rao, S., Solares, J. R. A., Hassaine, A., Ramakrishnan, R., Canoy, D., Zhu, Y., Rahimi, K., & Salimi-Khorshidi, G. (2020). BEHRT: Transformer for electronic health records. *Scientific Reports*, *10*(1), 7155. Advance online publication. DOI: 10.1038/s41598-020-62922-y PMID: 32346050

Li, Z., Wu, X., Du, H., Liu, F., Nghiem, H., & Shi, G. (2025). *A Survey of State of the Art Large Vision Language Models: Alignment, Benchmark, Evaluations and Challenges*. DOI: 10.1109/CVPRW67362.2025.00147

Lu, J., Batra, D., Parikh, D., & Lee, S. (2019). ViLBERT: Pretraining task-agnostic visiolinguistic representations for vision-and-language tasks. *Advances in Neural Information Processing Systems*, *32*, 13–23. DOI: 10.48550/arXiv.1908.02265

Lu, J., Batra, D., Parikh, D., & Lee, S. (2019). ViLBERT: Pretraining task-agnostic visiolinguistic representations for vision-and-language tasks. *Proceedings of the 33rd International Conference on Neural Information Processing Systems.* Curran Associates Inc., Red Hook, NY, USA, *Article 2,* 13–23.

Lu, Y., & Wang, A. (2025). Integrating language into medical visual recognition and reasoning: A survey. *Medical Image Analysis*, *103*, 103514. DOI: 10.1016/j.media.2025.103514 PMID: 40023891

Mamdouh, D., Attia, M., Osama, M., Mohamed, N., Lotfy, A., Arafa, T., Rashed, E. A., & Khoriba, G. (2025). Advancements in Radiology Report Generation: A Comprehensive Analysis. *Bioengineering (Basel, Switzerland)*, *12*(7), 693. DOI: 10.3390/bioengineering12070693 PMID: 40722385

Mccoy, L. G., Bihorac, A., Celi, L. A., Elmore, M., Kewalramani, D., Kwaga, T., Martinez-Martin, N., Prôa, R., Schamroth, J., Shaffer, J. D., Youssef, A., & Fiske, A. (2025). Building health systems capable of leveraging AI: Applying Paul Farmer's 5S framework for equitable global health. *BMC Global and Public Health*, *3*(1), 39. Advance online publication. DOI: 10.1186/s44263-025-00158-6 PMID: 40312417

Mehra, S., Singh, S. K., Kumar, S., Dubey, H., Arya, V., & Gupta, B. B. (2024). Transformative Approach for Prediction of Lung Disease Using Lung X-ray Images.

Merkow, J., Soin, A., Long, J., Cohen, J. P., Saligrama, S., Bridge, C., . . . Lungren, M. P. (2023, October). CheXstray: a real-time multi-modal monitoring workflow for medical imaging AI. In International Conference on Medical Image Computing and Computer-Assisted Intervention (pp. 326-336). Cham: Springer Nature Switzerland. DOI: 10.1007/978-3-031-43898-1_32

Mir, A. N., Rizvi, D. R., & Nissar, I. (2025). Enhancing medical image report generation using a self-boosting multimodal alignment framework. *Health Information Science and Systems*, *13*(1), 58. DOI: 10.1007/s13755-025-00378-y PMID: 41018682

Miró Catalina, Q., Vidal-Alaball, J., Fuster-Casanovas, A., Escalé-Besa, A., Ruiz Comellas, A., & Solé-Casals, J. (2024). Real-world testing of an artificial intelligence algorithm for the analysis of chest X-rays in primary care settings. *Scientific Reports*, *14*(1), 5199. DOI: 10.1038/s41598-024-55792-1 PMID: 38431731

Mongan, J., Moy, L., & Kahn, C. E.Jr. (2020). Checklist for Artificial Intelligence in Medical Imaging (CLAIM): A guide for authors and reviewers. *Radiology. Artificial Intelligence*, *2*(2), e200029. DOI: 10.1148/ryai.2020200029 PMID: 33937821

Moor, M., Huang, Q., Wu, S., Yasunaga, M., Dalmia, Y., Li, Y., Pfohl, S., Koreeda, Y., Rajpurkar, P., & Liang, P. (2023). Med-Flamingo: A multimodal medical few-shot learner. *Proceedings of Machine Learning Research*, *225*, 1–16. DOI: 10.48550/arXiv.2307.15189

Muralidharan, V., Adewale, B. A., Huang, C. J., Nta, M. T., Ademiju, P. O., Pathmarajah, P., Hang, M. K., Adesanya, O., Abdullateef, R. O., Babatunde, A. O., Ajibade, A., Onyeka, S., Cai, Z. R., Daneshjou, R., & Olatunji, T. (2024). A scoping review of reporting gaps in FDA-approved AI medical devices. *NPJ Digital Medicine*, *7*(1), 273. Advance online publication. DOI: 10.1038/s41746-024-01270-x PMID: 39362934

Nambiar, R., & Nanjundegowda, R. (2024a). Harnessing medical imaging applications: Survey on 3D deep learning models for image segmentation. In *Proceedings of the 2024 International Conference on Communication, Control, and Intelligent Systems (CCIS)* (pp. 1–6). IEEE. DOI: 10.1109/CCIS63231.2024.10932049

Nambiar, R., & Nanjundegowda, R. (2024b). A comprehensive review of AI and deep learning applications in dentistry: From image segmentation to treatment planning. [JRC]. *Journal of Robotics and Control*, *5*(6), 1744–1752.

Nambiar, R., & Nanjundegowda, R. (2025). Detection of missing tooth regions using deep learning in panoramic radiographs for dental implant planning. *Engineering, Technology &. Applied Scientific Research*, *15*(5), 28071–28076.

Nam, Y., Kim, D. Y., Kyung, S., Seo, J., Song, J. M., Kwon, J., Kim, J., Jo, W., Park, H., Sung, J., Park, S., Kwon, H., Kwon, T., Kim, K., & Kim, N. (2025). Multimodal large language models in medical imaging. *Korean Journal of Radiology*, *26*(10), 12479233. https://pmc.ncbi.nlm.nih.gov/articles/PMC12479233. DOI: 10.3348/kjr.2025.0599 PMID: 41015856

Nasra, P. (2024, August). Convolution Neural Network: A Proposed Method for Detecting Pneumonia from X-Ray Images. In *2024 Second International Conference on Intelligent Cyber Physical Systems and Internet of Things (ICoICI)* (pp. 1692-1697). IEEE. DOI: 10.1109/ICoICI62503.2024.10696221

Neshat, M., Ahmed, M., Askari, H., Thilakaratne, M., & Mirjalili, S. (2024). Hybrid Inception Architecture with Residual Connection: Fine-tuned Inception-ResNet Deep Learning Model for Lung Inflammation Diagnosis from Chest Radiographs. *Procedia Computer Science*, *235*, 1841–1850. DOI: 10.1016/j.procs.2024.04.175

Nissen, L., Zagar, P., Ravi, V., Zahedivash, A., Reimer, L. M., Jonas, S., . . . Schmiedmayer, P. (2025). Medicine on the edge: Comparative performance analysis of on-device LLMs for clinical reasoning. arXiv preprint arXiv:2502.08954.

Panwar, A., & Gupta, S. (2022). Deep learning models for early detection of pneumonia using chest X-ray images. In Proceedings of the International Conference on Paradigms of Communication, Computing and Data Sciences: PCCDS 2021 (pp. 701-709). Springer Singapore. DOI: 10.1007/978-981-16-5747-4_60

Pan, Z., Wang, H., Wan, J., Zhang, L., Huang, J., & Shen, Y. (2024). Efficient federated learning for pediatric pneumonia on chest X-ray classification. *Scientific Reports*, *14*(1), 23272. Advance online publication. DOI: 10.1038/s41598-024-74491-5 PMID: 39375440

Paola, J. D., Martikainen, J., Farahani, H., Lötjönen, K., & Rovamo, H. (2026). Drawn Futures: How Finland's Diverse Youth Visualise Tomorrow. *Journal of Community & Applied Social Psychology*, *36*(2), e70253. DOI: 10.1002/casp.70253

Papadimitriou, O., Kanavos, A., & Maragoudakis, M. (2023, July). Automated pneumonia detection from chest x-ray images using deep convolutional neural networks. In 2023 14th International Conference on Information, Intelligence, Systems & Applications (IISA) (pp. 1-4). IEEE. DOI: 10.1109/IISA59645.2023.10345859

Parashar, S., Lin, Z., Liu, T., Dong, X., Li, Y., Ramanan, D., & Kong, S. (2024). The neglected tails in vision-language models. In *Proceedings of the IEEE/CVF Conference on Computer Vision and Pattern Recognition* (pp. 12988-12997).

Parida, A., Jiang, Z., Packer, R. J., Avery, R. A., Anwar, S. M., & Linguraru, M. G. (2024). QUANTITATIVE METRICS FOR BENCHMARKING MEDICAL IMAGE HARMONIZATION. *Proceedings. IEEE International Symposium on Biomedical Imaging,* 2024, 1–5. DOI: 10.1109/ISBI56570.2024.10635289

Patel, J., Patel, D., & Raval, A. (2025). Artificial Intelligence for Predictive Modeling in CRISPR/Cas9 Gene Editing: A Survey of Methods and Design Strategies. *The Journal of Gene Medicine*, *27*(12), e70061. DOI: 10.1002/jgm.70061 PMID: 41367203

Patel, P., & Hiriyanna, G. S. (2022). Pneumonia detection in x-ray chest images based on cnn and data augmentation. *International Journal for Research in Applied Science and Engineering Technology*, *10*(7), 4639–4654. DOI: 10.22214/ijraset.2022.46031

Patidar, M., Pandey, G., & Koolagudi, S. G., S, K. K., & Chandra, V. (2024). Enhancing Paediatric Healthcare: Deep Learning-Based Pneumonia Diagnosis from Children's Chest X-rays. *IC3-2024: Proceedings of the 2024 Sixteenth International Conference on Contemporary Computing*, 128–135. https://doi.org/DOI: 10.1145/3675888.3676041

Peng, Y., Wang, H., Sonka, M., & Chen, D. Z. (2024). PHG-Net: Persistent homology guided medical image classification. In *2024 IEEE/CVF Winter Conference on Applications of Computer Vision (WACV)*. https://doi.org/DOI: 10.1109/WACV57701.2024.00741

Plaat, A., van Duijn, M., van Stein, N., Preuss, M., van der Putten, P., & Batenburg, K. J. (2025). Agentic large language models, a survey. arXiv preprint arXiv:2503.23037.

Pun, C. S., Lee, S. X., & Xia, K. (2022). Persistent-homology-based machine learning: A survey and a comparative study. *Artificial Intelligence Review*, *55*(7), 5169–5213. DOI: 10.1007/s10462-022-10146-z

Qinglong, L., Xiaodong, W., Song, X., Xiang, X., & Bo, P. (2025). Analysis of distribution network reliability based on distribution automation technology. *Energy Informatics*, *8*(1), 27. DOI: 10.1186/s42162-025-00478-9

Qiu, J., Wu, J., Wei, H., Shi, P., Zhang, M., Sun, Y., Li, L., Liu, H., Liu, H., Hou, S., Zhao, Y., Shi, X., Xian, J., Qu, X., Zhu, S., Pan, L., Chen, X., Zhang, X., Jiang, S., & Yuan, W. (2024). Development and Validation of a Multimodal Multitask Vision Foundation Model for Generalist Ophthalmic Artificial Intelligence. *NEJM AI, 1*(12). Advance online publication. DOI: 10.1056/AIoa2300221

Quidwai, M. A., & Lagana, A. (2024). *A RAG Chatbot for Precision Medicine of Multiple Myeloma*. Cold Spring Harbor Laboratory. DOI: 10.1101/2024.03.14.24304293

Radford, A., Kim, J. W., Hallacy, C., Ramesh, A., Goh, G., Agarwal, S., Sastry, G., Askell, A., Mishkin, P., Clark, J., Krueger, G., & Sutskever, I. (2021). Learning transferable visual models from natural language supervision. Proceedings of the 38th International Conference on Machine Learning (ICML), PMLR 139, 8748–8763.

Radford, A., Kim, J. W., Hallacy, C., Ramesh, A., Goh, G., Agarwal, S., Sastry, G., Askell, A., Mishkin, P., Clark, J., & Sutskever, I. (2021). Learning transferable visual models from natural language supervision. *Proceedings of the 38th International Conference on Machine Learning*, 139, 8748–8763. DOI: 10.48550/arXiv.2103.00020

Radford, A., Kim, J. W., Hallacy, C., Ramesh, A., Goh, G., Agarwal, S., & Sutskever, I. (2021, July). Learning transferable visual models from natural language supervision. In *International conference on machine learning* (pp. 8748-8763). PmLR.

Raffel, C., Shazeer, N., Roberts, A., Lee, K., Narang, S., Matena, M., Zhou, Y., Li, W., & Liu, P. J. (2020). Exploring the limits of transfer learning with a unified text-to-text transformer. [JMLR]. *Journal of Machine Learning Research, 21*(140), 1–67. https://dl.acm.org/doi/abs/10.5555/3455716.3455856

Raghu, N.. (2025). Blockchain-enhanced GAN image encryption scheme for cloud computing. In Joshi, H. (Eds.), *Intelligent systems and IoT applications in clinical health* (pp. 367–392). IGI Global Scientific Publishing., DOI: 10.4018/979-8-3693-8990-4.ch016

Rahujo, A., Atif, D., Inam, S. A., Khan, A. A., & Ullah, S. (2025). A survey on the applications of transfer learning to enhance the performance of large language models in healthcare systems. *Discover Artificial Intelligence, 5*(1), 90. DOI: 10.1007/s44163-025-00339-0

Rameez, M., & Logashree, M. J. (2024, October). Pneumonia Detection using Machine Learning Techniques. In 2024 8th International Conference on I-SMAC (IoT in Social, Mobile, Analytics and Cloud)(I-SMAC) (pp. 1803-1808). IEEE. DOI: 10.1109/I-SMAC61858.2024.10714803

Raminedi, S., Shridevi, S., & Won, D. (2024). Multi-modal transformer architecture for medical image analysis and automated report generation. *Scientific Reports*, *14*(1), 19281. DOI: 10.1038/s41598-024-69981-5 PMID: 39164302

Raval, A., Maheriya, A., Panchal, S., & Borisagar, K. (2024, August). Disentangled Attention Based Multi-Task Learning with Structural Estimations for Audio Feature Processing and Identification. In 2024 4th Asian Conference on Innovation in Technology (ASIANCON) (pp. 1-7). IEEE. DOI: 10.1109/ASIANCON62057.2024.10837983

Raval, A., & Borisagar, K. (2022, March). A Survey on Techniques and Methods of Recommender System. In *International Conference on Computational Intelligence in Data Science* (pp. 97-114). Cham: Springer International Publishing. DOI: 10.1007/978-3-031-16364-7_8

Raval, A., & Maheriya, A. (2023). A Survey on Deep Learning Methods for Addressing COVID-19 Issues. In *Information and Communication Technology for Competitive Strategies (ICTCS 2022) Intelligent Strategies for ICT* (pp. 61–73). Springer Nature Singapore. DOI: 10.1007/978-981-19-9304-6_7

Raval, A., & Oza, R. (2025). Advancing AI with Quantum Computing: Synergies Between Quantum Neural Networks and Quantum Reinforcement Learning. In *Quantum Machine Learning in Industrial Automation* (pp. 305–332). Springer Nature Switzerland. DOI: 10.1007/978-3-031-99786-0_14

Reddy, C. L., Mitra, S., Meara, J. G., Atun, R., & Afshar, S. (2019). Artificial Intelligence and its role in surgical care in low-income and middle-income countries. *The Lancet. Digital Health*, *1*(8), e384–e386. DOI: 10.1016/S2589-7500(19)30200-6 PMID: 33323217

Restrepo, D., Wu, C., Vásquez-Venegas, C., Matos, J., Gallifant, J., Celi, L. A., Bitterman, D. S., & Nakayama, L. F. (2024). *Analyzing Diversity in Healthcare LLM Research: A Scientometric Perspective*. Cold Spring Harbor Laboratory. DOI: 10.1101/2024.06.18.24309113

Rudin, C. (2019). Stop Explaining Black Box Machine Learning Models for High Stakes Decisions and Use Interpretable Models Instead. *Nature Machine Intelligence*, *1*(5), 206–215. DOI: 10.1038/s42256-019-0048-x PMID: 35603010

Ruggeri, G., & Nozza, D. (2023). A multi-dimensional study on bias in vision-language models. In J. Rogers, & N. Okazaki (Eds.), *Findings of the association for computational linguistics: ACL, 2023* (pp. 6445–6455). Association for Computational Linguistics. DOI: 10.18653/v1/2023.findings-acl.403

Ryu, J. S., Kang, H., Chu, Y., & Yang, S. (2025). Vision-language foundation models for medical imaging: A review of current practices and innovations. *Biomedical Engineering Letters*, *15*(5), 809–830. DOI: 10.1007/s13534-025-00484-6 PMID: 40917147

Sahiner, B., Chen, W., Samala, R. K., & Petrick, N. (2023). Data drift in medical machine learning: Implications and potential remedies. *The British Journal of Radiology*, *96*(1150), 20220878. DOI: 10.1259/bjr.20220878 PMID: 36971405

Saini, S. K., & Sunil, D. (2025). A Comprehensive Review Of Methodologies In Clinical Data-Driven Decision Support Systems For Healthcare. *International Journal of Environmental Sciences*, *11*(24s), 4204–4218. DOI: 10.64252/0e30q322

Sajed, S., Sanati, A., Garcia, J. E., Rostami, H., Keshavarz, A., & Teixeira, A. (2023). The effectiveness of deep learning vs. traditional methods for lung disease diagnosis using chest X-ray images: A systematic review. *Applied Soft Computing*, *147*, 110817. DOI: 10.1016/j.asoc.2023.110817

Salimparsa, M., Sedig, K., Lizotte, D. J., Abdullah, S. S., Chalabianloo, N., & Muanda, F. T. (2025). Explainable AI for Clinical Decision Support Systems: Literature Review, Key Gaps, and Research Synthesis. *Informatics (MDPI)*, *12*(4), 119. DOI: 10.3390/informatics12040119

Sarker, D., Sadi, M. T. H., Gomes, D., & Hasan, Md. M. (2025). Securing Patient Privacy and Data Protection by Federated Learning in AI-Driven Healthcare: In N. K. Mun, C.-S. Shieh, D. Ather, A. Panwar, & V. Jain (Eds.), *Advances in Computational Intelligence and Robotics* (pp. 317–352). IGI Global Scientific Publishing. DOI: 10.4018/979-8-3373-3306-9.ch012

Schuhmann, C., Beaumont, R., Vencu, R., Gordon, C. W., Wightman, R., Cherti, M., Coombes, T., Katta, A., Mullis, C., Wortsman, M., Schramowski, P., Kundurthy, S., Crowson, K., Schmidt, L., Dodge, J., & Jitsev, J. (2022). LAION-5B: An open large-scale dataset for training next generation image-text models. *Advances in Neural Information Processing Systems*, *35*, 25278–25294. DOI: 10.48550/arXiv.2210.08402

Shad, R., Cunningham, J. P., Ashley, E. A., Langlotz, C. P., & Hiesinger, W. (2021). Designing clinically translatable artificial intelligence systems for high-dimensional medical imaging. *Nature Machine Intelligence*, *3*(11), 929–935. DOI: 10.1038/s42256-021-00399-8

Shaikovski, G., Askari, A., Baras, J. S., Ciga, O., Gupte, S., Juyal, D., Kiani, A., Koshkin, A., Mehta, R., Pella, M., Russo, M., Salgado, R., Tosun, A. B., Trahearn, N., Zou, J., & Chen, T. Y. (2024). PathChat: A foundation model for human pathology. *Nature Medicine*, *30*(3), 776–785. DOI: 10.1038/s41591-024-02856-4

Sharma, H., Patel, R., & Singh, A. (2024). MAIRA-Seg: Enhancing radiology report generation with segmentation-aware multimodal large language models. arXiv:2411.11362. https://arxiv.org/abs/2411.11362

Sharshar, A., Khan, L. U., Ullah, W., & Guizani, M. (2025). Vision-language models for edge networks: A comprehensive survey. *IEEE Internet of Things Journal*, *12*(16), 32701–32724. DOI: 10.1109/JIOT.2025.3579032

Shi, D., Zhang, W., Yang, J., Huang, S., Chen, X., Xu, P., Jin, K., Lin, S., Wei, J., Yusufu, M., Liu, S., Zhang, Q., Ge, Z., Xu, X., & He, M. (2025). A multimodal visual–language foundation model for computational ophthalmology. *NPJ Digital Medicine*, *8*(1), 381. DOI: 10.1038/s41746-025-01772-2 PMID: 40542189

Siddiqi, R., & Javaid, S. (2024). Deep learning for pneumonia detection in chest x-ray images: A comprehensive survey. *Journal of Imaging*, *10*(8), 176. DOI: 10.3390/jimaging10080176 PMID: 39194965

Simon, B. D., Ozyoruk, K. B., Gelikman, D. G., Harmon, S. A., & Türkbey, B. (2024). *The future of multimodal artificial intelligence models for integrating imaging and clinical metadata: A narrative review*. Diagnostic and Interventional Radiology., DOI: 10.4274/dir.2024.242631

Singh, Y., Farrelly, C. M., Hathaway, Q. A., Leiner, T., Jagtap, J., Carlsson, G. E., & Erickson, B. J. (2023). Topological data analysis in medical imaging: Current state of the art. *Insights Into Imaging*, *14*(1), 58. Advance online publication. DOI: 10.1186/s13244-023-01413-w PMID: 37005938

Skaf, Y., & Laubenbacher, R. (2022). Topological data analysis in biomedicine: A review. *Journal of Biomedical Informatics*, *130*, 104082. DOI: 10.1016/j.jbi.2022.104082 PMID: 35508272

Sodero, S., Dhungana, N., & Sandoe, F. (2025). Vital mobilities of medical oxygen: Theorising oxygen justice. *Social Science & Medicine*, *364*, 117464.

Solomon, J., Dauber-Decker, K., Richardson, S., Levy, S., Khan, S., Coleman, B., Persaud, R., Chelico, J., King, D., Spyropoulos, A., & McGinn, T. (2023). Integrating Clinical Decision Support Into Electronic Health Record Systems Using a Novel Platform (EvidencePoint): Developmental Study. *JMIR Formative Research*, *7*, e44065. DOI: 10.2196/44065 PMID: 37856193

Srinivasulu, A., Agrawal, A., & Vedaiyan, R. (2025). Overcoming diagnostic and data privacy challenges in viral disease detection: An integrated approach using generative AI, vision transformers, explainable AI, and federated learning. *Frontiers in Virology*, *5*, 1625855. Advance online publication. DOI: 10.3389/fviro.2025.1625855

Sun, Y., Wen, X., Zhang, Y., Jin, L., Yang, C., Zhang, Q., Jiang, M., Xu, Z., Guo, W., Su, J., & Jiang, X. (2025). Visual-language foundation models in medical imaging: A systematic review and meta-analysis of diagnostic and analytical applications. *Computer Methods and Programs in Biomedicine*, *268*, 108870. DOI: 10.1016/j.cmpb.2025.108870 PMID: 40424873

Su, Z., Liu, X., Bou Hamdan, L., & Maroulas, V. (2025). Topological data analysis and topological deep learning beyond persistent homology: A review. *Artificial Intelligence Review*, *59*(2), 58. Advance online publication. DOI: 10.1007/s10462-025-11462-w PMID: 41743488

Swarup, L., R, P. D., Jain, R., N, R., Bewoor, L. A., & Kumar, V. M. (2024). MRI-based epilepsy seizure detection using combined approach of CNN with SVM networks. In *Proceedings of the 2024 IEEE 4th International Conference on ICT in Business Industry & Government (ICTBIG)* (pp. 1–6). IEEE. DOI: 10.1109/ICTBIG64922.2024.10911487

Tan, H., & Bansal, M. (2019). LXMERT: Learning cross-modality encoder representations from transformers. *Proceedings of the 2019 Conference on Empirical Methods in Natural Language Processing*, 5100–5111. DOI: 10.18653/v1/D19-1514

Tanno, R., Barrett, D. G. T., Sellergren, A., Ghaisas, S., Dathathri, S., See, A., Welbl, J., Lau, C., Tu, T., Azizi, S., Singhal, K., Schaekermann, M., May, R., Lee, R., Man, S., Mahdavi, S., Ahmed, Z., Matias, Y., Barral, J., & Ktena, I. (2025). Collaboration between clinicians and vision–language models in radiology report generation. *Nature Medicine*, *31*(2), 599–608. DOI: 10.1038/s41591-024-03302-1 PMID: 39511432

Teoh, J. R., Dong, J., Zuo, X., Lai, K. W., Hasikin, K., & Wu, X. (2024). Advancing healthcare through multimodal data fusion: A comprehensive review of techniques and applications. *PeerJ. Computer Science*, *10*, e2298. DOI: 10.7717/peerj-cs.2298 PMID: 39650483

Thakur, P. S., Khanna, P., Sheorey, T., & Ojha, A. (2022). Trends in vision-based machine learning techniques for plant disease identification: A systematic review. *Expert Systems with Applications*, *208*, 118117. DOI: 10.1016/j.eswa.2022.118117

Tong, R., Xu, T., Ju, X., & Wang, L. (2025). Progress in Medical AI: Reviewing Large LanguageModels and Multimodal Systems for Diagonosis. *AI Med*, *1*(1), 1–2. DOI: 10.71423/aimed.20250105 PMID: 40918416

Tralie, C., Saul, N., & Bar-On, R. (2018). Ripser.py: A lean persistent homology library for Python. *Journal of Open Source Software*, *3*(29), 925. DOI: 10.21105/joss.00925

Tran, J., Estevez, J. J., Howard, N. J., & Kumar, S. (2025). Barriers and Enablers Influencing the Implementation of Artificial Intelligence for Diabetic Retinopathy Screening in Clinical Practice: A Scoping Review. *Clinical & Experimental Ophthalmology*, *53*(7), 791–802. DOI: 10.1111/ceo.14567 PMID: 40515637

Tschandl, P., Rosendahl, C., & Kittler, H. (2018). The HAM10000 dataset, a large collection of multi-source dermatoscopic images of common pigmented skin lesions. *Scientific Data*, *5*(1), 180161. Advance online publication. DOI: 10.1038/sdata.2018.161 PMID: 30106392

Tu, T., Azizi, S., Driess, D., Mirchandani, S., Toda, K., Mai, P., Chang, J., Onoe, A., Sherber, S., Fletcher, A., Matias, Y., Schroeder, A. M., Adam, H., Tse, D., & Natarajan, V. (2024). Towards generalist biomedical AI. *NEJM AI*, *1*(3). Advance online publication. DOI: 10.1056/AIoa2300138

Tyagi, R. K., N, R., & Kumar, R. (2024). An innovative deep learning method for enhancing image resolution. In *Proceedings of the 2024 2nd World Conference on Communication & Computing (WCONF)* (pp. 1–6). IEEE. DOI: 10.1109/WCONF61366.2024.10692190

U.S. FDA. (2023). Good Machine Learning Practice (GMLP) guidelines for medical AI devices. Open Access. https://www.fda.gov

Ula, M., Muhathir, M., & Sahputra, I. (2022). Optimization of multilayer perceptron hyperparameter in classifying pneumonia disease through X-Ray images with speeded-up robust features extraction method. IJACSA). *International Journal of Advanced Computer Science and Applications*, *13*(10). Advance online publication. DOI: 10.14569/IJACSA.2022.0131025

Urooj, B., Fayaz, M., Ali, S., Dang, L. M., & Kim, K. W. (2025). Large Language Models in Medical Image Analysis: A Systematic Survey and Future Directions. *Bioengineering (Basel, Switzerland)*, *12*(8), 818. DOI: 10.3390/bioengineering12080818 PMID: 40868331

Vankayala, V.Venkata Naga Mahesh Kumar Vankayala. (2025). Auditing AI Access to Electronic Health Records: HIPAA Compliance, Challenges, Solutions, and Future Directions. *Journal of Computer Science and Technology Studies*, *7*(8), 458–464. DOI: 10.32996/jcsts.2025.7.8.51

Van, M.-H., Verma, P., & Wu, X. (2024). *On large visual language models for medical imaging analysis: An empirical study. In 2024 IEEE/ACM conference on connected health: applications, systems and engineering technologies. 172–176.*

Vemuri, S. S., Kotha, S., Voruganti, S., Kunam, P. R., Nandini, A., & Kumar Mishra, T. (2024, September). Pneumonia Detection from X-Ray Images Using Deep Transfer Learning. In International Conference on Computing, Communication and Learning (pp. 205-219). Cham: Springer Nature Switzerland.

Wadhwa, R. R., Williamson, D. F. K., Dhawan, A., & Scott, J. G. (2018). TDAstats: R pipeline for computing persistent homology in topological data analysis. *Journal of Open Source Software*, *3*(28), 860. DOI: 10.21105/joss.00860 PMID: 33381678

Wang, P., Lu, W., Lu, C., Zhou, R., Li, M., & Qin, L. (2025). Large Language Model for Medical Images: A Survey of Taxonomy, Systematic Review, and Future Trends. *Big Data Min. Anal.*, *8*(2), 496–517. DOI: 10.26599/BDMA.2024.9020090

Wang, X., Peng, Y., Lu, L., Lu, Z., Bagheri, M., & Summers, R. M. (2017). ChestX-ray8: Hospital-scale chest X-ray database and benchmarks. *Proceedings of the IEEE Conference on Computer Vision and Pattern Recognition*, 2097–2106. DOI: 10.1109/CVPR.2017.369

Wang, Y. (2024). Emotional Dependence Path of Artificial Intelligence Chatbot Based on Structural Equation Modeling. *Procedia Computer Science*, *247*, 1089–1094. DOI: 10.1016/j.procs.2024.10.131

Wang, Y., Yu, Z., Wang, J., Heng, Q., Chen, H., Ye, W., Xie, R., Xie, X., & Zhang, S. (2024). Exploring vision-language models for imbalanced learning. *International Journal of Computer Vision*, *132*(1), 224–237. DOI: 10.1007/s11263-023-01868-w

Wang, Z., Wu, Z., Agarwal, D., & Sun, J. (2022). MedCLIP: Contrastive learning from unpaired medical images and text. *Proceedings of the 2022 Conference on Empirical Methods in Natural Language Processing (EMNLP)*. https://doi.org/DOI: 10.18653/v1/2022.emnlp-main.256

Warner, E., Lee, J., Hsu, W., Syeda-Mahmood, T., Kahn, C. E., Gevaert, O., & Rao, A. (2024). Multimodal Machine Learning in Image-Based and Clinical Biomedicine: Survey and Prospects. *International Journal of Computer Vision*, *132*(9), 3753–3769. DOI: 10.1007/s11263-024-02032-8 PMID: 39211895

Weiner, E. B., Dankwa-Mullan, I., Nelson, W. A., & Hassanpour, S. (2025). Ethical challenges and evolving strategies in the integration of artificial intelligence into clinical practice. *PLOS Digital Health*, *4*(4), e0000810. DOI: 10.1371/journal.pdig.0000810 PMID: 40198594

Wu, J., He, K., Mao, R., Shang, X., & Cambria, E. (2025). Harnessing the potential of multimodal EHR data: A comprehensive survey of clinical predictive modeling for intelligent healthcare. *Information Fusion*, *123*, 103283. DOI: 10.1016/j.inffus.2025.103283

Wu, J., Wang, Y., Zhong, Z., Liao, W., Trayanova, N., Jiao, Z., & Bai, H. X. (2025). Vision-language foundation model for 3D medical imaging. *Npj Artificial Intelligence*, *1*(1), 17. DOI: 10.1038/s44387-025-00015-9

Xiao, J., Pisutsin, P., & Feroskhan, M. (2023). Collaborative Target Search With a Visual Drone Swarm: An Adaptive Curriculum Embedded Multistage Reinforcement Learning Approach. *IEEE Transactions on Neural Networks and Learning Systems*, •••, 1–15. DOI: 10.1109/TNNLS.2023.3331370 PMID: 37983144

Xinming, X. U., Haoxuan, L. I., Zhouyu, G. U. A. N., Dian, Z. E. N. G., Yiming, Q. I. N., Yang, W. E. N., & Weiping, J. I. A. (2025). Urgent needs, opportunities and challenges of virtual reality in healthcare and medicine in the era of large language models. *Virtual Reality & Intelligent Hardware*, *7*(5), 453–467. DOI: 10.1016/j.vrih.2025.08.001

Xue, C., Deng, Q., Li, X., Dou, Q., & Heng, P.-A. (2020). *Cascaded Robust Learning at Imperfect Labels for Chest X-ray Segmentation*. Springer., DOI: 10.1007/978-3-030-59725-2_56

Xu, K., Ba, J., Kiros, R., Cho, K., Courville, A., Salakhutdinov, R., Zemel, R., & Bengio, Y. (2015). Show, attend and tell: Neural image caption generation with visual attention. *Proceedings of the 32nd International Conference on Machine Learning*, 37, 2048–2057. DOI: 10.48550/arXiv.1502.03044

Xu, M., Yoon, S., Fuentes, A., & Park, D. S. (2023). A comprehensive survey of image augmentation techniques for deep learning. *Pattern Recognition*, *137*, 109347.

Yamada, Y., Lange, R. T., Lu, C., Hu, S., Lu, C., Foerster, J., . . . Ha, D. (2025). The ai scientist-v2: Workshop-level automated scientific discovery via agentic tree search. arXiv preprint arXiv:2504.08066.

Yang, S., Wu, X., Ge, S., Zhou, S. K., & Xiao, L. (2023). Radiology report generation with a learned knowledge base and multi-modal alignment. *Medical Image Analysis*, *86*, 102798. DOI: 10.1016/j.media.2023.102798 PMID: 36989850

Yang, X., Li, Y., Wang, J., Jia, Y., Yi, Z., & Chen, M. (2025). Utilizing multimodal artificial intelligence to advance cardiovascular diseases. *Precision Clinical Medicine*, *8*(3), pbaf016. Advance online publication. DOI: 10.1093/pcmedi/pbaf016 PMID: 40799363

Yang, Y., & Mei, G. (2022). Pneumonia recognition by deep learning: A comparative investigation. *Applied Sciences (Basel, Switzerland)*, *12*(9), 4334. DOI: 10.3390/app12094334

Yao, S., Zhao, J., Yu, D., Du, N., Shafran, I., Narasimhan, K. R., & Cao, Y. (2022, October). React: Synergizing reasoning and acting in language models. In The eleventh international conference on learning representations.

Yao, D., Xu, Z., Lin, Y., & Zhan, Y. (2023). Accurate and intelligent diagnosis of pediatric pneumonia using X-ray images and blood testing data. *Frontiers in Bioengineering and Biotechnology*, *11*, 1058888. Advance online publication. DOI: 10.3389/fbioe.2023.1058888 PMID: 37292095

Yao, S., Yu, D., Zhao, J., Shafran, I., Griffiths, T., Cao, Y., & Narasimhan, K. (2023). Tree of thoughts: Deliberate problem solving with large language models. *Advances in Neural Information Processing Systems*, *36*, 11809–11822.

Ye, J., Gong, S., Chen, L., Zheng, L., Gao, J., Shi, H., & Kong, L. (2024). Diffusion of thought: Chain-of-thought reasoning in diffusion language models. *Advances in Neural Information Processing Systems*, *37*, 105345–105374.

Yildirim, A. E., & Canayaz, M. (2023). A novel deep learning-based approach for prediction of neonatal respiratory disorders from chest X-ray images. *Biocybernetics and Biomedical Engineering*, *43*(4), 635–655. DOI: 10.1016/j.bbe.2023.08.004

Yi, Z., Xu, L., & Sun, J. (2025). A survey on multimodal large language models in radiology. *Information (Basel)*, *16*(2), 136. https://www.mdpi.com/2078-2489/16/2/136. DOI: 10.3390/info16020136

Zhang, C., Peng, B., Sun, X., Niu, Q., Liu, J., Chen, K., Li, M., Feng, P., Bi, Z., Liu, M., Zhang, Y., Song, X., Fei, C., Yin, C. H., Yan, L. K., He, H., & Wang, T. (2024). *From Word Vectors to Multimodal Embeddings: Techniques, Applications, and Future Directions For Large Language Models* (Version 3). arXiv. DOI: 10.48550/ARXIV.2411.05036

Zhang, Y., Jiang, H., Miura, Y., Manning, C. D., & Langlotz, C. P. (2020). *Contrastive Learning of Medical Visual Representations from Paired Images and Text* (Version 2). arXiv. DOI: 10.48550/ARXIV.2010.00747

Zhang, Z., Zhang, A., Li, M., & Smola, A. (2022). Automatic chain of thought prompting in large language models. arXiv preprint arXiv:2210.03493.

Zhang, P., Li, X., Hu, X., Yang, J., Zhang, L., Wang, L., & Gao, J. (2021). Vinvl: Revisiting visual representations in vision-language models. In *Proceedings of the IEEE/CVF conference on computer vision and pattern recognition* (pp. 5579-5588). DOI: 10.1109/CVPR46437.2021.00553

Zhang, S., Xu, Y., Usuyama, N., Xu, H., Bagga, J., Tinn, R., Preston, S., Rao, R., Wei, M., Valluri, N., Wong, C., Tupini, A., Wang, Y., Mazzola, M., Shukla, S., Liden, L., Gao, J., Crabtree, A., Piening, B., & Poon, H. (2025). A Multimodal Biomedical Foundation Model Trained from Fifteen Million Image–Text Pairs. *NEJM AI, 2*(1). Advance online publication. DOI: 10.1056/AIoa2400640

Zhang, X., Wu, C., Zhang, Y., Xie, W., & Wang, Y. (2023). Knowledge-enhanced visual-language pre-training on chest radiology images. *Nature Communications, 14*(1), 4542. DOI: 10.1038/s41467-023-40260-7 PMID: 37507376

Zhang, Y., Jiang, H., Miura, Y., Manning, C. D., & Langlotz, C. P. (2022). Contrastive learning of medical visual representations from paired images and text. *Proceedings of Machine Learning for Healthcare Conference*, 182, 2–25. DOI: 10.48550/arXiv.2010.00747

Zhang, Y., Jiang, H., Miura, Y., Manning, C. D., & Langlotz, C. P. (2023). Contrastive learning of medical visual representations from paired images and text. Proceedings of Machine Learning for Health (ML4H), 2023. https://arxiv.org/abs/2010.00747

Zhang, Y., Sun, R., Chen, Y., Pfister, T., Zhang, R., & Arik, S. (2024). Chain of agents: Large language models collaborating on long-context tasks. *Advances in Neural Information Processing Systems, 37*, 132208–132237.

Zhang, Z., & Jiang, A. (2024). Interactive dual-stream contrastive learning for radiology report generation. *Journal of Biomedical Informatics, 157*, 104718. DOI: 10.1016/j.jbi.2024.104718 PMID: 39209086

Zhou, K., Yang, J., Loy, C. C., & Liu, Z. (2022). Learning to prompt for vision-language models. *International Journal of Computer Vision, 130*(9), 2337–2348. DOI: 10.1007/s11263-022-01653-1

About the Contributors

Pethuru Raj, PhD is a chief architect at the Edge AI division of Reliance Jio Platforms Ltd. (JPL) Bangalore. Previously. Worked in IBM Global Cloud Centre of Excellence (CoE), Wipro consulting services (WCS), and Robert Bosch Corporate Research (CR). He had gained over 24 years of IT industry experience and nine years of research experience. He has finished the CSIR-sponsored PhD at Anna University, Chennai. He continued with the UGC-sponsored postdoctoral research in the Department of Computer Science and Automation, Indian Institute of Science (IISc), Bangalore. After that, he got two international research fellowships (JSPS and JST) to work as a research scientist for 3.5 years in two leading Japanese universities. He focuses on some of the emerging technologies, such as Multimodal Generative and Agentic AI, AI Model Optimization Techniques, the Internet of Things Use Cases, Cloud-native and Edge Computing Paradigms, Reliability Engineering, 6G Communication and Blockchain Technologies, Quantum-safe Cryptography Algorithms. He has authored and edited more than 65 technology books, published more than 60 research papers, contributed more than 55 book chapters, submitted a couple of international patents, completed a few IT architecture certifications (TOGAF and ITIL), delivered keynote addresses in 25 international confluences, conducted numerous technical sessions across colleges, universities, and institutes of eminence in India and abroad, participated as a panel member in IT industry symposiums, written several white papers for the IT companies, where he worked, articulated, built and deployed a few state-of-the-art IT products, solutions, and services for the organizations' growth. He has conducted over ten knowledge-sharing sessions to demystify several cutting-edge technologies and tools for software engineers and architects

B. Sundaravadivazhagan is a Postdoctoral Researcher in the Department of Engineering and Technology at Multimedia University, Malaysia. He earned his Ph.D. in Computer Science and Engineering from the Faculty of Information and Communication Engineering at Anna University, Chennai, India. Dr. Sundaravadivazhagan is a faculty member in the Department of Information Technology, College of Computing and Information Sciences, at the University of Technology and Applied Sciences-AL Mussanah, Oman. With over 23 years of academic and research experience, he is actively involved in three projects funded by Oman's Ministry of Higher Education Research and Innovation (MOHERI) through The Research Council (TRC). He holds professional memberships in ISACA and ISTE and is a Senior Member of IEEE. His research interests include cybersecurity, artificial intelligence, machine learning, deep learning, and cloud computing. He has published over 75 technical articles in journals and conferences globally, contributing significantly to the field. His extensive expertise and ongoing research continue advancing critical cybersecurity and intelligent systems technologies.

V. Kavitha is currently working as an Associate Professor, Department of Computer Science with Cognitive Systems, Sri Ramakrishna College of Arts & Science, Coimbatore, Tamil Nadu, India. She obtained her Ph.D Degree in2014 in the broad area of Data Mining. She has over 19 Yrs of teaching and research experience. She has been supervising research scholars, post-graduate end undergraduate students in the recent areas of Cyber Security. She has published more than 75 research papers in International as well as National Journals, International Conferences and Book chapters. She has delivered technical talk in the areas of Big Data Analysis and Cyber Security. Cyber Security, IoT Security, Artificial Intelligence, Machine Learning, Deep Learning are some of her research interests.

M. Baby Nirmala is working as an Associate Professor and Head in the PG & Research Department of Computer Science, Holy Cross College (Autonomous), Tiruchirappalli, Tamil Nadu, India. She has 24 years of teaching experience and 7 years of Industrial Experience. She was positioned as Head of the Department, Nodal officer for AICTE and Coordinator for various Clubs and programs. She has presented several papers in National and International Conferences and published number of research articles in Scopus indexed Journals and IEEE Xplore Library. She has authored 4 chapters in 3 books with Springer and IGI Global. She has organized 5 National and 11 International Conferences. She has served as a Consultant for many Government and Non-Government Organizations. Her areas of specialization are Data Engineering, Big data Analytics, Graph Analytics, Big data full stack development, Semantic Web, Data Science. Now she focuses on Generative, Explainable AI and Large Language models (LLMs).

***

Jaime Aguilar-Ortiz holds a Ph.D. in Mathematical Sciences (CINVESTAV–IPN, Mexico) and serves as a professor and researcher in the fields of Mathematics, Artificial Intelligence, and Project Management, with academic involvement also extending to the Universidad Politécnica Metropolitana de Hidalgo. He additionally leads innovation-driven initiatives as Director General of CICAINTE and TEDNOVA GROUP, bridging rigorous academic work with applied technological development and institutional impact. His prior scholarly and editorial contributions include the preparation and/or editing of a substantial body of books and educational resources spanning mathematics education, financial mathematics, programming, and technology-based learning, complemented by the creation of audiovisual materials, educational platforms, and serious-game applications aimed at strengthening learning outcomes. His academic production further includes dozens of peer-reviewed articles and book chapters addressing themes at the intersection of smart cities, education, and AI, together with sustained experience in research mentoring, curriculum development, and interdisciplinary collaboration. These achievements, combined with recognized academic credentials and a consistent record of knowledge dissemination and capacity building, position him as a strong editor for a high-impact scholarly volume with methodological rigor, cross-sector relevance, and measurable educational and societal value.

Ocotlán Diaz-Parra is a Professor and Researcher at Universidad Politécnica de Pachuca (UPP), a National Researcher under the Secretaria de Ciencia, Humanidades, Tecnología e Innovación program, and an Adjunct Researcher at the National Laboratory of Autonomous Vehicles and Exoskeletons (LANAVEX). His research interests include Smart Cities, Smart Water, Smart Education, Smart Government, Smart Healthcare, Smart Farming, Smart Energy, Smart Sports, Smart Food, Smart Tourism, Algorithmic Finance, Algorithmic Portfolio Management, Applications and Theory of Algorithms, Bio-inspired Algorithms, Combinatorial Optimization Problems, Compilers, Computational Intelligence, Computational Complexity Theory, Computational Financial Intelligence, Complexity of Algorithms, Complexity of Instances, Computational Statistics, Computer Networks, Computer Science Security, Cybercrimes, Data Mining, Education, Evolutionary Computation, Heuristic Optimization Techniques in Bioinformatics, Hybrid Evolutionary Algorithms, Hybrid Optimization Algorithms, Machine Learning, Meta-heuristics, Operations Research, Operations Management, Parallel & Distributed Computing, Production Planning and Logistics Optimization, Project Scheduling Problems, Software Engineering, and Transgenic Algorithms.

Carlos R. Domínguez-Mayorga holds a Ph.D. in Sciences specializing in Artificial Intelligence, with a foundational background in Physics and Mathematics.

His research focuses on Deep Learning, NLP, neural networks, and the development of predictive models. He has an extensive track record in scientific publications and graduate program management, applying cutting-edge data science techniques to engineering and sustainability projects.

Sabrina Edralin serves as the Instructional Designer in the field of Crop Sciences. She has designed and developed online courses to equip crop science professionals with foundational knowledge, best practices, and techniques throughout the entire life cycle. Additionally, Edralin's academic publications encompass lifelong learning and a range of health-related topics such as uveal melanoma, wastewater management, and sustainable design thinking through biomimetic approaches and ML/AI analysis. Edralin is currently a doctoral researcher in Education, Policy, Organization, and Leadership with concentrations in Human Resource Development and Global Studies in Education. Edralin's academic accolades include a Master's of Education in Curriculum & Instruction and an MBA in Leadership and Management.

M.Murali is currently working as Professor in Department of Computing Technologies, SRM Institute of Science and Technology, Kattankulathur 603203, India. He Completed his M.Tech degree in 2002 and Ph.D. in 2013. His research interests include Generative AI, Computer Vision, Deep Learning.

Raghu N has Ten years of experience in Academic and Research. He received the Ph.D. (2020) in Electronics Engineering from Jain University, and B.E. in Electronics and Telecommunications Engineering from VTU University, Karnataka. His research interests were in RF Communication and Image Processing. He has published his research findings in various Scopus indexed Journals and International conferences. He is a member of various professional bodies.

George A. Papakostas received the Diploma, M.Sc., and Ph.D. degrees in electrical and computer engineering from the Democritus University of Thrace (DUTh), Greece, in 1999, 2002, and 2007, respectively. Currently, he is a tenured Full Professor with the Department of Informatics, DUTh, Kavala, Greece. He has 15 years of experience in large-scale systems design, as a senior software engineer and a technical manager. He is also the Head of the Machine Learning and Vision (MLV) Research Group. He has (co)authored more than 250 publications in indexed journals, international conferences, and book chapters, one book (in Greek), two edited books, and eight journal special issues. His publications have more than 6000 citations with H-index is 42 (Google Scholar). His research interests include machine learning, computer/machine vision, pattern recognition, and computational intelligence. He is a member of the IAENG, MIR Labs, EUCogIII, and the Technical

Chamber of Greece (TEE). He served as a reviewer for numerous journals and conferences.

R.S. Vinod Kumar received his BE in Electronics and Communication Engineering in 1991 and ME in Communication Systems in 2000, both from the Madurai Kamaraj University, Tamil Nadu, India. He pursued his PhD from the Anna University, Chennai, India, in 2015. His areas of research are multiresolution patch-based texture synthesis, steganography, and medical imaging. He is presently working as a Professor and the Head of the Department of Electronics and Communication Engineering, Noorul Islam Centre for Higher Education, Kumaracoil, Tamil Nadu, India

Jorge A. Ruiz-Vanoye is a Professor and Researcher at Universidad Politécnica de Pachuca (UPP), a National Researcher under the Secretaria de Ciencia, Humanidades, Tecnología e Innovación program, and an Adjunct Researcher at the National Laboratory of Autonomous Vehicles and Exoskeletons (LANAVEX). Additionally, he holds the title of Lecturer-level Researcher for the Agency for the Quality of the University System of Catalonia (Generalitat de Catalunya). His research interests include Smart Cities, Smart Water, Smart Education, Smart Government, Smart Healthcare, Smart Farming, Smart Energy, Smart Sports, Smart Food, Smart Tourism, Algorithmic Finance, Algorithmic Portfolio Management, Applications and Theory of Algorithms, Bio-inspired Algorithms, Combinatorial Optimization Problems, Compilers, Computational Intelligence, Computational Complexity Theory, Computational Financial Intelligence, Complexity of Algorithms, Complexity of Instances, Computational Statistics, Computer Networks, Computer Science Security, Cybercrimes, Data Mining, Education, Evolutionary Computation, Heuristic Optimization Techniques in Bioinformatics, Hybrid Evolutionary Algorithms, Hybrid Optimization Algorithms, Machine Learning, Meta-heuristics, Operations Research, Operations Management, Parallel & Distributed Computing, Production Planning and Logistics Optimization, Project Scheduling Problems, Software Engineering, and Transgenic Algorithms.

Kazi Tanvir is a Bangladeshi computer-science lecturer and early-career researcher whose work joins machine learning, explainable AI and bioinformatics. He currently teaches in the Department of Computer Science at American International University-Bangladesh (AIUB). Kazi Tanvir has an MSc in Data Science at Vellore Institute of Technology (VIT), Vellore, Tamil Nadu, India. He has completed his BSc in Computer Science and Engineering majoring in Computational Theory from American International University-Bangladesh (AIUB). He has passed his Secondary and Higher Secondary from Birshrestha Noor Mohammad Public

College, Dhaka. He aims to become a successful researcher in his domain. His fields of interest are Data Science, Image Processing, and Biostatistics. He has taken part in various international conferences and also have published some papers, data, book chapters and patents.

Trejo-Macotela holds a Ph.D. in Electronics from the National Institute of Astrophysics, Optics and Electronics (INAOE) and is Professor and Senior Researcher at Universidad Politécnica de Pachuca (UPP). He is a National Researcher of the Secretariat of Science, Humanities, Technology and Innovation (SECIHTI) of Mexico and adjunct member of LANAVEX. His prolific academic output comprises slightly more than 60 publications in domains including smart cities, embedded IoT systems, telecommunications, electronics, aquaculture, artificial intelligence, bio-inspired algorithms, combinatorial optimisation, and educational technologies.

Vipin Tyagi is a distinguished academician, researcher and author, currently serving as Dean (Academics and Research) at Jaypee University of Engineering and Technology in Guna, Madhya Pradesh. With a rich background in Computer Science, his expertise spans across Image Processing, Cyber Forensics and Speech Recognition. Prof. Tyagi has a prolific publication record, contributing significantly to his fields of interest. His scholarly work includes numerous journal articles, conference papers, and books. Some of his notable publications are in the areas of image forgery detection, image denoising and content-based image retrieval. He has authored and edited several books and papers in the field of Computer Science, such as "Digital Image Forgery Detection: Techniques, Challenges and Applications", "Predictive Computing and Information Security" and "Content-Based Image Retrieval: Ideas, Influences, and Current Trends" published by Springer Singapore. His book "Understanding Digital Image Processing" using MATLAB, published by Taylor and Francis is highlighted by Mathworks at: https://in.mathworks.com/academia/books/understanding-digital-image-processing-tyagi.html His scholarly work has earned him a respectable h-index and numerous citations in the academic community.

Clark Xu is the Principal Scientist at the Mayo Clinic, Artificial Intelligence & Discovery. Prior he served as a Senior Staff Researcher at the University of Wisconsin-Madison, School of Medicine and Public Health. His research interests include threat intelligence, cyber defense, attack vectors, homeland security, and common vulnerabilities and exposures. His national security projects include the Air Force UP GovCloud (Cloud One), the Army Integrated Visual Augmentation System (IVAS), and the NIH COVID-19 Rapid Acceleration of Diagnostics (RADx). As an applied scientist in artificial intelligence and machine learning, his research passion is to advance the state-of-the-art in the United States' national health and defense capabilities. He holds an MS degree in Computer Science from the Georgia Institute of Technology and a BA degree in Mathematics from Vassar College. He has published research work in premier journals and conferences such as IEEE, OUP, and SFN. He is also a certified CISSP, HCISSP distinguished SME with ISC2 and a member of the Society for Neuroscience.

Index

A

B

C

D

E

H

L

M

P

S

T

V

W

www.ingramcontent.com/pod-product-compliance
Lightning Source LLC
LaVergne TN
LVHW081535300926
849161LV00006B/1440